Phytonutrients

Phytonutrients

Edited by

Andrew Salter

The University of Nottingham

Helen Wiseman

King's College, London

Gregory Tucker

The University of Nottingham

WILEY-BLACKWELL

A John Wiley & Sons, Ltd., Publication

This edition first published 2012 © 2012 by Blackwell Publishing Ltd

Wiley-Blackwell is an imprint of John Wiley & Sons, formed by the merger of Wiley's global Scientific, Technical and Medical business with Blackwell Publishing.

Registered Office
John Wiley & Sons, Ltd, The Atrium, Southern Gate, Chichester, West Sussex, PO19 8SQ, UK

Editorial Offices
9600 Garsington Road, Oxford, OX4 2DQ, UK
The Atrium, Southern Gate, Chichester, West Sussex, PO19 8SQ, UK
2121 State Avenue, Ames, Iowa 50014-8300, USA

For details of our global editorial offices, for customer services and for information about how to apply for permission to reuse the copyright material in this book please see our website at www.wiley.com/wiley-blackwell.

Library of Congress Cataloging-in-Publication Data

Phytonutrients / edited by Andrew Salter, Helen Wiseman, Gregory Tucker.
    p. cm.
  Includes bibliographical references and index.
  ISBN 978-1-4051-3151-3 (hardcover : alk. paper)
1. Phytonutrients. 2. Phytochemicals. 3. Food–Composition. I. Salter, Andrew M.
II. Wiseman, Helen. III. Tucker, G. A. (Gregory A.)
  QK861.P49 2012
  572′.2–dc23
                                        2011045493
A catalogue record for this book is available from the British Library.

Wiley also publishes its books in a variety of electronic formats. Some content that appears in print may not be available in electronic books.

Set in 10/12.5pt Times by SPi Publisher Services, Pondicherry, India
Printed and bound in Malaysia by Vivar Printing Sdn Bhd

1 2012

Contents

Preface

Plants have been a major source of nutrition for humans ever since the start of our evolution, although more recently we have become more reliant on animal-based foods. This has led to some challenging situations in terms of diet and health and we are encouraged, through schemes such as the 5-A-Day campaign, to consume more plant-based foods. Plants can provide us with almost all of our dietary requirements and this includes macronutrients such as carbohydrates and lipids as well as the wide range of essential micronutrients such as vitamins and minerals. It is also becoming increasingly evident that many other phytochemicals, whilst perhaps not essential, are nonetheless beneficial to our health. These would include the carotenoids, polyphenols and phytoestrogens.

There has long been an interest amongst plant scientists in the enhancement of nutrients within crops. Traditionally this has been brought about by breeding or modifications to agronomic or horticultural practice. More recently this has also been achieved through the application of genetic engineering, for example to enhance levels of vitamins such as vitamin A and folate, or through manipulation of biosynthetic pathways to introduce novel nutrients into plants such as the production of long chain polyunsaturated fatty acids. Such modifications to the plants metabolism often require an intricate knowledge of the metabolic pathways and more specifically their control. Acquisition of this knowledge is greatly facilitated by the rapid progress being made in the areas of transcriptomics, proteomics and systems biology.

These phytonutrients are normally presented in the diet in the form of a complex food matrix. Understanding the interactions between this matrix and the digestive system is a key part of modelling the fate of nutrients in the diet. The plant cell wall for instance can represent a barrier to the release of nutrients and its 'digestibility' in the gastrointestinal tract is a significant factor in determining the bioaccessibility of nutrients. Similarly, the fate of nutrients in terms of how they are able to cross the gut lumen and their subsequent metabolism within the body are also key factors in determining bioavailability and functionality, respectively.

This book contains contributions from both plant scientists and nutritionists. The plant science perspective is primarily about how nutrients are made within the plant and how this may be manipulated to enhance their levels or availability. The nutrition perspective is more on how these food matrices behave during digestion and, more specifically, the functionality of nutrients within the body. It is hoped therefore that this book will be of interest to researchers and students in both of these disciplines. Indeed one of its aims is to encourage understanding, dialogue and collaboration between these two often disparate fields of expertise.

Contributors

John Brameld

Nutritional Sciences Division, University of Nottingham, Sutton Bonington Campus, Loughborough, Leicestershire, LE12 5RD, UK.

John Brameld is currently Associate Professor of Nutritional Biochemistry at the University of Nottingham. His main interests relate to the regulatory effects of nutrients on gene expression in relation to cell/tissue development, metabolism and function.

Martin R. Broadley

Plant and Crop Sciences Division, University of Nottingham, Sutton Bonington Campus, Loughborough, Leicestershire, LE12 5RD, UK.

Dr Martin Broadley is a Reader in Plant Nutrition at the University of Nottingham. Martin's research focus is on mineral dynamics in soil-plant systems, including the use of agronomic and genetics-based understanding of mineral improvement of crops (biofortification).

Judith Buttriss

British Nutrition Foundation. High Holborn House, 52-54 High Holborn, London WC1V 6RQ.

Professor Judith Buttriss is the Director General at the British Nutrition Foundation, a post she has held since 2007; prior to this she was the Foundation's Science Director since 1998. She is a public health nutritionist with an interest in a broad range of nutrition topics.

David Gray

Food Sciences Division, University of Nottingham, Sutton Bonington Campus, Loughborough, Leicestershire, LE12 5RD, UK.

Dr David Gray gained his PhD in the field of plant lipid biochemistry and is now an Associate Professor in Food Chemistry. His research includes an exploration of novel ways of delivering healthy oils to foods, with minimum loss to oil quality and minimum impact on the environment.

Úrsula Flores-Perez

Centre for Research in Agricultural Genomics (CRAG) CSIC-IRTA-UAB, Campus UAB Bellaterra, 08193 Barcelona, Spain.

Dr. Flores-Perez obtained her PhD degree at CRAG, where she developed her interest in the regulation of plant carotenoid biosynthesis and biotechnology. She is currently a postdoctoral fellow working on plastid import mechanisms at the Department of Biology, University of Leicester, University Road, Leicester LE1 7RH, UK.

Manuel Rodriguez-Concepcion
Centre for Research in Agricultural Genomics (CRAG) CSIC-IRTA-UAB, Campus UAB Bellaterra, 08193 Barcelona, Spain.
Dr. Rodriguez-Concepcion is a Research Professor at CRAG, where he leads a group working on the regulation of isoprenoid and carotenoid biosynthesis. His research has unveiled a number of molecular mechanisms used by plant cells to control the supply of carotenoid precursors and their channelling to the carotenoid pathway at transcriptional and post-transcriptional levels.

Stéphane Ravanel
Laboratoire de Physiologie Cellulaire Végétale, UMR5168 CNRS- UMR1200 INRA – CEA-Université Joseph Fourier Grenoble I, Institut de Recherches en Technologies et Sciences pour le Vivant – CEA-Grenoble, 17 rue des Martyrs, 38054 Grenoble Cedex 9, France.
Dr Stéphane Ravanel is a plant biochemist and molecular biologist with a long-standing interest in the metabolism of amino acids and folates.

Fabrice Rébeillé
Laboratoire de Physiologie Cellulaire Végétale, UMR5168 CNRS- UMR1200 INRA – CEA-Université Joseph Fourier Grenoble I, Institut de Recherches en Technologies et Sciences pour le Vivant – CEA-Grenoble, 17 rue des Martyrs, 38054 Grenoble Cedex 9, France.
Dr Fabrice Rébeillé is a plant biochemist and physiologist who has been conducting research on photorespiration before studying folate metabolism.

Andrew Salter
Nutritional Sciences Division, University of Nottingham, Sutton Bonington Campus, Loughborough, Leicestershire, LE12 5RD, UK.
Andy Salter is Professor of Nutritional Biochemistry. His major interests lie in the mechanisms whereby dietary fatty acids regulate lipid and lipoprotein metabolism and development of atherosclerosis.

Jeremy P E Spencer
Molecular Nutrition Group, School of Chemistry, Food and Pharmacy, University of Reading, Reading, RG2 6AP, UK.
Professor Spencer is Leader of the Food Chain and Health sub-theme "Plant Bioactives and Health" within Food and Nutritional Sciences at Reading University. His interests are focused on investigating the molecular mechanisms that underlie the accumulating body of epidemiological, and medical anthropological evidence, on a positive correlation between the consumption of diets rich in fruits and vegetables and a decreased risk of neurodegenerative disorders.

Gregory Tucker
Nutritional Sciences Division, University of Nottingham, Sutton Bonington Campus, Loughborough, Leicestershire, LE12 5RD, UK.
Greg Tucker is Professor of Plant Biochemistry at Nottingham University. A major area of interest is the molecular basis of quality in fruit and vegetables. This includes

methods to extend the shelf life of these commodities and the impact that this may have on nutritional composition.

Katerina Vafeiadou
Molecular Nutrition Group, School of Chemistry, Food and Pharmacy, University of Reading, Reading, RG2 6AP, UK.
Dr Katerina Vafeiadou is a research fellow at the Hugh Sinclair Unit of Human Nutrition, University of Reading. Dr Vafeiadou has previously carried out research on the effects of dietary flavonoids on both cardiovascular and neurodegenerative diseases, with main focus on flavonoids role in the prevention of inflammation and endothelial dysfunction. Dr Vafeiadou is currently working for a Food Standards Agency project which investigates the impact of replacing dietary saturated fats with either monounsaturated fats or polyunsaturated fats on cardiovascular risk.

David Vauzour
Norwich Medical School, Faculty of Medicine and Health Sciences, University of East Anglia, Norwich, NR4 7TJ, UK.
Dr David Vauzour is a Senior Research Associate at Norwich Medical School, University of East Anglia. Dr Vauzour has carried out many investigations on the influence of phytochemicals on brain health through their interactions with specific cellular signalling pathways pivotal in protection against neurotoxins, in preventing neuroinflammation and in controlling memory, learning and neuro-cognitive performances.

Philip J. White
The Scottish Crop Research Institute, Invergowrie, Dundee, DD2 5DA, UK.
Professor Philip J. White is a Senior Research Scientist at Scottish Crop Research Institute (which became The James Hutton Institute w.e.f. April 2011). Philip's research comprises a wide range of subjects within the field of plant mineral nutrition, ranging from molecular genetic through to agronomic scales. He has previously held positions at the Universities of Edinburgh and Cambridge, and Horticulture Research International. He is a Special Professor in Plant Ion Transport at the University of Nottingham, and a Visiting Associate Professor at the Comenius University, Bratislava.

Helen Wiseman
Nutritional Sciences, Diabetes and Nutritional Sciences Division, King's College London, Franklin-Wilkins Building, 150 Stamford Street, London, SE1 9NH.
Dr Helen Wiseman leads the Phytochemical Research Group at King's College London. Dr Wiseman has carried out numerous investigations of the potential health effects of dietary phytochemicals, such as flavonoids, including possible protection against cardiovascular disease, cancer and loss of cognitive function, which may be exerted via a wide range of mechanisms including effects on gene expression, regulatory microRNA and post-translational modification and modulation of cell signalling pathways.

Abbreviations

AA	ascorbic acid
ACP	acyl carrier protein
ADC	4-amino-4-deoxychorismate
AdoMet	*S*-adenosylmethionine
AICAR	aminoimidazole carboxamide ribonucleotide
AICART	aminoimidazole carboximide ribonucleotide transformylase
ALA	alpha linolenic acid
ANR	anthocyanidin reductase
ANS	anthocyanidin synthase
BCO	β-carotene-15,15′-oxygenase
cAMP	cyclic AMP
CHD	coronary heart disease
CHI	chalcone flavanone isomerase
CHS	chalcone synthase
CHYB	carotenoid β-ring hydroxylase
CHYE	carotenoid ε-ring hydroxylase
CI	confidence interval
COMT	catechol-*O*-methyltransferases
CRTISO	carotenoid isomerase
CYP	cytochrome P450
CVD	cardiovascular disease
DAG	diacylglycerol
DAHP	D-arabino-heptulosonic acid 7-phosphate
DFE	dietary folate equivalents
DFR	dihydroflavonol reductase
DHA	docosahexaenoic acid
DHA	dehydroascorbate (Chapter 5)
DHAA	dehydroascorbic acid
DHF	dihydrofolate
DHFR	dihydrofolate reductase
DHPS	dihydropteroate synthase
DHQ	3-dehydroquinic acid
DMAPP	dimethylallyl diphosphate
DMPBQ	dimethylphytylbenoquinol
E-4-P	D-erythrose-4-phosphate

EGCG	epigallocatechin gallate
EPSP	3-enolpyruvylshikimic acid 3-phosphate
ER	endoplasmic reticulum
ERK	extracellular signal-related kinase
EPA	eicosapentoenoic acid
F3H	Flavanone 3-hydroxylase
FAS	fatty acid synthase complex
FCL	5-formyl-THF cycloligase
FGGH	folylpolyglutamate γ-glutamyl hydrolase
FPGS	folylpolyglutamate synthetase
FS	flavone synthase
FTCD	glutamate formiminotransferase/formimino-THF cyclodeaminase
FTHFS	10-formyl-THF synthetase
GAR	glycinamide ribonucleotide
GART	glycinamide ribonucleotide transformylase
GBSS	granule bound starch synthase
GDC	glycine decarboxylase
GI	gastrointestinal tract
GGPP	geranylgeranyl pyrophosphate
GGR	geranylgeranyl reductase
GH	glycosyl hydrolase
GLA	gamma linolenic acid
GLUT	glucose transporter
GSH	glutathione
GSHPx	glutathione peroxidise
GT	glycosyl transferase
GTPCHI	GTP-cyclohydrolase I 7,8-dihydroneopterin (DHN) triphosphate
HBA	hydroxybenzoic acids
HCA	hydroxycinnamic acids
HDL	high density lipoproteins
HO-1	haem oxygenase 1
HPPK	hydroxymethyldihydropterin pyrophosphokinase
IFS	isoflavone synthase
IMP	inosine monophosphate
IPP	isopentenyl diphosphate
JNK	c-jun amino-terminal kinase
KPHMT	ketopantoate hydroxymethyl transferase
LA	linoleic acid
LAR	leucoanthocyanidin reductase
LCYB	lycopene cyclase B
LCYE	lycopene cyclase E
LDL	low density lipoprotein
MAPK	MAP kinase signalling pathway
MATE	multidrug and toxin extrusion transporter
MDHA	monodehydroascorbate

MEP	methylerythritol 4-phosphate pathway
MGGBQ	2-methy-6-phytylbenzoquinol
MPBQ	2-methy-6-phytylbenzoquinol
MRP	multidrug resistance-associated proteins
MS	methionine synthase
MTF	methionyl-tRNA transformylase
MTHFC	5,10-methenyl-THF cyclohydrolase
MTHFD	5,10-methylene-THF dehydrogenase
MUFA	monounsaturated fatty acid
NSP	non starch polysaccharide
NTD	neural tube defects
ODA	octadecatetraenoic acid
pABA	para-aminobenzoic acid
pABAGlu$_n$	*p*-aminobenzoyl(poly)glutamate
PAL	phenylalanine ammonia lyase
PC	phosphatidylcholine
PDP	phytyl pyrophosphate
PDS	phytoene desaturase
PE	phosphatydyl ethanolamine
PEP	phosphoenolpyruvate
PMP	phytol monophosphate
PPAR	peroxisome proliferator activated receptor
PS1	photosystem 1
PSY	phytoene synthase
PUFA	polyunsaturated fatty acid
QTL	quantitative trait loci
RALDH	NAD$^+$-dependent retinal dehydrogenase
RDA	recommended dietary allowance
RDH	retinol dehydrogenase
ROS	reactive oxygen species
RR	relative risk
SBE	starch branching enzyme
SDE	starch debranching enzyme
SFA	saturated fatty acid
SHMT	serine hydroxymethyl transferase
SVCT	sodium vitamin C co-transporters
TAG	triacyl glycerol
TAL	tyrosine ammonia lyase
TG	triglycerides
THF	tetrahydrofolates
TS	thymidylate synthase
UFGT	UDP glucose-flavonoid 3-*O*-glucosyl transferase
UGT	UDP-glucuronosyltransferases
VAD	vitamin A deficiency
VDE	violaxanthin de-epoxidase

VLDL	very low density lipoproteins
XET	xyloglucan endo transglycosylase
ZDS	ζ-carotene desaturase
ZEP	zeaxanthin eopxidase

Chapter 1

Plant foods and health

Judith Buttriss

Introduction

The purpose of this introductory chapter is to pave the way for subsequent chapters by looking at the historical context of plant food consumption, reviewing the contribution plant foods make to intakes of essential nutrients (e.g. fibre, vitamins, minerals, protein and essential fatty acids), examining the evidence linking plant food intake to health, summarising current recommendations and policy regarding plant food intake, and comparing these recommendations with current intakes.

Historical changes in the plant content of the human diet

Throughout human history, communities and societies have developed a diversity of dietary patterns and habits that have taken advantage of the food plants and animals available to them as a result of personal skills, climate, geography, trade and economic status. It is a basic premise the diets that persisted were capable of providing sufficient energy and essential nutrients to support growth and reproduction. They may not, however, have been conducive to optimal health.

Archaeological investigations have been used to predict what the diet of early man was like. Nestle (1999) cites Eaton and Konner (1985) who proposed that by the time of the emergence of modern *Homo sapiens* 45 000 years ago (Table 1.1), meat intake was high, but lean, and plant foods provided levels of vitamin C that exceed current recommendations. The diets of those modern day communities who survive primarily through hunting and gathering have also been used as a source of information, although the extent to which the diets of such communities simulate those of early man can only be speculated. Estimates suggest that most of the modern day hunter-gatherer communities lived in areas where plant foods grew readily, one exception being the indigenous people living in the Arctic whose traditional diets were dominated by meat and who relied almost completely on hunting for much of the year (Eaton and Konner 1985). Also, anthropologists have examined the diets of closely related primates for clues about the possible diets of our distant

Phytonutrients, First Edition. Edited by Andrew Salter, Helen Wiseman and Gregory Tucker.
© 2012 Blackwell Publishing Ltd. Published 2012 by Blackwell Publishing Ltd.

Table 1.1   Stages of evolution of human diets

	Time period elapsed (years)
Pleistocene: Stone Age	1.6 million
Homo sapiens: Archaic	400 000
Neanderthal	80 000
Modern	45 000
Holocene: Agriculture	10 000
Industrial revolution	200
Global food economy	50

Adapted from Eaton and Konner (1985).

ancestors. In general, primates seem to eat whatever is convenient, mainly plants but also insects, eggs, crustaceans and carrion (Nestle 1999). Recent documentary evidence has captured film of chimpanzees and other primates hunting and killing animals as prey, which has subsequently been shown on wildlife television programmes in the UK.

Archaeology has provided considerable evidence for meat consumption by early man, including characteristic marks on fossilised animal bones and stone artefacts consistent with meat eating. However, this information must be considered in context: bones are better preserved than vegetable matter and hence reliance on such evidence is likely to underestimate plant food consumption (Nestle 1999).

Plant foods can be categorised in many ways but the method used here can be seen in Table 1.2. It has been suggested that the plant foods gathered by our early ancestors were those that did not require digging with hands or sticks, such as fruits, leaves and stems, and seeds in pod-like structures (e.g. peas, beans) that would have provided protein. There is also early evidence of the cultivation and storage of legumes such as broad beans in the Middle East, where 'farming' is said to have begun, and among cave dwellers living as far apart as Mexico and Peru, and north-east Thailand (Toussaint-Samat 1992). Similar evidence exists for collection of wild chick peas, lentils and peas, followed by their cultivation.

In hot, humid areas where top soil is poor, root systems grow near to the surface and will have been easy to forage. In more temperate climates, such as the Middle East, a stick or similar pointed implement would probably have been required and its use was perhaps the first step towards farming. The digging stick is thought to have been the ancestor of the hoe and the plough (Toussaint-Samat 1992). Roots and tubers, gathered or cultivated, have been a dietary staple in tropical zones since early times, providing energy and being easy to acquire. A limited number are popular now but many other examples exist in nature. The sweet potato, for example, comes from the equatorial forests of South America but is thought to have reached Polynesia 2000 years ago, perhaps via early trade (Toussaint-Samat 1992). The potato and sweet potato reached the shores of Europe as part of a present to Queen Isabella of Spain from Christopher Columbus. The potato itself was not popular and had to wait until the eighteenth century before it came into its own, but the versatile sweet potato was a success in Elizabethan England, perhaps because of its sweet taste at a time when sugar was scarce and very expensive (Toussaint-Samat 1992). Following the example of the native Indians in North America, European colonists made sweet potato one of their national dishes. The Jerusalem artichoke, another tuber, is also well travelled.

Table 1.2 Categorisation of plant derived foods and drinks

Group	Examples
Fruits	
Tree Fruits	Apples, pears, plums, apricots, peaches, cherries, citrus fruit, dates, pineapple, mango, papaya, fig, olive
Soft fruits	Strawberries, raspberries, blackberries, cranberries, currants
Other	Melons, grapes, kiwi, bananas
Vegetables	
Root crops*	Potatoes, sweet potatoes, yam, cassava
	Carrots, turnips, swedes, parsnips
Cabbage family	Cabbage, broccoli, Brussels sprouts
Onion family	Onions, leeks, garlic
Salad vegetables	Lettuce, celery, cucumbers
Tomato family	Tomatoes, sweet peppers, chilli peppers, aubergine
Mushrooms and fungi	Mushroom varieties, Quorn™
Other	Squashes, sprouted seeds, sea vegetables
Cereals (grains)	Wheat, barley, maize (corn), millet, oats, rice, rye
Tree nuts and seeds	Walnuts, cashews, almonds, chestnuts, pecans, brazils, hazelnuts, pistachio, pine kernels, sesame seeds, pumpkin seeds
Pulses (legumes)	Soya beans and products e.g. tofu, red kidney beans, butter beans, chick peas, lentils, peanuts (groundnuts)
Beverages	Tea, coffee, cocoa, wine, spirits, beer
Oils	Seed oils e.g. sunflower oil, corn oil, rapeseed oil, linseed oil; olive oil, soya oil, peanut oil; evening primrose oil, borage oil
Other	Chocolate
Herbs, spices, condiments	Sage, rosemary, thyme, ginger, pepper, cumin, mustard, tomato-based sauces

*Potato, sweet potato and yam are classified as starchy foods, rather than vegetables, in many food guidance models.
From Buttriss 2003.

It was found growing wild in North America and transported across the Atlantic in the seventeenth century and is said to be the only food plant that has been introduced to Europe from North America (Toussaint-Samat 1992). The yam, of a different botanical family to the sweet potato, grows naturally in tropical forests all over the world and is relatively rich in protein. Tapioca, a popular milk pudding ingredient in the recent past, is derived from cassava. The cassava shrub is protected from parasites by the cyanide compounds (prussic acid) it contains in the skin of its tubers, which need to be carefully prepared before consumption because even a tiny quantity of the bitter cassava juice causes instant death. The complex methods for its preparation must presumably have been identified by trial and error among people with very limited dietary options.

There is also early evidence of the consumption of onions, which have the advantage that they can be eaten raw. They grow wild in a large part of the Middle East and the Indian subcontinent, and it is suggested they were used to relieve the monotony of frugal diets. Labourers working on the Great Pyramid were paid in onions, garlic and parsley, and onions accompanied Egyptian mummies into their tombs (Toussaint-Samat 1992). The onion has been widely used over the centuries and was taken on long sea voyages in the hope that it might prevent scurvy. Garlic, also a member of the allium family, is thought to have come from a desert area of Central Asia and is surrounded by a remarkably rich and ancient body of folklore.

The discovery and study of Palaeolithic refuse tips has been facilitated because grains found there were preserved from the ravages of time by carbonisation (parching) during their processing to remove the inedible husk. This primitive form of 'cooking' in stone age culture remained in use in the Middle Ages (Toussaint-Samat 1992). Perhaps the development of such techniques and the identification of areas where wild cereals grew in abundance or could be cultivated were triggers for people to become 'settled' in one place rather than living a more nomadic life, thus experiencing a less tenuous lifestyle and greater life expectancy. Early evidence shows that initially the cereals cultivated were identical to the wild types, but even as early as 10 000 BC there is evidence from Jericho of selection of the forms of barley and wheat that less readily shed their seed on ripening, allowing it to be harvested more effectively. Indeed there is evidence from all around the world of early cereal cultivation thousands of years ago, for example in the Dordogne in France in 8000 BC, Japan in 7500 BC, Mexico in 6000 BC, Denmark, China and Siberia in 4000 BC, and India in 3000 BC. By AD 100, rye and oat cultivation was widespread across Europe, joining wheat which had been in cultivation in many parts of Europe for some time (Toussaint-Samat 1992). The spread of cereal growing provides information about the migration of the people who consumed it, as they took their customs with them.

The most commonly consumed cereal grains in the human diet are wheat, rice and maize, although barley, oats, rye, millet and sorghum are more common in some countries than others, consumption patterns being largely determined by climate and cultural differences (Southgate 2000).

Current dietary patterns in developed countries have been largely shaped by the changes in food production that began with the industrial revolution during the 1800s. These dietary patterns have been fuelled by a global food economy in which food is now transported long distances, enabling a diverse range of plant foods to be available in shops all year round and removing the dependency on local, seasonal produce.

In developing countries in the twenty-first century, plant-based diets are associated with extreme poverty and poor health and, when economic conditions improve, low-income populations tend to increase their consumption of meat, and display fewer signs of nutritional deficiency (Nestle 1999). However, as such countries become still more prosperous and 'westernised' they begin to share the disease patterns prominent in Europe, North America and Australasia, characterised by obesity, type 2 diabetes, cardiovascular disease and particular forms of cancer such as colon cancer. In such populations, nutrition policy focuses on restoring the balance between foods derived directly from plants, such as fruits, vegetables, wholegrain cereal products and pulses, and, on the other hand, foods derived from animals, which can be relatively high in saturated fatty acids though good sources of essential vitamins and minerals, and processed foods rich in fat, sugar or salt.

It has also recently become apparent that the diversity of plant foods collected in the wild and consumed in developing countries is greater than previously thought. For example, East African food systems are based on a rich diversity of traditional cereals, legumes, leafy vegetables, indigenous fruits (and animal source foods) that are cultivated or gathered from the wild (Johns and Eyzaguirre 2006). Retention of traditional food habits based on local knowledge and biodiversity is important for food security.

Changing composition of dietary constituents in the past 50 years

Improvements in agricultural practices and the development of new products have led to a change in both the composition of individual foods and the patterns of food consumption all over the world. Plants and animals used as food exhibit marked variations in composition, against which the effects of changes in production and processing need to be judged. Changes that have occurred in connection with new developments in farming and food processing often fall well within this natural variation (Paul 1977).

There are many factors that influence the composition of plants, the most important being genetic inheritance, growing conditions (light intensity, heat, moisture and fertilisers) and maturity when harvested. After harvesting, changes may also take place during storage and distribution. Furthermore, particularly with vegetables, nutrient content can be affected by cooking processes. Therefore, changes in the nature of the crops grown and growing conditions will have had an impact on their composition. For example, the vitamin C content of tomatoes is enhanced by direct sun, being outdoors, fast ripening, and use of potassium and manganese fertiliser, and is higher in the outer part of the fruit. It is decreased by shade, being under glass, slow ripening and use of nitrogen fertiliser (Paul 1977).

The major drivers for changes in food choice have been innovations in food processing. Although processes such as canning, freezing and drying are not new, continuous improvements have been made to these processes over recent decades and these techniques have been joined in recent years by other packaging and processing innovations. In particular, over the past 50 years almost ubiquitous home ownership of fridges and freezers has had a major impact on the types of foods that can be consumed all year round. Processing improvements have also enabled storage losses to be minimised, especially of labile nutrients such as vitamin C.

By the late 1970s, consumption of processed potato products had also increased, from contributing up to 2% of total potato consumption in 1955 to 30% (Paul 1977). This was of interest with regards to the vitamin C content of potatoes, which falls progressively during storage and varied between products available at that time.

In addition to changes in the type of a particular product bought, new products were coming onto the market, for example soya-based meat substitutes. These were designed to replace meat in the diet but had a different amino acid profile, notably lower methionine.

Thirty years on, these changes have been overtaken by a huge range of new processes, formulations and products, making it even more challenging to maintain good quality food composition data. Food composition databases are essential to the work of a variety of different users, including those involved in nutritional research, health care professionals, the food industry, regulatory bodies and caterers.

Since 2005, the British Nutrition Foundation has been a partner in a project known as EuroFIR (European Food Information Resource Network of Excellence), which has created a pan-European databank of food composition information (Williamson and Buttriss 2007). The EuroFIR network has comprised around 50 organisations across Europe and beyond. Its work continues through EuroFIR Nexus (a further 2 year grant from the European Commission, 2011–12) and a not-for-profit organisation established in Brussels. A feature of the work of EuroFIR has been to develop a comprehensive database of published information about bioactive substances in plant foods. More information and progress to date with this database and the projects as a whole can be found at http://www.eurofir.eu.

Plants – nutrients and other constituents

Before discussing the evidence linking plant food intake with health, it is helpful to consider the range of different nutrients available to us from the plant kingdom and the plethora of other components, sometimes referred to as bioactive substances or phytochemicals, that may confer health benefits. A summary of these and examples of their plant food sources can be found in Table 1.3.

A summary of the evidence linking plant food intake and health

A substantial number of epidemiological studies have shown that people who consume a diet rich in fruits, vegetables and other plant foods (e.g. nuts and pulses) are at reduced risk of developing cardiovascular disease (CVD), i.e. coronary heart disease and stroke, and to a lesser extent cancer (Margetts and Buttriss 2003; Stanner et al. 2004; Hung et al. 2004; He et al. 2007; Crowe et al. 2011). As a result of their analysis of two large US cohorts, Hung and colleagues (2004) propose that the benefits, especially in relation to cancer, may have been overstated. This has been confirmed by the World Cancer Research Fund/American Institute for Cancer Research (WCRF/AICR) report published in 2007, which reported that the overall evidence for fruits and vegetables had reduced in strength as new research had been published since their report of 1997. However, with regard to dietary fibre and colon cancer, the evidence of a protective effect has strengthened and is now regarded as convincing (WCRF/AICR 2010).

The beneficial effects of diets rich in plant foods have also been reported for other chronic conditions, namely age-related macular degeneration (AMD) (Goldberg et al. 1998), cataract (Brown et al. 1999a), chronic obstructive pulmonary disease (e.g. asthma and bronchitis) (Miedema et al. 1993) and dementia (Morris et al. 2006). However, the associations are typically less strong and, as discussed later in more detail, little is known for certain about the mechanisms by which plant foods exert their apparent effects.

These associations have led to efforts to identify the mechanisms underpinning these health effects and the active components within plant foods, as mentioned earlier. There are several plausible reasons why there may be an association between fruit and vegetable consumption and a reduced risk of chronic disease, apart from possible confounders associated with other factors such as non-smoking and physical activity (Lampe 1999). These include changes to detoxification enzymes; stimulation of the immune system; reduction

Table 1.3 Nutrients and other constituents of plant-derived foods and drinks

Plant constituent	Main plant derived sources in the UK
Minerals	
Calcium	Bread (flour is fortified in the UK), pulses, green vegetables, (and if eaten regularly, dried fruit, nuts and seeds)
Chromium	Whole grains, and to a lesser extent legumes and nuts
Copper	Bread and cereal products, vegetables
Iodine	Sea vegetables, e.g. kelp, beer
Iron	Vegetables, pulses; to a lesser extent potatoes and dried fruit Fortified breakfast cereals and foods made from fortified flour are also important sources
Magnesium	Cereals and products (especially wholegrain), green vegetables, nuts and seeds
Manganese	Tea is a major source Other sources include wholegrain cereals, vegetables, nuts and seeds
Molybdenum	Vegetables, bread and other cereal products Also present in pulses
Potassium	Particularly abundant in vegetables, potatoes, fruit (especially bananas), and juices It is also found in bread, nuts and seeds
Selenium	Cereals, concentration being dependent on soil type
Zinc	Cereal products such as bread, especially wholemeal Other plant sources include bead and lentils, nuts, sweetcorn and rice Absorption is relatively poor from phytate-rich cereals
Vitamins	
Folate	Green leafy vegetables (raw or lightly boiled), especially sprouts and spinach; green beans and peas, potatoes; fruit, especially oranges
Niacin	Potatoes Also present in fortified cereals and bread
Riboflavin	Fortified breakfast cereals
Thiamin	All cereals, potatoes Also present in vegetables
Vitamin B6	Potatoes and breakfast cereals
Vitamin C	Richest sources are citrus fruit, citrus fruit juices, kiwi fruit, soft fruits Other sources include green vegetables, other fruit, peppers, potatoes (especially new potatoes)
Vitamin E	Vegetable oils, wholegrain cereals, vegetables (especially dark green leafy types), fruit, vegetable oils, cereals
Vitamin K	Green leafy vegetables are the richest source Also in other vegetables, fruit, vegetable oils and cereals
Other nutrients	
Dietary fibre	All cereals (especially wholegrain), vegetables, fruit, pulses, nuts
Fatty acids MUFA	Rich sources are olive oil and rapeseed oil Also present in other seed and nut oils
PUFA (n-6) PUFA (n-3)	Rich sources are sunflower, safflower and corn oils Also present in other seed and nut oils

(Continued)

Table 1.3   (Cont'd)

Plant constituent	Main plant derived sources in the UK
	There are no plant sources of the long chain n-3 fatty acids (EPA and DHA) associated with hear health, but the essential fatty acid α-linolenic acid is present in large amounts in linseed (flax) oil, grapeseed and rapeseed oils, walnut oil and walnuts It is also present in green leafy vegetables, soybeans (and soya oil) and hazelnuts
Other plant substances	
Carotenoids α-carotene	Carrots, butternut squash, oranges, tangerines; other sources include passion fruit andkumquats
β-carotene Lycopene	Orange vegetables (eg carrots), green leafy vegetables (e.g. spinach), tomato products; other sources include apricots, guava, mangoes, orange melons, passion fruit Tomato and tomato products
Flavonoids, eg flavanols, flavan-3-ols, flavones, flavanones, anthocyanidins	Tea, red wine, onions, apples are major sources of this large family of compounds Cocoa and hence dark chocolate also provide members of this family, primarily flavan-3-ols But sources of specific types of compounds also include grapes, berries and cherries (flavonols, anthocyanidins); parsley, thyme and celery (flavones); citrus fruit (flavanones)
Glucosinolates	Brassica vegetables eg sprouts, cabbage, broccoli
Phytoestrogens (isoflavones, lignans)	Soya, seeds, e.g. linseed, other pulses, grains, nuts
Sterols and stanols	Naturally present in vegetable oils eg soya oil Also present in cereals, nuts and vegetables
Sulphur-containing compounds	Onions, leeks, garlic, chives (also see glucosinolates)
Terpenoids other than carotenoids	Herbs and spices, e.g. mint, sage, coriander, rosemary, ginger

Adapted from Buttriss (2003).

of platelet aggregation; an effect on cholesterol synthesis, blood pressure or hormone metabolism; and antioxidant effects.

A popular explanation within the scientific community, and more recently among the general public, is that dietary antioxidants, including vitamins C and E, the carotenoids (e.g. beta-carotene, lycopene and lutein), selenium, and flavonoids may prevent carcinogenesis and the atherosclerosis associated with heart disease and stroke by blocking oxidative damage to DNA, lipids and proteins, as discussed in more detail later. Normal oxidative metabolism produces large quantities of potentially damaging oxidants (free radicals) that can damage cells and tissues in a number of ways, including disruption of normal repair mechanisms. The delicate balance between pro- and antioxidants determines the degree of oxidative stress, and this has been implicated in the pathophysiology of many chronic diseases, including heart disease, diabetes, cancer and the ageing process (Jackson 2003).

In relation to a potential protective role for antioxidant nutrients, a substantial amount of work has been done in the areas of CVD and cancer, and some of this is summarised here. To date, much of the research has concerned fruits and vegetables, although many of the compounds of interest are to be found in other plant-derived foods, such as tea, cocoa, cereals, wine and herbs.

Associated with this research effort, there has been interest in the use of health claims on foods. A European Commission (EC) regulation on nutrition and health claims was agreed in December 2006. It applies to all nutrition and health claims made in commercial communications, i.e. labelling, presentation or advertising of foods, and aims to provide a high level of consumer protection whilst allowing the European Union market to function effectively. The regulation came into force on 1 July 2007. It describes how nutrition and health claims should be used, and the procedures that need to be followed to obtain authorisation of a claim by the EC (http://ec.europa.eu/food/food/labellingnutrition/claims/community_register/index_en.htm).

This regulation will provide a list of permitted nutrition and health claims that can be used by food operators across the EU and the process for assessing claims is ongoing. Ultimately, only health claims that are on this list will be permitted for use in the EU, although there are interim measures in place to give manufacturers and retailers time to adapt to the new rules.

Overall any claim made should be truthful and not attempt to mislead consumers. Nor should it call into question the safety or nutritional content of other foods or the adequacy of a balanced diet. The claim itself must apply to the food as eaten, prepared according to the manufacturer's instructions, and the effects described in the claim must be understandable to the average consumer.

The science underpinning each potential health claim is being assessed by the European Food Safety Authority (EFSA). A large number of potential claims have been submitted for consideration and many of these have received negative opinions. The EC makes the final decision on whether or not to approve the claim, as they must take consumer understanding as well as the science into account, but it is very unlikely that approval will be given to any of those claims for which EFSA has specified that a cause and effect relationship has not been established or that the constituent in question has not been sufficiently characterised.

Coronary heart disease and stroke

Fruits and vegetables

Armstrong and Doll were among the first to note associations between population food patterns, based on UK National Food Survey data, and data concerning mortality from coronary heart disease (CHD) (Armstrong and Doll 1975). CHD rates were higher in areas where fruit and vegetable consumption was lowest. Across Europe, countries whose populations consumed the most fruits and vegetables have been shown to have lower rates of CHD, and analyses of trends over time suggest an inverse relationship between declines in fruit and vegetable consumption and increasing rates of CHD.

The Women's Health Study in the USA has shown that women who eat more fruit and vegetables had a lower cardiovascular risk, particularly in relation to myocardial infarction

(Liu et al. 2000a). Similar results have been reported in a cohort study of Swedish men (Strandhagen et al. 2000). A factor analysis using data from the Health Professionals' Follow-up Survey (Hu et al. 2000) showed that men following a 'prudent diet', characterised by higher intake of vegetables, fruit, legumes, wholegrains, fish and poultry, were less likely to develop coronary heart disease. Knekt et al. (1996) found that intake of apples and onions and intake of flavonoids were inversely linked to coronary mortality in a Finnish cohort. A more recent analysis (Knekt et al. 2000) has shown that apples remain protective against thrombotic or embolic stroke, after adjustment for intake of quercetin. This suggests that there may be other bioactive substances in apples that need further investigation.

In their meta-analysis of cohort studies investigating the relationship between ischaemic heart disease and markers of fruit and vegetable consumption (both the foods themselves and related nutrients), Law and Morris concluded that the risk of ischaemic heart disease is about 15% lower at the 90th than at the 10th centile of fruit and vegetable intake (Law and Morris, 1998).

After an average of 8.4 years of follow up of more than 313 000 men and women in the EPIC study, those consuming at least eight (80g) portions of fruit and vegetables a day had a 22% lower risk of fatal IHD than those consuming fewer than three portions a day (Crowe et al. 2011); a one portion (80g) increment was associated with a 4% lower risk.

Bobak et al. (1999) compared men in the Czech Republic, Bavaria and Israel and suggested that differences in fruit and vegetable intakes may explain differences in risk factors between eastern and western Europe. Ness and Powles reviewed the literature linking fruit and vegetable consumption with risk of CHD (Ness and Powles 1997) and compared this with the literature on stroke (Ness and Powles 1999). They found that in nine out of ten ecological studies, two of three case-control studies and six out of sixteen cohort studies there was a significant inverse association between coronary heart disease and intake of fruit and vegetables (or a nutrient used as a marker of intake) (Ness and Powles, 1997). For stroke, three out of five ecological studies, and six of eight cohort studies showed an association of this type (Ness and Powles, 1999). The authors concluded that although studies showing no effect may be under-reported, the results were consistent with a strong protective effect of fruit and vegetables for stroke and a weaker protective effect for coronary heart disease.

Using data from the Nurses' Health Study and the Health Professionals Follow-up study, an analysis by Hu (2003) identified relative risks of coronary artery disease associated with different categories of fruits and vegetables (Table 1.4). Again stronger support for an association with stroke was evident, especially for total fruit, citrus fruit and vitamin C rich fruits and vegetables (Hu 2003).

Joshipura et al. (1999) examined intakes of specific fruits and vegetables, as well as overall fruit and vegetable intake, in two large cohorts of US men and women, followed for 8 and 14 years respectively, and free of cardiovascular disease, cancer and diabetes at baseline. After controlling for standard cardiovascular risk factors, those in the highest quintile of fruit and vegetable intake (median 5.1 servings per day in men and 5.8 in women) had a relative risk for ischaemic stroke of 0.69 compared with those in the lowest quintile. An increment of one serving per day of fruit or vegetables was associated with a 6% lower risk of ischaemic stroke. Green leafy vegetables, cruciferous vegetables and

Table 1.4 Multivariate relative risks (RRs) of coronary artery disease based on a comparison of the highest and the lowest quintiles of fruit and vegetable intakes in the pooled analyses of the Nurses' Health Study and the Health Professionals' Follow-up Study

Food	RR (95% CIs)	
	Coronary artery disease	Stroke
All fruit	0.80 (0.69, 0.92)	0.69 (0.52, 0.91)
All vegetables	0.82 (0.71, 0.94)	0.90 (0.68, 1.18)
Total citrus fruit	0.88 (0.77, 1.00)	0.72 (0.47, 1.11)
Citrus fruit juice	1.06 (0.85, 1.32)	0.65 (0.51, 0.84)
Cruciferous vegetables	0.86 (0.75, 0.99)	0.71 (0.55, 0.93)
Green leafy vegetables	0.72 (0.63, 0.83)	0.76 (0.58, 0.99)
Vitamin C rich fruit and vegetables	0.91 (079, 1.04)	0.68 (0.52, 0.89)
Legumes	1.06 (0.91, 1.24)	1.03 (0.77, 1.39)
Potatoes (including French fries)	1.15 (0.78, 1.70)	1.18 (0.90, 1.54)

RRs adjusted for standard cardiovascular disease risk factors.
Source: Hu (2003).

citrus fruit including fruit juice contributed most to the apparent protective effect. A particular role for citrus fruit in reducing CHD risk has also been reported in the PRIME study of subjects in France and Northern Ireland (Dauchet et al. 2004).

Van't Veer and colleagues (2000) carried out a review of 250 observational studies (case-control and prospective) on cardiovascular disease and cancer, in which measurements were made of fruit and vegetable intake (excluding potatoes). The authors noted that, overall, testing the efficacy of fruits and vegetables in population trials is hampered by methodological factors such as 'blinding' (i.e. it is not possible to conceal the true exposure from either subjects or researchers), compliance and study duration. Relative risks (RR) or odds ratios (OR) (depending on the type of study) for high versus low intake of fruit and vegetables were calculated. The proportion of cases attributable to low consumption was estimated using three scenarios: best guess, optimistic (using stronger RRs) and conservative (using weaker RRs and eliminating the contribution of smoking and/or drinking). These RRs usually represented risk for subjects in the highest versus the lowest category of intake, typically a difference of about 150 g/day of fruit and vegetables. These estimates represent the overall effect of beneficial and adverse properties of fruits and vegetables. The researchers calculated the proportion of cases of CVD that could be prevented in the Dutch population if current average intakes of 250 g/day were increased to 400 g/day (the World Health Organisation recommendation). The 'best guess' estimate for cardiovascular disease was 16% (8000 cases annually), ranging from 6% (conservative) to 22% (optimistic).

A meta-analysis of nine independent cohorts (comprising 257 551 individuals and adjusted for major confounding factors), with an average follow-up of 13 years, reported a 11% reduction in risk of stroke in those consuming three to five servings of fruits and vegetables per day compared to less than three servings, and a reduction in risk of 26% in those consuming more than five servings (see Figure 1.1) (He et al. 2006). The authors

	Servings per day		Relative risk (95% CI)
Joshipura et al[6] (women)	3–5		0.89 (0.66–1.20)
	>5		0.70 (0.58–0.85)
Joshipura et al[6] (men)	3–5		0.77 (0.49–1.20)
	>5		0.78 (0.57–1.06)
Hirvonen et al[7]	3–5		0.85 (0.78–0.93)
	>5		0.74 (0.58–0.95)
Bazzano et al[8]	3–5		0.94 (0.83–1.07)
	>5		0.70 (0.55–0.89)
Johnsen et al[9]	3–5		0.86 (0.66–1.12)
	>5		0.73 (0.54–0.99)
Sauvaget et al[10]	3–5		0.90 (0.82–0.99)
	>5		0.75 (0.69–0.82)
Steffen et al[11]	3–5		1.24 (0.96–1.61)
	>5		0.94 (0.54–1.63)
Keli et al[15]	3–5		0.82 (0.54–1.24)
	>5		0.75 (0.45–1.24)
Gillman et al[16]	3–5		0.60 (0.39–0.92)
	>5		0.49 (0.30–0.79)
Pooled relative risk	3–5		**0.89 (0.83–0.97)**
	>5		**0.74 (0.69–0.79)**

0.2   0.5   1.0   2.0   5.0
Relative risk

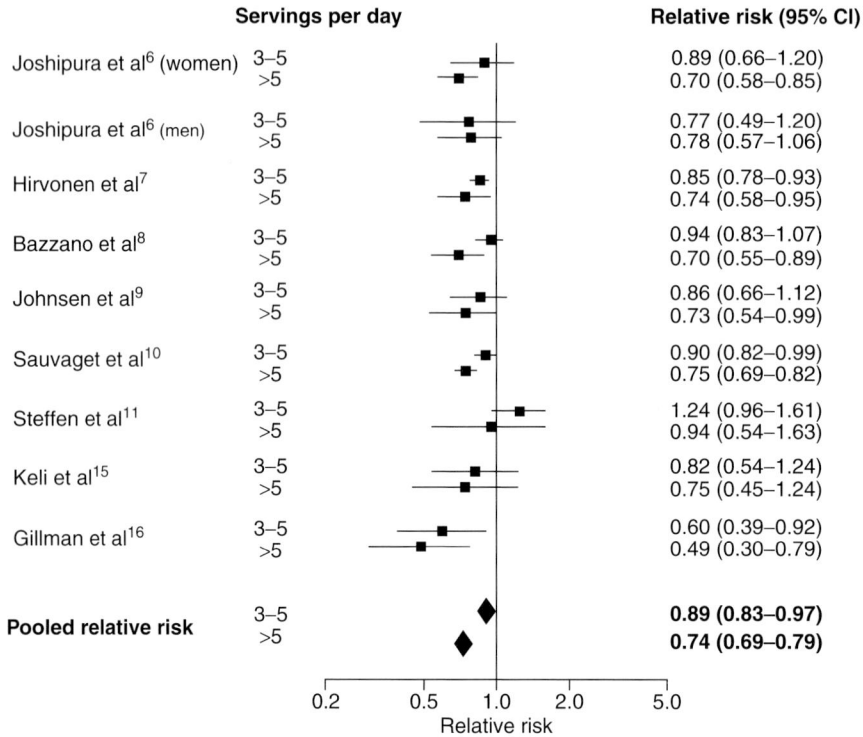

Figure 1.1   Risk of stroke for 3–5 and 5+ servings of fruit and vegetables per day compared with less than 3 servings. Size of the squares is proportional to weight of the studies in the meta-analysis. Source: He *et al.* 2006.

speculate that the mechanism of effect may concern potassium, or possibly folate or dietary fibre, all of which are present in these foods.

A meta-analysis of 13 independent cohorts, followed prospectively, found that both fruits and vegetables had a significant protective effect on CHD risk and that increased consumption of fruits and vegetables from less than three to more than five servings a day was associated with a 17% reduction in CHD risk (He et al. 2007).

A number of studies have compared vegetarians with non-vegetarians. Key et al. (1996) studied a cohort of health-conscious men and women, 43% of whom said they were vegetarian. They found that daily consumption of fresh fruit was associated with significantly lower deaths from ischaemic heart disease after adjustment for smoking (rate ratio 0.76), deaths from cerebrovascular disease (rate ratio 0.68) and with significantly lower all-cause mortality (rate ratio 0.79). In a subsequent study, Key et al. (1998) conducted a pooled analysis of data from five major cohort studies in the USA, UK and Germany. Vegetarians (defined as not eating any fish or meat) had a 24% lower mortality rate from ischaemic heart disease than non-vegetarians (Key et al. 1998). This reduction in risk was greatest for the younger age groups; for example, the rate ratio for premature death from ischaemic heart disease (under the age of 65 years) was 0.55 and for those aged 65–79 it was 0.69 (Key et al. 1998). Although plant foods may contribute to this effect, the habits of vegetarians tend to differ in a number of ways from the general population, for example they are typically more health conscious, less likely to smoke and more likely to be physically active.

Two of the most important risk factors for CVD are raised serum cholesterol and hypertension. Many experimental studies have explored the effects of changing diet on these two risk factors, although there are relatively fewer trials that have assessed the effects of changing food patterns. The most widely quoted study that has changed dietary patterns is the DASH trial (Appel et al. 1997). This study showed that a diet rich in fruits and vegetables, low in fat and incorporating low-fat dairy products, without changes in salt or weight loss, could lower blood pressure. Reducing salt had an additional benefit (Sacks et al. 2001). Other trials have broadly supported the results from DASH showing that moving dietary patterns towards a more plant-based food intake is associated with lower blood pressure.

Fruit and vegetable consumption has also been associated inversely with low-density lipoprotein (LDL)-cholesterol concentrations in men and women, for example in cross-sectional studies (Djousse et al. 2004). Subjects in the highest fruit and vegetable groups had LDL concentrations that were 6–7% lower than those in the lowest groups, an effect that the authors suggest may be attributable to dietary fibre (propionic acid derived from fermentation of fibre in the large bowel has been shown to reduce blood cholesterol). For a review on fibre and health, see Lunn and Buttriss (2007). However results of other studies have been inconsistent. For example, a similar response (a 7.3% reduction) was seen in the Indian Diet Heart Study, a 12-week intervention study (Singh et al. 1992), whilst no significant effect was reported in the 8-week DASH trial (Obarzanek et al. 2001).

Much less work has focused on bioactive substances in plants but a trial by Hodgson et al. (1999) showed that giving isoflavones (found in soya beans for example) did not reduce blood pressure compared with the response to a placebo, highlighting a need for caution in extrapolating from the effects of foods to specific compounds and vice versa.

The Lyon Diet Heart Study (de Lorgeril et al. 1999) showed that various modifications to a 'Mediterranean'-type diet, in patients who survived a first myocardial infarction, led to a statistically significant reduction in the occurrence of subsequent cardiac death and non-fatal myocardial infarction over a 4-year period. The dietary changes included fruit and vegetable intakes and the type of fat consumed. The percentage energy from fat in the diet of the control group was 33.6% compared with 30.4% in the experimental group; these fat intakes are well below current UK levels. No details on the exact dietary differences or the increase in plant-based food intake were given, but the authors noted that there seemed to be good compliance with dietary advice over the 4 years of follow-up.

Pulses and nuts

There have been relatively few studies that have looked specifically at the effects of pulses and nuts and risk of CHD and stroke. Participants in the National Health and Nutrition Examination Survey (NHANES) epidemiological follow-up study who ate more legumes (including dry beans, as well as peanuts and peanut butter) had a lower risk of CHD and CVD (Bazzano et al. 2001). No association was found between legume consumption and stroke in the two Boston cohort studies (Joshipura et al. 1999). Using a series of meta-analyses of prospective cohort studies, Hu (2003) compared the relative effects of fruit and vegetables, nuts and wholegrains on cardiovascular risk.

Table 1.5 Impact of wholegrain consumption on cardiovascular disease risk

Risk Factor or end point	Study and no. of subjects	Outcome	Reference
Death rates from CVD	Iowa Women's Health Study (baseline data from 1984, follow-up to 1995) 34 333 women	HR of all CVD across quintiles of whole-grain intake was 0.82 (95% CI 0.66. 1.01; $P = 0.02$) HR for deaths from CHD across quintiles of whole-grain intake was 0.82 (95% CI 0.63, 1.06; $P = 0.03$) HR for deaths from stroke and other CVD were not significantly different across quintiles of whole-grain intake.	Jacobs et al. (1999)
Incidence and deaths from IHD	California Seventh-day Adventists (baseline data from 1976, 6-year follow-up) 13 857 men, 20 341 women	RR of fatal IHD was lower (0.89; $P < 0.005$) and non-fatal IHD was lower (0.56; $P < 0.01$) in those who preferred wholegrain bread compared with those who preferred white bread	Fraser (1999)
Incidence and deaths from CHD	Nurses' Health study (baseline data from 1984, average 10-year follow-up) 75 521 women	RR for cases of CHD across quintiles of whole-grain intake was 0.47 (95% CI 0.27, 0.79; $P = 0.006$) for never smokers, and was 0.79 (95% CI 0.62, 1.01 $P = 0.07$) for the full cohort	Liu et al. (2000b)
Incidence of Ischaemic stroke	Nurses' Health study (baseline data from 1984, average 12-year follow-up) 75 521 women	RR of incident IHD across quintiles of whole-grain intake was 0.69 (95% CI 0.50, 0.98; $P = 0.03$)	
Death rates from CHD and CVD	Bread eaters in Norwegian County Study (data from 1977 to 1994) 16 933 men, 16 915 women	HR of death from CHD across quintiles of wholegrain bread consumption was 0.75 (95% CI 0.65, 0.88, $P = 0.006$) HR of CVD across quintiles of wholegrain bread consumption was 0.77 (95% CI 0.60 0.98 $P = 0.016$)	Jacobs et al. (2001)
Incidence of coronary artery and ischaemic stroke	Atherosclerosis Risk in Communities cohort (baseline data in 1987–9, 11-year follow-up) 11 940 subjects	HR of incident coronary artery disease across quintiles of whole-grain intake was 0.72 (95% CI 0.53, 0.97; $P = 0.05$) HR of incident ischaemic stroke across quintiles of whole-grain intake was 0.75 (95% CI 0.46, 1.22; $P = 0.15$)	Steffen et al. (2003)
Non-Fatal myocardial infarction and fatal CHD	Health Professionals Follow-up study (data from 1986 to 2000) 42 850 men	HR of CHD between highest and lowest quintile of whole-grain intake was 0.82 (95% CI 0.70, 0.96; $P = 0.01$	Jensen et al. (2004)

Source: Seal (2006).

Legumes, including soya and its products, have been associated in clinical studies with decreased serum cholesterol. Anderson et al. (1995) reported that their meta-analysis of 38 studies, which provided an average of 47 g/day of soya protein, showed an average reduction in total and LDL cholesterol of 0.6 and 0.56 mmol/L, respectively. It should be noted that despite a wide range of soya protein intakes (17–124 g/day) in these studies, no dose–response effect was evident. Also, only seven of the studies used intakes of soya protein of 25 g or less. Achievement of an intake of 25 g within the context of the UK diet would require replacement of dietary items at each meal with soya-derived foods, e.g. soya drink or tofu (BNF 2002).

A review of five large cohort studies (the Adventist Health Study, the Iowa Women's Health Study, the Nurses' Health Study, the Cholesterol and Recurrent Events (CARE) Study and the Physicians' Health Study) showed that eating nuts more than once a week was associated with a decreased risk of CHD in both men and women (RRs varied from 0.45 to 0.75) (Kris-Etherton et al. 2001). They also reviewed 11 clinical trials of the effects of diets containing nuts on lipid and lipoprotein endpoints: they concluded that it was not possible to attribute the lipid-lowering effect to nuts alone because of the complex nature of most of the dietary interventions. Four clinical trials compared the lipid lowering effects of diets with or without nuts, and suggested that the diets with nuts had a greater effect. As well as being low in saturates, nuts contain fibre, various micronutrients and other bioactive substances such as phytosterols, recognised for their lipid lowering properties (see later). There has been particular interest in almonds (Berryman et al. 2011) and also walnuts (EFSA 2011a). Potential mechanisms, including a vasodilatory effect via the arginine-nitric oxide pathway have been summarised (Hu 2003; Berryman et al. 2011).

Cereals

Cereal grains and their products are an important part of most diets around the world (Truswell 2002). Several prospective cohort studies have specifically explored the association between wholegrain cereals and risk of CVD (Pietinen et al. 1996; Jacobs et al. 1999; Liu et al. 1999; Steffen et al. 2003; Jensen et al. 2004) and these studies have been reviewed (Seal 2006; see Table 1.5). The consensus from these studies is that people who eat a healthy diet, of which wholegrain cereals form a part, have a lower risk of CVD and that the effect is independent of an effect of dietary fibre (see Seal 2006; Seal et al. 2006). In another meta-analysis of seven studies, a pooled average of 2.5 servings per day versus 0.2 servings per day was associated with a 21% lower risk of CVD events. Nevertheless, the exact mechanism remains unclear and analysis is complicated because wholegrain consumption is often a marker of a healthy diet in other respects (Mellen et al. 2008).

To date there have been few large intervention studies to support the epidemiological findings. The Wholeheart Study, a 16-week intervention in 100 subjects, found no effect on LDL cholesterol of enhanced wholegrain consumption (3 × 20 g servings per day or 3 rising to 6 servings per day compared to control), and no effect on blood pressure or other markers of CVD risk (Brownlee et al. 2010). In another (12-week) intervention that assessed the effects of three daily portions of wholegrain foods (provided as only wheat or a mixture of wheat and oats) on cardiovascular risk factors in over 200 relatively high-risk subjects, systolic blood pressure and pulse pressure were significantly reduced by 6 and 3 mmHg respectively (Tighe et al. 2010). Other CVD markers were largely unchanged. The reduction in systolic blood pressure was judged to be sufficient to reduce the incidence of coronary artery disease and stroke by ≥15% and 25%, respectively.

Recently, evidence from meta-analysis has emerged that consumption of wholegrains may be associated with weight control and reduced obesity, especially central adiposity (Harland and Garton 2008).

In contrast to the relatively small number of studies on wholegrains, there have been many studies, including large prospective cohort studies and smaller intervention studies, that have considered interactions between dietary fibre intake and risk of cardiovascular disease. Individuals consuming high-fibre diets (13–14.7 g/1000 kcal) have a substantially (15–59%) reduced their risk of developing coronary heart disease compared with those consuming the lowest amounts of fibre (3–6 g/1000 kcal). Several large-scale cohorts have estimated the effect on coronary heart disease risk of increasing fibre intake (see Lunn and Buttriss 2007 for a review). An increase in intake of 6g/day of dietary fibre has been shown to be associated with a 33% reduction in risk of coronary heart disease in women and a 24% reduction in men (Khaw and Barrett-Connor 1987). A similar study reported a 19% decrease when fibre intake was increased by 10g/d (Rimm et al. 1996). A pooled analysis of 10 prospective cohort studies reported a 14% decrease in the risk of CHD for each 10 g/day increase in dietary fibre intake (Pereira et al. 2004). Intervention trials have also demonstrated the effectiveness of dietary fibre in modifying blood lipid concentrations.

Some of the strongest associations have been in studies focusing on particular fibre components, e.g. oat bran or oatmeal. It has been estimated that consumption of at least 3 g/day of soluble fibre from oats lowers blood cholesterol levels by 0.13 mmol/L in people whose blood cholesterol levels were less than 5.9 mmol/L i.e. only moderately elevated. EFSA has published a positive opinion regarding the association between beta glucan consumption and maintenance of healthy cholesterol levels (EFSA 2011b). Similar cholesterol lowering effects have been reported when other viscous fibres – such as guar gums, pectin and psyllium – are fed (Brown et al. 1999b; Lunn and Buttriss 2007).

There is now emerging evidence that the type or source of dietary fibre is especially relevant in terms of CHD prevention. A review by Flight and Clifton (2006) has demonstrated the importance of cereal grains in reducing CHD risk and a recent analysis (He et al. 2010) reported an association between the bran component of wholegrain foods and reduced CVD specific mortality (and all cause mortality) in women with type 2 diabetes. Viscous, soluble fibres such as gums, psyllium and beta-glucan are believed to reduce cholesterol concentrations by altering cholesterol and bile acid absorption, and by effects on hepatic lipoprotein production and cholesterol synthesis. But when the whole grain is considered, mechanisms involving the other components of whole grains, e.g. magnesium, folate or vitamin E, cannot be discounted; indeed there may be a complex interplay between other components present in plant foods.

Cereal grains (and soya beans, flaxseed, fruits and vegetables) also contribute lignans, rye being a particularly rich source. These are converted to enterolactones by gut bacteria and have been suggested to have beneficial health effects (see Seal 2006).

Antioxidant nutrients

Dietary antioxidants have been the focus of much research interest with respect to CVD (Buttriss et al. 2002; Stanner et al. 2004; Bruckdorfer 2005).

Although there are some exceptions, cross-sectional studies comparing different populations within one country or between different countries have found that the incidence of CVD, particularly in Europe, is inversely associated with plasma levels of beta-carotene, vitamin E and, to a lesser extent, vitamin C (see Stanner et al. 2004). For example, plasma vitamin C concentration was inversely related to mortality from all causes and from CVD and ischaemic heart disease in men and women in the Norfolk cohort of the European Prospective Investigation into Cancer and Nutrition (EPIC) (Khaw et al. 2001). Risk of death during the 4-year study period in the top vitamin C quintile was about half the risk in the lowest quintile, the association being continuous through the whole distribution of concentrations. A 20 μmol/L difference in vitamin C, approximately equivalent to a 50 g/day difference in fruit and vegetable intake, was associated with a 25% fall in the risk of all-cause mortality, which was independent of other risk factors. The authors concluded that a small increase in fruit and vegetables, amounting to an extra daily serving, has encouraging prospects in helping to prevent disease.

Some case-control studies have also reported similar relationships between cardiovascular risk and nutrient status. For example, subjects with CVD have been shown to have lower levels of plasma vitamin E and selenium than subjects without CVD (Beaglehole et al. 1990), and lower leucocyte concentrations of vitamin C have been reported in subjects with angiographic coronary artery disease compared with controls (Riemersma et al. 1990). However, case-control studies cannot exclude the possibility of changes in nutritional status as a consequence of the disease. A more convincing source of evidence is prospective studies in which nutrient status is measured years before the onset of the disease. Several large studies of this type have considered the relationship between dietary antioxidant nutrients or vitamin supplements and the incidence of CVD. They have generally identified a trend towards decreasing risk of CVD incidence or mortality with higher dietary intake of vitamin E, beta-carotene and vitamin C, and with higher plasma levels of these vitamins, each of which is largely derived from plant foods (see Stanner et al. 2004 for a review). It is of note that the studies that investigated dietary supply of vitamins were generally more convincing than those that investigated the impact of supplements.

In their review of relative risks for CHD, Tavani and La Vecchia (1999) found that whilst case-control studies and six cohort studies suggested inverse associations between beta-carotene and relative risk of CHD, four more recent cohort studies showed no association. Four randomised controlled trials of beta-carotene supplementation were found to give relative risks close to unity for the association. The authors concluded that the apparent benefit in observational studies may be linked to consumption of foods rich in beta-carotene rather than beta-carotene itself (Tavani and La Vecchia, 1999).

In their meta-analysis of cohort studies, in which a 15% reduction in risk of ischaemic heart disease between the top and bottom deciles of fruit and vegetable consumption was estimated, Law and Morris (1998) concluded that intakes of beta-carotene or vitamin E are unlikely to be important but that the combined effect of potassium, folate and possibly fibre in fruit and vegetables could account for the difference in risk.

The findings of prospective studies investigating the link between low selenium intake/ status and heart disease have been more mixed, and an association has only been found in countries where selenium status has been low until recently, such as Finland (Salonen et al. 1982; BNF 2001).

Although not perfect, intervention trials are usually considered to be a superior type of study design because this approach is able to measure causal relationships between diet and a health outcome. A number of large studies have been conducted and some of the most positive evidence comes from the Cambridge Heart Antioxidant Study (CHAOS), which showed that vitamin E treatment significantly reduced the rate of non-fatal heart attacks although it had relatively little effect on CVD deaths (Stephens et al. 1996). Other smaller trials have also demonstrated the benefit of antioxidant supplementation in groups of high risk patients but the majority of primary and secondary prevention trials have failed to detect any benefit of supplementation with vitamin E or other dietary antioxidants (see Stanner et al. 2004). Examples include the Heart Protection Study of a cocktail of vitamins in 20 000 UK adults with CHD (Heart Protection Study Collaborative Group 2002), the HOPE trial of almost 10 000 subjects aged 55 years and over that showed no effect of dietary supplementation on the risk of stroke (Health Outcomes Prevention Evaluation (HOPE) Study Investigators 2000) and the Alpha Tocopherol Beta Carotene Prevention Study (ATBC), in which supplemental beta-carotene actually increased the incidence of cerebral haemorrhage in a high risk group (Leppala et al. 2000) and led to an increase in fatal heart attacks (see Stanner et al. 2004).

In summary, systematic reviews and meta-analyses of trials (e.g. Marchioli et al. 1999; Asplund 2002; Morris and Carson 2003; Vivekananthan et al. 2003) have concluded that despite evidence from observational studies suggesting an association between occurrence of CVD and low intakes or plasma levels of antioxidant nutrients, supplementation with single antioxidants or cocktails has not been found to be of benefit in either primary or secondary prevention trials. So, despite considerable effort in the antioxidant nutrients field, it remains unclear as to which components of fruits and vegetables are responsible for their apparent protective effect in CVD risk reduction.

Other bioactive substances

This failure to demonstrate an effect for antioxidant nutrients in CVD risk reduction has led researchers to look at other plant components with antioxidant properties, such as flavonoids, in the search for a protective mechanism in CVD. But, to date, the findings have not been particularly consistent and the stronger findings have often been associated with case-control studies, which are generally regarded to be less convincing than prospective studies. However, more progress has been made in other fields, such as cognitive function, as described later.

A number of studies have investigated associations between flavonoids and CHD. An ecological study of middle-aged men from 16 different cohorts showed an inverse association between flavonoid intake and coronary mortality (Hertog et al. 1995). Also, in some, but not all, prospective studies, a diet rich in the flavonoids (found mainly in apples, onions, tea and wine) has been associated with a reduced risk of subsequent heart disease (Hollman and Katan 1999). The Iowa postmenopausal women's study reported flavonoid intake to be associated with a decreased risk of death from CHD after adjustment for age and energy intake. Of the foods contributing to flavonoid intake, only broccoli was strongly associated with a decreased risk (Yochum et al. 1999); there was no association between flavonoid intake and stroke. In a review of prospective epidemiological studies, Hollman and Katan (1999) found that intake of flavonols and flavones was inversely associated with subsequent CHD in most but not all studies.

The findings of subsequent studies have continued to be inconsistent. A meta-analysis of seven prospective cohort studies (including 105 000 people aged 30–84 years), designed to overcome the fact that many studies have been small, suggested a 20% reduction of risk of CHD deaths when the top and bottom tertiles of intake were compared (RR 0.80, 95% CI 0.69–0.93) (Huxley and Neil 2003). Mean duration of follow-up of subjects was 6–26 years. In four of the seven studies, intake was assessed at baseline using a food frequency questionnaire validated against 7-day weighed intakes and in the remaining studies the information was obtained from an interview with a trained dietitian. A cross-sectional analysis with the SU.VI.MAX cohort in France suggested, perhaps confusingly, that women with a high intake of flavonoids were at lower risk and men at higher risk of CVD (Mennen et al. 2004).

Other studies have focused on flavonoid-rich foods or on specific classes of flavonoids. Sesso et al. (2003) reported non-significant inverse associations for CVD risk and tea consumption (four or more cups per day), broccoli and apples, although their interpretation has been criticised (Donovan 2004). Conversely, others have reported a stronger association (Arts et al. 2001a).

There has also been interest in flavonols present in cocoa, red wine and tea in the context of a possible beneficial effect on endothelial function and hence cardiovascular health. To date there have been some clinical trials (in healthy volunteers and in subjects with cardiovascular risk markers) that have been suggestive of a beneficial effect on endothelial function but they have typically been short term (see Kay et al. 2006; Heiss et al. 2006, Hodgson 2006 for reviews). Whilst these findings are promising, longer term studies and mechanistic investigations are needed to establish whether these short-term effects on endothelial function translate into long-term cardiovascular health benefits.

As reported earlier, case-control studies frequently provide more optimistic findings than studies with more robust designs such as prospective cohort studies, although these too can be sources of measurement error. A case control study in Italy looked at the impact of intake of specific flavonoids on risk of myocardial infarction and reported a reduced risk with high intakes of anthocyanins, which are abundant in berries (Tavani et al. 2006) and another in Greece reported an inverse association between CHD risk and flavan-3-ols, which are largely found in tea and wine; they reported that an increase in intake of about 24 mg/day corresponded to a 24% reduction in risk (Lagiou et al. 2004).

A major difficulty with such studies is delivering an accurate assessment of flavonoid intakes given the limitations of current food composition databases in this respect, the diversity of flavonoid compounds and the general problems associated with assessing dietary intakes. Accessibility to high quality data on plant bioactives is being addressed by the EU-funded project *EuroFIR* (www.eurofir.eu).

Antioxidant hypothesis

In conclusion, the results of the various trials concerning the link between antioxidants and CVD are generally not supportive of the oxidation hypothesis. Bruckdorfer (2005) has suggested various possible explanations of this:

- The habitual diets of many of the subjects studied are unlikely to have been low in the antioxidant vitamins studied, and supplementation may saturate body tissues. For example, intakes as low as 100 mg/day will saturate body tissues in most individuals.
- The limited range of antioxidants selected for the studies may not have been the most appropriate because antioxidants are not necessarily interchangeable in terms of their effect in quenching free radical reactions.
- The oxidation process is initiated at an early stage in the atherosclerosis process; supplementation later on in the process may not be able to reverse the process.
- Antioxidants may be unable to enter the necrotic core of unstable atherosclerotic plaques, which pose the highest risk for CVD, making late antioxidant therapy ineffective. Evidence that antioxidants do have beneficial effects on vasomotor tone suggests that the intimal regions may be more accessible.
- Under conditions where free transitional metal ions or delocalised iron-containing proteins are available, antioxidants can exert pro-oxidant properties and may promote further damage.
- The role of oxidation processes in the development of atherosclerosis may be a contributing one rather than a central one.

It is quite plausible that mechanisms other than those involving antioxidants potentially may be responsible for some of these observations, for example displacement or binding of potentially toxic compounds, enzyme inhibition or activation, selective interaction within cell signalling cascades or a direct effect on gene expression within tissues. There is ongoing work focusing on other potential mechanisms by which flavonoids might exert a beneficial effect on cardiovascular health, including platelet reactivity and increased fibrinolysis (Holt et al. 2006) and potentially anti-inflammatory effects (Selmi et al. 2006). In addition, non-antioxidant nutrients found in plants may be involved. For example, it is also now recognised that dietary folate/folic acid intake is inversely associated with blood levels of homocysteine, a recognised risk factor for CHD, but despite a number of large trials totalling about 14 000 participants, there is no clear evidence of the benefit of B vitamin supplementation on the risk of vascular disease (Clarke, 2009).

Phytosterols and –stanols

In contrast there is now a large body of evidence to support a link between consumption of plant stanols and plant sterols and cholesterol lowering (Caswell et al. 2008), and associated health claims have been approved (http://ec.europa.eu/food/food/labellingnutrition/claims/community_register/index_en.htm).

Conclusions for coronary heart disease and stroke

Plant-based diets are associated with a lower risk of CVD (e.g. CHD and stroke). Fruit and vegetable consumption is generally associated with other health-promoting activities, e.g. being physically active and not smoking, as well as a higher consumption of wholegrain cereals. Adjustment for such factors does not explain the association between high fruit and vegetable intake and lowered risk, although adjustment often attenuates the strength of the association. There is evidence of a dose–response relationship that is consistent with current recommendations to increase intakes of these foods. It is difficult to separate out the role of diet in general and of specific nutrients in particular, and so the causal mechanism(s) associated with this dietary pattern remain to be established. Most epidemiological research has focused on a number of individual antioxidants studied in relative isolation (see previous sections) and it is likely that at the very least there is a complex interaction between the many components found in plant foods, and the rest of the diet, that may have an integrated effect on CHD risk.

Cancer

The COMA Working Group on The Nutritional Aspects of Cancer (Department of Health, 1998) systematically reviewed the data on associating diet with various forms of cancer. This subject was also reviewed by the World Cancer Research Fund (WRCF) and the American Institute of Cancer Research (AICR) in 1997 and again in 2007 (WCRF 1997; WRCF and AIRC 2007).

Fruit and vegetables

These major reviews used different methodologies and the WCRF/AICR reviews looked at the available data from a global perspective. Although the conclusions of the UK report were more guarded, the two reports reached similar conclusions in the majority of cases, as shown in Table 1.6.

In summary, the UK COMA Working Group concluded that, overall, there is moderate evidence that higher vegetable consumption will reduce the risk of colorectal cancer, and that higher fruit and vegetable consumption will reduce the risk of gastric cancer. There is weak evidence, based on fewer data, that higher fruit and vegetable consumption will reduce the risk of breast cancer. These cancers combined represent about 18% of the cancer burden in men and about 39% of the cancer burden in women in the UK, so even a small reduction in relative risk can have important public health benefits in terms of the reduction in the absolute numbers of people affected. The data generally show a graded reduction in risk associated with higher fruit and vegetable consumption. The overall picture supported the hypothesis that the consumption of fruits and vegetables protects against the development of some cancers. On the basis of their conclusions, the COMA Working Group recommended that fruit and vegetable consumption in the UK should increase. They did not specify by how much, but said that any increase would be expected to carry benefits.

Table 1.6 Summary of the conclusions of the WCRF/AICR and COMA reports on the possible effect of fruit and vegetable consumption on decreasing cancer risk

Cancer site	Committee on Medical Aspects of Food and Nutrition Policy, UK, 1998	World Cancer Research Fund/American Institute of Cancer Research, 1997	World Cancer Research Fund/American Institute of Cancer Research, 2007 (fruit)	World Cancer Research Fund/American Institute of Cancer Research, 2007 (non-starchy vegetables)
Mouth and pharynx	Weakly consistent for fruit, inconsistent for vegetables	Convincing	Probable	Probable
Larynx	Moderately consistent, limited data	Probable	Probable	Probable
Oesophagus	Strongly consistent	Convincing	Probable	Probable
Lung	Moderately consistent for fruit, weakly consistent for vegetables	Convincing, particularly for green vegetables and carrots	Probable	Limited–suggestive
Stomach	Moderately consistent	Convincing, particularly for raw vegetables, allium vegetables and citrus fruit	Probable	Probable, limited–suggestive for pulses
Pancreas	Strongly consistent, limited data	Probable	Limited–suggestive, probable for foods containing folate	Probable for foods containing folate
Liver	Not included in the review	Possible for vegetables, not fruit	Limited–suggestive	–
Colorectum	Moderately consistent for vegetables, inconsistent and limited data for fruit	Convincing for vegetables, limited and inconsistent data for fruit	Limited–suggestive	Limited–suggestive

Breast	Moderately consistent for vegetables, weakly consistent for fruit	Probable	—	—
Ovary	Insufficient data	Possible	—	Limited–suggestive
Endometrium	Insufficient data	Possible	—	Limited–suggestive
Cervix	Strongly consistent, limited data	Possible	—	Limited–suggestive for carrots
Prostate	Moderately consistent, especially raw and salad type for vegetables	Possible for vegetables	Probable for foods containing lycopene and foods containing selenium	Probable for foods containing lycopene, foods containing selenium and for pulses
Kidney	Not included in the review	Possible for vegetables	—	—
Bladder	Moderately consistent, limited data	Probable	—	—

Note: According to WCRF's assessment process, judgements of 'convincing' (none found for these foods) and 'probable' usually generate public health goals and recommendations for individuals. Other categories such as 'limited–suggestive' (i.e. limited amounts of information that can only be regarded as suggestive of a causative relationship) are not considered sufficient.

Sources: DH (1998); WCRF (1997, 2007).

Table 1.7 Summary analysis of the meta-analyses on fruit and vegetables and the risk of some cancers in case control and cohort studies

	Vegetables		Fruits	
	Case control	**Cohort**	**Case control**	**Cohort**
Mouth and pharynx	NS	?	↓	?
Larynx	NS	?	↓	?
Oesophagus	↓	?	↓	?
Breast	↓	NS	NS	NS
Lung	↓	NS	↓	↓
Bladder	NS	NS	↓	↓
Stomach	↓	NS	↓	NS
Colorectum	↓	NS	↓	NS

↓ Significant protective effect; NS, non-significant protective effect; ? inconclusive.
Source: Riboli and Norat (2003).

One of the weaknesses of the evidence base at the time the COMA and the first WCRF reviews were conducted and published was the relative reliance on case-control data and the relative lack of cohort studies for some cancer sites, the latter being viewed as a more robust study design, although it is still subject to measurement errors. Where cohort data did exist, they typically seemed to be weaker than those derived from the case-control studies (Table 1.7). Over the intervening years, more cohort studies have been completed and perhaps as a result the evidence base supporting a role for fruit and vegetables in cancer prevention has been somewhat weakened in some cases, as summarised in Table 1.6 (the column referring to the more recent WCRF review; i.e. a reduction for some cancer sites from convincing to probable).

A meta-analysis by Riboli and Norat (2003) discusses the relatively limited supportive evidence from cohort compared to case-control studies and they report that cohort studies do not support the hypothesis of a protective effect of fruit and vegetable consumption on colorectal cancer risk and suggest that the most promising way of reducing risk is to increase physical activity levels and avoid overweight. Indeed, the recent update from WCRF on colon cancer has provided support for this approach (WCRF and AICR 2010). However, Riboli and Norat (2003) do not discard the possibility that the lack of significance could be indicative of a lack of statistical power of the published cohort studies because of random error in the measurement of diet rather than because of the lack of a biological association.

Furthermore, over recent years, data has become available from the unique European Prospective Investigation into Cancer and Nutrition (EPIC), which has investigated dietary and other determinants of cancer and other diseases in nine European countries. The study began in 1992 and involves 406 303 subjects including two cohorts in the UK (Oxford and Norfolk). In the EPIC-Norfolk cohort of the study, additional data have been collected to enable assessment of determinants of chronic disease. Data from the study suggest that plasma ascorbic acid is inversely related to cancer mortality in men but not women (Khaw et al. 2001). Findings for fruits and vegetables are shown in Table 1.8.

Table 1.8   Findings from EPIC for plant foods and cancer, by main cancer site

Cancer site	Publications	Main results
Prostate	Key et al. (2004)	No association of fruits and vegetables with prostate cancer risk.
Lung	Miller et al. (2004)	Inverse association with fruit intake. No association with vegetables.
Colon and rectum	Bingham et al. (2003) Bingham et al. (2005) Jenab et al. (2004)	Inverse relation of dietary fibre with colorectal cancer incidence with the greatest protective effect in the left colon, and least in the rectum. No individual food source of fibre is significantly more protective than others. Confirmation of the above after adjustment for folate and longer follow up. Inverse association with nuts and seeds in women, but not men.
Breast	van Gils et al. (2005) Grace et al. (2004) Keinan-Boker et al. (2004)	No statistically significant decreased risks for fruits and vegetables. One study found positive association with isoflavones in EPIC-Norfolk cohort. But no association was found with these phytoestrogens in the EPIC-Utrecht cohort. Further analyses with pooled data are on-going.
Ovaries	Schulz et al. (2005)	No protective effect overall but some evidence of an effect of garlic/onions.

The recent update from WCRF on colon cancer risk concurred with the 2007 WCRF report that the evidence that fruits and non-starchy vegetables protect against colorectal cancer risk is limited (WCRF 2010).

Some pooling analyses have also been indicative of a weakening of the evidence base regarding the impact of fruits and vegetables on cancer risk. A pooled analysis of cohort studies suggests there is no significant association between breast cancer risk and fruit and vegetable consumption (totals and subcategories) (Smith-Warner et al. 2003), a finding that is supported by data from EPIC (van Gils et al. 2005). A similar study of 12 cohort studies found no significant association between fruit and vegetable intake and ovarian cancer (Koushik et al. 2006).

Inverse associations between fruit and vegetable consumption and lung cancer have been consistently reported. A recent analysis pooling eight prospective cohort studies indicates that the modest reduction on cancer risk that remains once smoking is taken into account is largely attributable to fruit, not vegetables (Smith-Warner et al. 2003). EPIC has also demonstrated a significant inverse association between fruit consumption and lung cancer (the hazard ratio for the highest consumption quintile relative to the lowest being 0.60). Again there was no association with total vegetable intake or consumption of vegetable subtypes (Miller et al. 2004). The primary focus remains the reduction of tobacco use.

Legumes and nuts

Very few studies have specifically investigated the relationship between the consumption of legumes or nuts and the risk of cancers, and the evidence is often difficult to interpret. The WCRF Report (WCRF, 1997) identified 58 epidemiological studies that reported results for pulses and cancer risk, either for specific pulses or pulses in general. There was no clear picture: 50% reported a reduced risk of cancer, 38% reported an increased risk and 12% reported no association. The 2007 report concluded that the evidence for pulses (in relation to stomach and prostate cancer specifically) is no more than limited-suggestive (WCRF 2007). Very few studies have looked specifically at the association between nut consumption and cancer risk and WCRF concluded that there was no evidence to suggest that nuts might protect against some cancers (WCRF 1997).

Foods containing fibre

The evidence for a role of dietary fibre in cancer protection has strengthened in recent years. The 2007 WCRF Panel concluded that such foods probably reduce the risk of colon cancer, and for oesophageal cancer the evidence was considered limited-suggestive. Recently, an update by WCRF of colon cancer risk, taking into account recently published studies, has concluded that the evidence for a protective effect from foods containing dietary fibre is now convincing (WRCF and AICR 2010). A meta-analysis revealed a 10% decrease in colorectal cancer for each 10 g of fibre consumed (12% for men and 8% for women). Intakes in Britain are currently 14.9 g/day in men and 12.8 g/day in women (Department of Health, 2011) and so fall short of the 18 g/day recommendation. A statistically significant 10% decrease in colorectal cancer risk with cereal fibre intake was found in meta-analysis. The reduction in risk with other sources of fibre was in the same direction but did not achieve statistical significance. For wholegrains, there was a 21% decreased risk per three servings a day for colorectal cancer and 16% decreased risk for colon cancer (WCRF and AICR 2010). Fibre exerts various effects in the gastrointestinal tract (such as increasing transit time and providing substrates for short chain fatty acid production via fermentation) but the specific mechanism of effect in cancer protection is still not understood. Fibre intake is also strongly correlated with folate intake but the WCRF update found that adjustment for folate did not typically affect the risk reduction attributed to fibre.

Vitamins

Case-control and prospective studies have consistently shown an inverse association between intake of carotenoids and risk of lung and stomach cancer (Department of Health 1998). Some prospective nested case-control studies have also shown an inverse association between plasma level and risk of lung cancer, with levels in the range 0.34–0.53 µmol/L conferring the lowest risk (National Academy of Sciences 2000). However, this association was no longer significant after adjusting for beta-cryptoxanthin. A recent pooling project of seven studies of beta-carotene and lung cancer failed to reveal a significant association (Mannisto et al. 2004). WCRF regards the evidence as probable for an inverse association between carotenoids and cancers of the mouth, pharynx, larynx and lung; between beta-carotene specifically and oesophageal cancer; and between lycopene and prostate cancer (WRCF 2007).

Vitamin C intake from food alone has been shown to be associated inversely with lung cancer risk in a pooling project of eight studies (Cho et al. 2006) but there was no association with total vitamin C intake. Most observational studies have also reported an inverse association between vitamin C status and cancer risk, particularly for the non-hormone-dependent cancers, and two large studies (NHANES II and EPIC) have found an inverse association between plasma vitamin C and cancer risk in men but not in women (Loria et al. 2000; Khaw et al. 2001). WCRF reported a probable inverse association between vitamin C intake and risk of oesophageal cancer (WRCF 2007).

The findings of intervention trials, which have the potential to identify causative relationships, have been summarised by Stanner et al. (2004). Beta-carotene supplements seem to offer no protection against cancer and may actually increase risk among smokers. There is no published evidence from randomised controlled trials of a role for high-dose vitamin C in cancer prevention, perhaps because dietary supply has been adequate in the subjects studied. There is also little evidence for a beneficial effect of vitamin E supplementation. However, there is some evidence to suggest that an adequate supply of selenium is important for cancer prevention, based on an association between increased risk of cancer at several sites in subjects with low baseline plasma selenium status in a selenium supplementation trial. WCRF reported a limited-suggestive inverse association between vitamin E and risk of oesophageal and prostate cancers and between selenium intake and risk of stomach and colorectal cancers. The inverse association between selenium and prostate cancer was considered probable (WRCF 2007).

COMA (Department of Health 1998) and authorities in the USA (see Krinsky and Johnson 2005) recommended the avoidance of beta-carotene supplements as a means of protecting against cancer and the need to exercise caution in the use of high doses of puri-fied supplements of other micronutrients as they cannot be assumed to be without risk.

Since publication of the COMA report, several studies have been published showing inverse associations between cancer risk and higher folate consumption (Kim 2006), for example in relation to colon (Giovannucci et al. 1998) and breast cancers (Sellers et al. 2001). A significantly lower risk of colorectal cancer was reported in the highest versus lowest category of food folate intake in a metanalysis of seven cohort studies, although the trend was non-significant for total folate (i.e. including folic acid supplements) (Sanjoaquin et al. 2005). Similar relationships also exist for folate status (although the results are not totally consistent) and reduced colorectal cancer risk, and data from intervention trials suggest that supplementation can improve surrogate endpoint markers for colorectal cancer (Kim 2006). Animal studies are also generally supportive but emphasise that the timing is critical and provision once cancer development is underway can promote the process (Kim 2006). These findings have been interpreted as suggestive of a dual modulatory role for folate. However, there is little evidence for other cancer sites, for example a pooling project on lung cancer found no association (Cho et al. 2006).

This subject has been reviewed recently by the UK's Scientific Advisory Committee (SACN 2006). SACN concluded that prospective studies suggest a trend towards a protec-tive effect of folate intake on colon cancer risk, in particular, but noted that some studies did not adjust for all likely confounding factors, such as fibre. The association was typically less strong for total folate intake (including folic acid from supplements). WRCF concluded that an inverse association between folate intake and pancreatic cancer was probable and was limited-suggestive between oesophageal and colorectal cancers (WRCF 2007).

Other plant-derived substances

Some of the more promising data comes from studies of glucosinolates. Alongside a variety of bioactive substances, these compounds are found in cruciferous (including brassica) vegetables such as sprouts, broccoli and cabbage. When these vegetables are chewed, crushed or sliced, isothiocynates and indoles are formed from the glucosinolates (they can also be formed less efficiently by the gut flora) and these have been shown in animal studies to inhibit chemically-induced colon cancer but recent prospective cohort studies have been inconsistent (see Lynn et al. 2006). Indeed, a series of seven cohort studies summarised by Lynn et al. revealed little evidence of a protective effect of cruciferous vegetable intake, although habitual intakes were low and measurement by a food frequency questionnaire may have led to poor assessments of intake. It has been suggested that there may be gene–nutrient interactions, and clinical studies have confirmed a possible effect in some subsets of the population, dependent on glutathione-S-transferase genotype (Seow et al. 2002). Possible mechanisms for the effects of cruciferous vegetables have been reviewed recently (Lynn et al. 2006) and include modulation of drug metabolising enzymes, induction of apoptosis (controlled cell death), cancer cell cycle arrest and antioxidant effects.

Several studies have investigated associations with flavonoids. There was no association found between the intake of five major flavonoids and mortality from total cancer, lung cancer, colorectal cancer or stomach cancer in an analysis of data from the Seven Countries Study after 25 years of follow-up (Hertog et al. 1995), or with mortality from cancer at all sites (Hertog et al. 1994) or epithelial cancer sites (Arts et al. 2001b) in the Zutphen Elderly Study. Sacks et al. (2006) concluded that the efficacy and safety of using isoflavones to prevent or treat cancer of the breast, endometrium or prostate is not established; evidence from clinical trials is meagre and cautionary with regard to possible adverse effects. Therefore, despite plausible mechanisms, there is little observational evidence for a beneficial effect of flavonoids against cancer. WCRF has reported a limited-suggestive inverse association between quercetin and lung cancer risk (WRCF 2007).

Conclusions for cancer

According to the comprehensive analysis by WCRF, the only convincing inverse association is between dietary fibre intake and reduced risk of colorectal cancer. This association has been strengthened in the light of recently published cohort studies (WRCF and AICR 2010). In addition there are a number of inverse associations between plant foods and cancer risk that are probable. Contrary to the view 10 years ago, the evidence linking fruit and non-starchy vegetables with cancer risk education has weakened and the relationship is now considered to be limited with regard to colorectal cancer, though probable for cancers of the upper gastrointestinal tract (fruit and vegetables) and lung (fruit).

As with CVD, in contrast to popular belief and despite considerable effort, it remains unclear whether antioxidants in fruits and vegetables are responsible for the apparent protective effect of these foods for some cancers. Not all work has focused on the direct antioxidant properties of components present in these foods and evidence is accumulating to support other potential mechanisms as discussed earlier in the context of CVD. It has been suggested that plant-derived substances may be able to protect against genomic damage resulting in aberrant gene expression, either by up-regulating repair of the damage or resulting in the removal of damaged cells via apoptosis (see Mathers 2006).

Type 2 diabetes

The US Health Professionals' Follow-up Study of 42 504 men has shown that a 'prudent' dietary pattern was associated with a marginally decreased risk of type 2 diabetes (van Dam et al. 2002). The prudent dietary pattern was characterised by high consumption of vegetables, legumes, fruit, wholegrains, fish and poultry. Another US cohort study found that low consumers of fruits and vegetables were more likely to develop diabetes (Ford and Mokdad, 2001).

A recent meta-analysis of six cohort studies revealed a 14% reduction in risk of type 2 diabetes in association with a greater intake of green leafy vegetables (Carter et al. 2010). Similar associations were found in the US Nurses' Health Study for leafy green vegetables and also fruit (Bazzano et al. 2008).

Results from the 10-year follow-up of US Nurses showed that women who were in the top fifth for wholegrain cereal intake had a 38% lower risk of developing diabetes than women in the lowest fifth for intake; the effects were not explained by dietary fibre intake or intake of magnesium or vitamin E (Liu et al. 2000b). Also, in the Health Professionals' Follow-up Study cohort, the relative risk of type 2 diabetes was 0.58 in the highest compared to the lowest quintile of wholegrain intake (Fung et al. 2002). The association was reduced to 0.7 when adjustment was made for BMI, but remained highly significant. A similar protective effect was reported in Finland (Montonen et al. 2003).

It is well known that people with diabetes are vulnerable to oxidative stress. There have been a number of short-term clinical trials to assess whether isolated flavonoid compounds could influence lipoprotein vulnerability to oxidation. Results have been mixed, with some studies showing an effect (e.g. Lean et al. 1999) and others not (e.g. Blostein-Fujii et al. 1999). There have been many studies that have assessed the hypoglycaemic effect of compounds found in many different foods; the relevance of these studies to humans is not clear.

Age-related macular degeneration and cataract

Age-related macular degeneration (AMD) and cataracts are eye disorders that are increasingly common among older people (Fletcher 2009). Macular degeneration is the leading cause of irreversible blindness in people over the age of 65 years. The macula is the central part of the retina and in the early stages of the disease begins to accumulate lipid deposits known as drusen, ultimately resulting in atrophy associated with distortion and finally loss of vision (especially in the central area of vision). Cataracts result from glycosidation of lens proteins, which leads to opacities forming within the lens. Although the aetiology of cataracts varies and they can develop at any stage of life, the vast majority develop in elderly individuals and so are sometimes referred to as senile cataracts.

The tissues of the lens and the retina are subject to oxidative stress throughout life as a result of the combined exposure to light and oxygen. It has been proposed that antioxidants may prevent cellular damage by reacting with free radicals produced during the process of light absorption (Christen et al. 1996). Indeed, laboratory and animal studies have demonstrated the important role of antioxidants in the lens and retina. Epidemiological studies have also suggested that dietary antioxidants (e.g. vitamins C and E, carotenoids and, more recently, lutein and zeaxanthein) may provide protection against cataracts and AMD (see Fletcher 2009). Although there is less consistency for individual antioxidants, the data from both animal and human studies suggest that vitamin C, carotenoids, lutein and zeaxanthein play a critical role.

This evidence supports general dietary recommendations concerning the importance of fruits and vegetables, especially citrus fruit and other rich sources of vitamin C, and vegetables rich in lutein and zeaxanthein, such as spinach, broccoli, kale, lettuce and red and orange peppers. For example, a 10-year study of almost 40 000 female subjects found a modest but significant reduction in cataract risk of 10–15% when the highest quintile of fruit and vegetable consumption was compared with the lowest (Christen et al. 2005). In contrast, evidence is lacking that the use of vitamin supplements is of proven benefit in the prevention of age-related eye disease (Fletcher, 2009).

In summary, the evidence is suggestive that increased fruit and vegetable intakes are associated with a lower risk of AMD and with cataracts in older people. It is not yet clear which components and which vegetables are protective; confounding cannot be ruled out in explaining some of the associations previously reported.

Age-related cognitive decline

A prospective cohort study of almost 4000 subjects over 65 years of age has suggested that high vegetable consumption, especially leafy green vegetables (median 2.8 servings per day), but not high fruit intake, was associated with a slower rate of cognitive decline (Morris et al. 2006). Similar results were observed in the Nurses' Health Study (Kang et al. 2005). An interesting finding was a significantly reduced risk of Alzheimer's disease associated with the consumption of fruit and vegetables juices, especially among ApoE4 carriers (Dai et al. 2006), a genotype reported to be potentially influential in several other studies (see Gillette-Guyonnet et al. 2007) in which higher intakes of fruits and vegetables (and fish) were associated retrospectively with reduced risk of cognitive decline or dementia. Nevertheless, several recent reviews have reported inconsistent associations or a lack of an association between various aspects of diet and cognitive decline (Nooyens et al. 2011, Plassman et al. 2010). This is likely to be due, at least in part, to study design to date and the need for prospective studies of adequate duration, appropriately rigorous collection of dietary data and RCTs that are appropriately focused.

Chronic obstructive pulmonary disease

Chronic obstructive pulmonary disease (COPD) is an all-inclusive and non-specific term that refers to a defined set of breathing-related symptoms, characterised by airflow obstruction. Asthma is defined as a chronic inflammatory airway disorder. The criteria used to define COPDs in general have not always been applied in the same way in all epidemiological studies, making interpretation of data more difficult.

Bearing definition problems in mind, there have been a number of reviews of the links between nutrition and COPDs (Schunemann et al. 2001; Romieu and Trenga 2001; Trenga et al. 2001; Denny et al. 2003). Schunemann et al. (2001) concluded that the largest body of literature exists for a protective effect of vitamin C and fresh fruit and vegetable intake. The review concluded that the evidence is insufficient to recommend the use of any supplements, but the data do support the recommendation to eat more fruits and vegetables. Denny et al. (2003) concluded that people who have a diet rich in fruit and vegetables have a lower risk of poor respiratory health and a recent study reported the benefit of a 'prudent diet' (high consumption of fruit, vegetables, fish and wholegrain cereals) with regard to COPD and impaired lung function, especially in male smokers (Shaheen et al. 2010).

An analysis from EPIC, using a nested case-control approach, has shown that symptomatic asthma is associated with a low dietary intake of fruit, vitamin C and manganese, and low plasma vitamin C levels in adults (Patel et al. 2006), replicating previous findings in other groups and suggesting that nutrition might be a modifiable risk factor for asthma, the prevalence of which has increased considerably in recent years.

A population-based case-control study in South London showed that, after adjusting for potential confounding factors, apple consumption was inversely associated with asthma (odds ratio 0.84, 95% CI 0.75–0.97) (Shaheen et al. 2001). The authors concluded that there is a need for a better understanding of how flavonoids or other constituents of apples might influence respiratory health. Shaheen et al. (2001) also found that a higher intake of selenium was inversely associated and the authors commented on the declining intake of selenium in the UK population, which they speculate may be expected to lead to an increased prevalence of asthma in the future.

Currently, it would be premature to attribute causality to any particular food or food constituent.

Osteoporosis and bone health

There is epidemiological data that suggests that a diet rich in plant foods is also beneficial to bone health (see Lanham-New and Loveridge 2007). Further support comes from the DASH trials (Lin et al. 2003), which are suggestive of conservation of calcium at least in part by a high potassium intake. A recent systematic review concerning fruit and vegetable intake and bone health in women aged 45 and over reported that any benefits remain unclear (Hamidi et al. 2011). The findings of studies investigating the ability of soya to slow postmenopausal bone loss are inconsistent (Sacks et al. 2006).

Plant foods and health: overall conclusions

Eating patterns characterised by an abundance of fruit, vegetables and other plant foods are associated with a moderately reduced risk of chronic disease (e.g. CVD – especially stroke – and cancer), and to a much lesser extent of other conditions such as age-related eye defects and possibly cognitive decline. Researchers from Harvard (Hung et al. 2004) suggested some years ago that the benefits of fruits and vegetables may have been over-stated, and this now seems to be the case, especially for cancer. Much of the supportive evidence derives from case-control studies, which are potentially affected by methodo-logical biases such as recall bias and selection bias. Selective reporting and publication may also have exacerbated the situation. Evidence from prospective cohort studies, regarded as more robust in design, has typically been less strong. However, these findings do not preclude the benefits of specific plant foods.

One possible explanation for the lack of association with cancer risk in some studies is that the category 'fruits and vegetables' is too broad to capture effects exerted by specific constituents found only in subclasses of fruits and/or vegetables. It is also important to recognise that the methods used in large-scale studies, such as food frequency question-naires, can be relatively ineffective in providing a precise measure of the intake of specific foods, and this can lead to an underestimation of the strength of associations.

The search for the active components in these foods has met with limited success. Research initially focused on the antioxidant vitamins C and E and beta-carotene, although a few studies have also looked at other carotenoids and some of the other plant bioactives (e.g. flavonoids, glucosinolates, phytosterols). In relation to plant bioactives, promising and generally consistent results have been reported for animal studies and for *in vitro* studies, but to date convincing evidence from human intervention and epidemio-logical studies is sparse, and this is reflected in the paucity of authorised health claims emerging from the health claims process in Europe.

Evidence is now accumulating that flavonoids might exert neuro-modulatory effects that are independent of classical antioxidant capacity through interaction with various protein kinase and lipid kinase signalling cascades, which regulate transcription factors and gene expression involved in both synaptic plasticity and cerebrovascular blood flow (Spencer, 2010a, b). Recent evidence demonstrates the reversal of age-related memory deficits following supplementation of animals with anthocyanin-rich blueberry extract (Andres-Lacueva et al. 2005). Such findings, though still preliminary, are of particular importance in the context of our ageing population.

As was mentioned at the start of the section 'A summary of the evidence linking plant food intake and health', the use of health claims on foods and beverages in Europe is now regulated. So far in 2011, claims about plant stanols and sterols and cholesterol lowering and about the effect of a tomato extract on platelet aggregation have been approved by the EC. In addition, claims on walnuts and endothelial function and on beta-glucan and main-tenance of healthy cholesterol levels have received positive opinions from EFSA. However, many other claims including those on dietary fibre, soy protein, nuts other than walnuts, and plant antioxidants have received negative opinions to date (see EFSA 2011c for more details).

Recommendations and current policy on plant food intake

Fruit and vegetables

The World Health Organisation (WHO) recommends a minimum intake of 400 g of fruits and vegetables per day (WHO 2002), and this recommendation has been adopted globally in the context of ensuring a healthier dietary pattern. A joint FAO/WHO workshop in 2004 in Japan concluded that there is strongly suggestive evidence that there is potential for increased consumption of fruits and vegetables to reduce the risk of CHD, stroke and type 2 diabetes, but further research is needed to evaluate the effects of specific fruits (WHO/FAO 2005). The evidence for a role for fruit and vegetable consumption in obesity prevention, weight management and cancer prevention is weaker and further research is needed to evaluate these associations. The workshop also concluded that messages about fruit and vegetables need to be integrated into food-based dietary guidelines, to be country specific and culturally relevant, and coordinated with other messages about healthy diets. Intervention strategies need to be multidisciplinary and coordinated, and should comprise a balance of components to stimulate growth in both supply and demand of fruits and vegetables. Evaluating such projects is essential in order to learn what works and what does not and to avoid wasting time and resources on inappropriate approaches.

There have been efforts in many countries around the world to increase fruit and vegetable intake, including many national campaigns. The first such scheme began in California in 1988 as an initiative of the US National Cancer Institute and the local health services, and preceded the WHO advice. It advised eating three to seven plant foods per day. This developed into the national US '5-a-day' scheme. The most recent advice in the USA focuses on the message to eat five to nine servings of fruits and vegetables each day and the most recent guidance, the 'My Plate' model (Figure 1.2a), shows separate categories for grains, protein, vegetables and fruits, with more emphasis placed on vegetables than fruit. There is also a UK equivalent (Figure 1.2b).

Table 1.9 lists the websites for schemes from other countries (some current, some historical). The Australian scheme, for example, specifies two servings of fruit as well as five servings of vegetables, whereas others provide a composite target figure.

Use of the UK '5 a day' logo and associated portion counter is governed by criteria that take account of portion size. Currently, the logo can only be used on fresh and frozen produce, dried fruits and pure juices, but criteria for composite foods are under development, which are expected to take into account fat, sugar and salt content. A key difference between these two schemes is that the US scheme includes potatoes whereas the UK one does not. The UK 5 A DAY scheme emphasises variety and embraces fresh, frozen, tinned and juiced fruits and vegetables, and pulses.

Most UK retailers have also developed their own logos to link with the campaign. In the UK, there is the Department of Health's '5 a day' campaign and the associated School Fruit and Vegetable Scheme, whereby in England children aged 4–6 years have been entitled to a piece of free fruit or vegetable at school each day. Related school fruit schemes have also operated in other parts of the UK. The scheme in England has now been evaluated (see www.5aday.nhs.uk). One of the findings was that over a quarter of children and their families ate more fruit at home after their school joined the scheme.

(a)

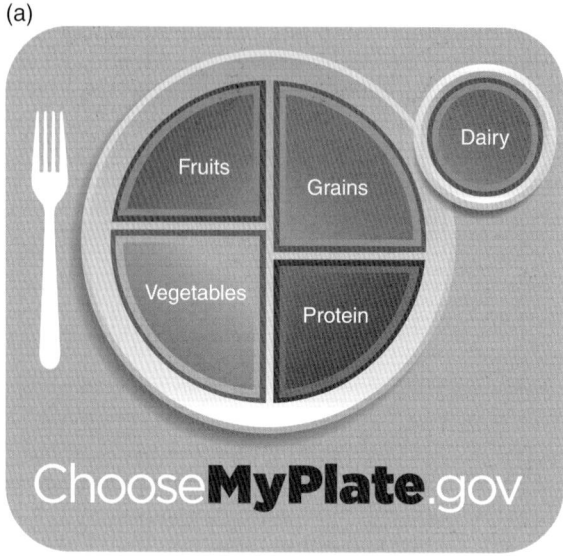

(b)

The eatwell plate

FOOD STANDARDS AGENCY

food.gov.uk

Use the eatwell plate to help you get the balance right. It shows how much of what you eat should come from each food group.

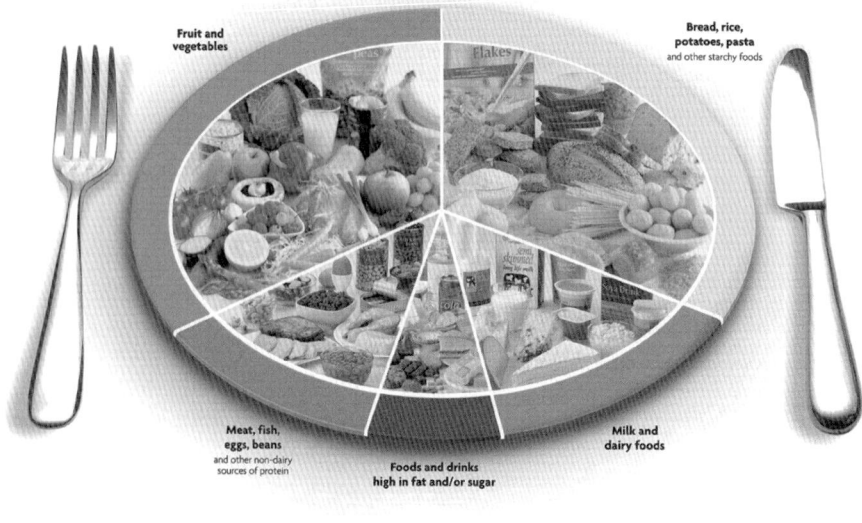

Fruit and vegetables

Bread, rice, potatoes, pasta and other starchy foods

Meat, fish, eggs, beans and other non-dairy sources of protein

Foods and drinks high in fat and/or sugar

Milk and dairy foods

Figure 1.2   (a) US model (source: USDA 2011). (b) UK model (source: Department of Health in association with the Welsh Government, the Scottish Government and the Food Standards Agency in Northern Ireland).

Table 1.9   Worldwide schemes to increase fruit and vegetable consumption

Country	Website
UK	www.5aday.nhs.uk
Australia	www.gofor2and5.com.au
USA	www.5aday.org
USA	www.5aday.gov
New Zealand	www.5aday.co.nz
Canada	www.5to10aday.com
Germany	www.5amtag.de
Japan	www.5aday.net
France	www.10parjour.net/site/pages/home/index.php
Mexico	www.cincopordia.com.mx
Chile	http://www.5aldiachile.cl/
Argentina	http://www.5aldia.com.ar/esp_home/index.php
Spain	www.5aldia.org

Wholegrain foods

The growing body of evidence suggesting a beneficial effect of wholegrains on the risk of CVD, type 2 diabetes and some cancers (see Seal 2006) has been used in the US, in particular, to propose recommendations for daily wholegrain consumption, based on a definition from the American Association of Cereal Chemists (AACC 2005), that: wholegrains shall consist of the intact, ground, cracked or flaked caryopsis, whose principal anatomical components – the starchy endosperm, geum and bran – are present in the same relative proportions as they exist in the intact caryopsis. For composite foods, it has been suggested that the product should contain >51% wholegrain by weight (with reference to the amount typically consumed per day) in order for a wholegrain claim to be made. There has been far less interest in this type of approach at a policy level in the UK or indeed Europe.

Current consumption patterns

The National Food Survey (NFS) collected data on UK household food purchases/supplies every year from 1942 until 2000. It was initiated to monitor household food supplies during World War II and the early years of the survey (not featured in the table) reflect the constraints of rationing. For example, in 1942, total fruit was only 197 g/person/week but potatoes were 1877 g/person/week and bread 1718 g/person/week. Household supplies of bread and potato remained high for the following decade but have gradually declined subsequently. (http://www.defra.gov.uk/statistics/foodfarm/food/familyfood/nationalfood survey/). Trends between 1954 and 1999 are illustrated in Table 1.10.

Around 2000, there was a change in methodology for the survey (Speller, 2000; Burgon, 2007, 2009) and it is now known as the Family Food Survey. Data collected between 1975 and 2000 has been adjusted to enable trends over this period to be compared

Table 1.10 Trends in plant food consumption 1954–1999 (g/person/week)

	1954	1959	1964	1969	1974	1979	1984	1989	1994	1999
Total vegetables (all types, excluding potatoes, beans and pulses)	714	807	996	807	980	1004	980	1041	968	975
Total fruit (all types excluding juice)	575	832	686	848	633	664	628	692	712	766
Fruit juice	7	12	16	15	30	63	150	214	240	284
Pulses and beans	149	86	101	112	111	125	133	135	117	119
Nuts and nut products	12	10	11	7	7	11	12	13	16	13
Potatoes (fresh and frozen products)	1792	1561	1407.3	1457	1357	1311	1234	1151	997	872
Bread	1596	1341	1190	1070	946	891	866	833	758	717
Rice	24		15	14	16	20	28	30	37	68
Breakfast cereals	45	49	57	75	81	96	117	126	134	134
Pasta	–	–	–	–	–	–	–	–	–	79

Source: DEFRA (2000); MAFF (1955, 1960, 1965, 1970, 1975, 1980, 1985, 1990, 1995, 2000).

Table 1.11 Trends in intake between 1975 and 2009. Data for 1975 and 1990 are adjusted to reflect the methodology used since 2000

	1975	1990	2000	2006	2007	2008	2009
Total fruit and vegetables (excluding potatoes)	1868	2170	2336	2454	2421	2317	2246
Total fruit (excluding juice)	738	962	1189	1313	1281	1199	1143
Fresh fruit	511	624	765	855	855	790	762
Processed fruit and fruit products	228	338	424	458	426	409	381
Fruit juices (ml)	42	225	332	366	340	325	302
Total vegetables (excluding potatoes)	1131	1208	1147	1142	1140	1118	1103
Fresh green vegetables	341	287	246	221	224	203	201
Other fresh vegetables	405	475	506	566	566	557	552
Processed vegetables excluding potatoes	385	446	395	355	350	358	350
Fresh and processed potatoes	1378	1199	1002	810	781	776	761
Rice	17	32	69	87	94	90	92
Bread	1029	859	782	692	677	659	656
Breakfast cereals	82	121	135	135	130	130	133
Pasta	15	32	73	87	92	91	91

Source: DEFRA (2010, 2011).

with newer data (Table 1.11). Over this period, fruit and fruit juice purchases have risen considerably but peaked around 2006 and have been falling since then. Total vegetable purchases (excluding potatoes) have remained fairly constant but fresh have been replaced to some extent by processed vegetables. Purchases of fresh and processed potatoes have almost halved during this period from 1378 to 761 g/person/ week, and bread has continued to fall. There have been increases in purchases of pasta, rice and breakfast cereal since 1975, reflecting changes in meal patterns.

To some extent, the trends in bread and potatoes reflect the downward trend in total energy intake that has been a characteristic of dietary patterns, and will have affected dietary fibre intakes. Current intakes in the UK are 14.9 g/day in men aged 19–64 years and 12.8 g/day in women (Department of Health, 2011).

Despite the recent interest in wholegrains and health, intake remains low. For example, low intakes exist in the USA where there has been specific advice to increase intake to three servings per day and the latest advice is to 'make at least half of your grains who-legrains' (USDA 2011).

Similarly, in the UK, Lang et al. (2003) reported that about one-third of adults failed to consume wholegrains on a daily basis and over 97% consumed less than three servings per day. In studies in the USA and UK, in which careful analysis was made of absolute wholegrain intake by young people, intake was only 7 g/day (Thane et al. 2005; Harnack et al. 2003). Bread and breakfast cereals were the main contributors.

Table 1.12 Achievement of the 5-a-day target

Average daily consumption of fruit and vegetables*	Age (years)					
	Boys	Men		Girls	Women	
	11–18	19–64	65+	11–18	19–64	65+
Mean portions per day	3.1	4.2	4.7	2.7	4.1	4.2
% achieving ≥ 5-a-day	13	32	39	7	29	35

*Excludes potatoes and potato products. All fruit juice limited to 150 g/day; baked beans and other pulses consumption limited to 80 g/day; tomato puree multiplied by 5; dried fruit multiplied by 3. Children under 11 years have not been included as the 80 portion is only appropriate for older children and adults. Source: Department of Health (2011).

Whereas the Family Food Survey provides information on household purchases, the UK's National Diet and Nutrition Survey (NDNS) provides information about the intakes of individuals rather than estimated consumption at the household level. The most recent survey, which combines years one and two of the new rolling survey, provides for the first time the contribution of fruits and vegetables from composite dishes, as a result of a project to disaggregate composite dishes in the NDNS database. Using this approach, vegetable intakes (excluding potatoes) are reported to be 189 g/day for men and 186 g/day for women, in contrast to 140 g and 159 g respectively when composite dishes are not taken into account (Department of Health, 2011). Current fruit intakes are much less affected by use of this methodology and are 99g/day for men and 103g/day for women (Department of Health 2011). This equates to fruit and vegetable intakes of 288 g/day for men and 289 g/day for women (Department of Health 2011) compared to an average of about 250 g in the 1980s (Gregory et al. 1990).

Current intakes of fruits and vegetables in Britain and other developed countries are generally lower than the five plus daily servings typically recommended (equivalent to at least 2800g/week). Explanations for resistance to dietary advice to increase the consumption of fruit, vegetables and wholegrain cereals generally stem from issues related to taste, convenience, cost, access, cultural values and education (Buttriss et al. 2004).

At present, men in Britain are eating an average of 4.2 portions of fruits and vegetables (excluding potatoes and potato products) per day and women an average of 4.1 portions per day (Department of Health, 2011) rather than the recommended 5 or more portions (Table 1.12). Overall, 32% of men and 29% of women consumed five or more portions of fruit and vegetables per day (Department of Health, 2011). Intakes in children aged 11–18 are poorer, with only 13% of boys and 7% of girls achieving five portions a day.

The NDNS series also provides information on regional and socioeconomic differences in consumption, the most recent being from 2000–2001. In this dataset there were no statistically significant regional differences for fruit and vegetables: values ranged from 2.6 portions a day for men and 2.7 for women in the Northern region of England to 3.0 and 3.2 respectively for the South East (Henderson et al. 2002). Scotland no longer had the lowest intakes, at 2.9 and 3.0 for men and women respectively.

Men and women living in households in receipt of state benefits consumed a significantly lower number of portions of fruit and vegetables than those in non-benefit households: 2.1 portions compared with 2.8 for men, and 1.9 compared with 3.1 for women (Henderson et al. 2002). About a third, 35% of men and 30% of women, in benefit households had eaten no fruit during the 7-day recording period, and 4% and 6% respectively had eaten no vegetables. The NDNS of school age children (conducted in the 1990s) revealed that children in the lowest income groups are around 50% less likely to eat fruit and vegetables than those in the highest income groups (Gregory et al. 2000).

Conclusions

Throughout human history, communities have developed a diversity of dietary patterns, influenced to a large extent by the foods available in their locality, but usually heavily reliant on plant foods. Such foods, in combination, are capable of providing a diverse range of nutrients. More recently, they have been recognised as providers of an even wider diversity of non-nutrient bioactive substances that are speculated to have health promoting properties.

Diets rich in fruits, vegetables and other plant foods have been shown to be associated with a lower risk of diseases such as CVD (especially stroke) and some types of cancer. These associations persist after adjustment for lifestyle factors often associated with high consumption of such foods (e.g. being physically active and not smoking and having a higher consumption of wholegrain cereals), although the strength of the association is often attenuated. There is also evidence of a dose–response relationship that is consistent with the current recommendations to increase intakes of these foods. It is difficult to separate out the role of diet in general and of specific nutrients in particular, and so the causal mechanism(s) associated with this dietary pattern remain to be established. Most epidemiological research has focused on a number of individual antioxidants studied in relative isolation and it is likely that at the very least there is a complex interaction between the many plant food components and the rest of the diet, that may have an integrated effect on cardiovascular and other chronic diseases.

The strongest association between plant food intake (particularly fruit and vegetable intake) and cancer risk comes from case-control studies. The publication of data from prospective (cohort) studies, which are considered to be more robust, suggests that associations between fruit and vegetable intake and cancer risk may have been overstated. Some evidence also exists for certain eye disorders (e.g. age-related macular degeneration), chronic obstructive pulmonary disease and age-related cognitive decline.

Despite considerable research effort, the specific constituents responsible for these associations have yet to be identified. Animal and *in vitro* experiments have suggested a role in health promotion for a number of plant constituents, particularly those with antioxidant properties, but these findings have generally not been replicated in human intervention trials. The evidence that antioxidants such as vitamins E and C and beta-carotene are responsible for the beneficial effects of fruit and vegetables is at best equivocal, despite popular belief. Not all work has focused on the direct antioxidant properties of the components present in these foods and evidence is accumulating to support other potential mechanisms. It has been suggested that plant-derived substances may be able to protect against genomic damage resulting in aberrant gene expression, either by up-regulating repair of the damage or the removal of damaged cells by apoptosis. Dietary fibre has recently been shown to be of particular importance in the reduction of colorectal cancer risk (the evidence now being described as convincing) but the specific mechanism is as yet unclear.

As a prelude to randomised controlled trials, there is a need for soundly constructed prospective studies and parallel mechanistic studies, designed to identify the active components in plant foods and their mode of action. Identification of these would enable dietary advice to be more specific. However, in the meantime, regular consumption of a diversity of fruits, vegetables and other plant foods such as wholegrains remains an important message.

Around the world, recommendations exist to increase fruit and vegetable consumption to at least five servings per day. Yet at the current time, typical intakes fall well short of this target in developed countries, meaning that there are considerable opportunities for growers and others in the food chain to encourage intake through a readily available supply of high quality products.

Acknowledgement

I wish to thank Bethany Hooper for her assistance in researching information for use in this chapter.

References

AACC (American Association of Cereal Chemists) (2005) *Definition/Reports.* Available at: http://www.aaccnet.org/definitions/wholegrain.asp (accessed November 2006)

Anderson, J.W., Johnstone, B.M. and Cook-Newell, M.E. (1995) Meta-analysis of the effects of soy protein intake on serum lipids. *New England Journal of Medicine* **333**: 276–382.

Andres-Lacueva, C., Shukitt-Hale, B., Galli, R.L., Jauregui, O., Lamuela-Raventos, R.M. and Joseph, J.A. (2005) Anthocyanins in aged blueberry-fed rats are found centrally and may enhance memory. *Nutritional Neuroscience* **8** (2), 111–20.

Appel, L.J., Moore, T.J., Obarzanek, E., Vollmer, W.M., Svetkey, L.P. Sacks, F.M., Bray, G.A., Vogt, T.M., Cutler, J.A., Windhauser, M.M., Lin, P.H. and Karanja, N. (1997) A clinical trial of the effects of dietary patterns on blood pressure. DASH Collaborative Research Group. *New England Journal of Medicine* **336**, 1117–24.

Armstrong, B. and Doll, R. (1975) Environmental factors and cancer incidence and mortality in different countries, with special reference to dietary practices. *International Journal of Cancer* **15**: 617–31.

Arts, I.C., Hollman, P.C., Freskens, E.J., Bueno de Mesquita, M.B. and Kromhout, D. (2001a) Catechin intake might explain the inverse relation between tea consumption and ischaemic heart disease: the Zutphen Elderly Study. *American Journal of Clinical Nutrition* **74**, 227–32.

Arts, I.C., Hollman, P.C., Bueno de Mesquita, H.B., Feskens, E.J. and Kromhout, D. (2001b) Dietray catechins and epithelial cancer incidence: the Zutphen Elderly study. *International Journal of Cancer* **92**, 298–302.

Asplund, K. (2002) Antioxidant vitamins in the prevention of cardiovascular disease: a systematic review. *Journal of Internal Medicine* **251**, 372–92.

Bazzano, L.A., He, J., Ogden, L.G., Vupputun, S., Loria, C., Myers, L. and Whetton, P.K. (2001) Legume consumption and risk of coronary heart disease in US men and women: NHANES I Epidemiologic Follow-up Study. *Archives of Internal Medicine* **161**, 2573–8.

Bazzano, L.A., Li, T.Y., Joshipura, K.J. and Hu, F.B. (2008) Intake of fruit, vegetables, and fruit juices and risk of diabetes in women. *Diabetes Care* **31**,1311–17.

Beaglehole, R., Jackson, R., Watkinson, J., Scragg, R. and Yee, R.L. (1990) Decreased blood selenium and risk of myocardial infarction. *International Journal of Epidemiology* **19**, 918–22.

Berryman, C.E., Preston, A.G., Karmally, W., Deckelbaum, R.J. and Kris-Etherrton, P.M. (2011) Effects of almond consumption on the reduction of LDL-cholesterol: a discussion of potential mechanisms and future research directions. *Nutrition Reviews* **69**, 171–85.

Bingham, S.A., Day, N.E., Luben, R., Ferrari, P., Slimani, N., Norat, T., Clavel-Chapelon, F., Kesse, E., Nieters, A., Boeing, H., Tjonneland, A., Overvad, K., Martinez, C., Dorronsoro, M., Gonzalez, C.A., Key, T.J., Trichopoulou, A., Naska, A., Vineis, P., Tumino, R., Krogh, V., Bueno-de-Mesquita, H.B., Peeters, P.H., Berglund, G., Hallmans, G., Lund, E., Skeie, G., Kaaks, R. and Riboli, E. (2003) Dietary fibre in food and protection against colorectal cancer in the European Prospective Investigation into Cancer and Nutrition (EPIC): an observational study. *Lancet* **361**, 1496–501.

Bingham, S.A., Norat, T., Moskal, A., Ferrari, P., Slimani, N., Clavel-Chapelon, F., Kesse, E., Nieters, A., Boeing, H., Tjonneland, A., Overvad, K., Martinez, C., Dorronsoro, M., Gonzalez, C.A., Ardanaz, E., Navarro, C., Quiros, J.R., Key, T.J., Day, N.E., Trichopoulou, A., Naska, A., Krogh, V., Tumino, R., Palli, D., Panico, S., Vineis, P., Bueno-de-Mesquita, H.B., Ocke, M.C., Peeters, P.H., Berglund, G., Hallmans, G., Lund, E., Skeie, G., Kaaks, R. and Riboli, E. (2005) Is the association with fibre from foods in colorectal cancer confounded by folate intake? *Cancer Epidemiology, Biomarkers and Prevention* **14**, 1552–6.

Blostein-Fujii, A., DiSilvestro, R.A., Frid, D. and Katz, C. (1999) Short term citrus flavonoid supplementation of type II diabetic women: no effect on lipoprotein oxidation tendencies. *Free Radical Research* **30**, 315–20.

Bobak, M., Hense, H.W., Kark, J., Kuch, B., Vojtisek, P., Sinnreich, R., Gostomzyk, J., Bui, M., von Eckardstein, A., Junker, R., Fobker, M., Schulte, H., Assmann, G. and Marmot, M. (1999) An ecological study of determinants of coronary heart disease rates: a comparison of Czech, Barvarian and Israeli men. *International Journal of Epidemiology* **28**, 437–44.

Bonithon-Kopp, C., Kronborg, O., Giacosa, A., Rath, U. and Faivre, J. (2000) Calcium and fibre supplementation in prevention of colorectal adenoma recurrence: a randomised intervention trial. European Cancer Prevention Organisation Study Group. *Lancet* **356**, 1300–306.

BNF (2001) *Briefing Paper. Selenium and Health.* London: British Nutrition Foundation.

BNF (2002) *Briefing Paper. Soya and Health.* London: British Nutrition Foundation.

Brown, L., Rimm, E.B., Seddon, J.M., Giovannucci, E.L., Chasan-Taber, L., Spiegelman, D., Willett, W.C. and Hankinson, S.E. (1999a) A prospective study of carotenoid intake and risk of cataract extraction in US men. *American Journal of Clinical Nutrition* **70**, 517–24.

Brown, L., Rosner, B., Willett, W.W. and Sacks, F.M. (1999b) Cholesterol lowering effects of dietary fibre: a metanalysis. *American Journal of Clinical Nutrition* **69**, 30–42.

Brownlee, I.A., Moore, C., Chatfield, M., Richardson, D.P., Ashby, P., Kuznesof, S.A., Jebb, S.A. and Seal, C.J. (2010) Markers of cardiovascular risk are not changed by increased whole-grain intake: the WHOLEheart study, a randomised, controlled dietary intervention. *British Journal of Nutrition* **104**, 125–34.

Bruckdorfer, K.R. (2005) Oxidative stress. In: *Cardiovascular Disease: Diet, Nutrition and Emerging Risk Factors. Report of a British Nutrition Foundation Task Force.* (ed. S. Stanner). Oxford: Blackwell.

Burgon, C. (2007) Introduction to the Expenditure and Food Survey. *Nutrition Bulletin* **32**, 283–6.

Burgon, C. (2009) Family food – an introduction to data sources and uses. *Nutrition Bulletin* **34**, 2220–24.

Buttriss, J. (2003) Introduction: plant foods and health. In: *Plants: Diet and Health. Report of a British Nutrition Foundation Task Force.* (ed. Goldberg, G.). Oxford: Blackwell.

Buttriss, J.L., Hughes, J., Kelly, C.N.M. and Stanner, S. (2002) Antioxidants in food: a summary of the review conducted for the Food Standards Agency. *Nutrition Bulletin* **27**, 227–36.

Buttriss, J., Stanner, S., McKevith, B., Nugent, A.P., Kelly, C., Phillips, F. and Theobold, H.E. (2004) Successful ways to modify food choice: lessons from the literature. *Nutrition Bulletin* **29**, 333–43.

Carter, P., Gray, L.J., Troughton, J., Khunti, K. and Davies, M.J. (2010) Fruit and vegetable intake and incidence of type 2 diabetes mellitus: systematic review and meta-analysis. *British Medical Journal* **341**, c4229.

Caswell, H., Denny, A. and Lunn, J. (2008) Plant sterol and stanol esters. *Nutrition Bulletin* **33**, 368–73.

Cho, E., Hunter, D.J., Spiegelman, D., Albanes, D., Beeson, W.L., van den Brandt, P.A., Colditz, G.A., Feskanich, D., Folsom, A.R., Fraser, G.E., Freudenheim, L., Giovannucci, E., Goldbohm, R.A., Graham, S., Miller, A.B., Rohan, T.E., Sellers, T.A., Virtamo, J., Willett, W.C. and Smith-Warner, S.A. (2006) Intakes of vitamins A, C, and E and folate and multivitamins and lung cancer: a pooled analysis of 8 prospective studies. *International Journal of Cancer* **118**, 970–78.

Christen, W.G., Glynn, R.J. and Hennekens, C.H. (1996) Antioxidants and age-related eye disease. Current and future perspectives. *Annals of Epidemiology* **6**, 60–66.

Christen, W.G., Liu, S., Schaumberg, D.A. and Buring, J.E. (2005) Fruit and vegetable intake and the risk of cataract in women. *American Journal of Clinical Nutrition* **81**, 1417–22.

Clarke, R. (2009) Healthy ageing: the brain. In: *Healthy Ageing: The Role of Nutrition and Lifestyle* (eds Stanner, S. Thompson, R. and Buttriss, J.), pp. 125–42. Chichester: Wiley-Blackwell.

Crowe, F.L., Roddam, A.W., Key, T.J., Appleby, P.N., Overad, K., Jakobsen, M.U., Tjonneland, A., Hansen, L., Boeing, H., Weikert, C., Linseisen, J., Kaaks, R., Trichopouyou, A., Misirli, G., Lagiou, P., Sacerdote, C., Pala, V., Palli, D., Tumino, R., Panico, S., Bueno-de-Mesquita, H.B., Boer, J., van Gils, C.H., Beulens, J.W.J., Barricarete, A., Rodriguez, L., Larranaga, N., Sanchez, M.J., Tormo, M.J., Buckland, G., Lund, E., Hedblad, B., Melander, O., Jansson, J.H., Wennberg, P., Wareham, N.J., Slimani, N., Romieu, I., Jenab, M., Danesh, J., Gallo, V., Norat, T. and Riboli, E. (2011) Fruit and vegetable intake and mortality from ischaemic heart disease: results from the European Prospective Investigation into Cancer and Nutrition (EPIC)-Heart study. *European Heart Journal* **32**, 1235–43.

Dai, Q., Borenstein, A.R., Wu, Y., Jackson, J.C. and Larson, E.B. (2006) Fruit and vegetable juices and Alzheimer's disease: the Kame Project. *American Journal of Medicine* **119**, 751–9.

van Dam, R.M., Rimm, E.B., Willett, W.C., Stampfer, M.J. and Hu, F.B. (2002) Dietary patterns and risk for type 2 diabetes mellitus in U.S. men. *Annals of Internal Medicine* **136**, 201–9.

Dauchet, L., Ferrieres, J., Arveiler, D., Yarnell, J.W., Grey, F., Ducimetiere, P., Ruidavets, J.B., Haas, B., Evans, A., Bingham, A., Amouyel, P. and Dallongeville, J. (2004) Frequency of fruit and vegetable consumption and coronary heart disease in France and Northern Ireland: the PRIME study. *British Journal of Nutrition* **92**, 963–72.

Denny, S.I., Thompson, R.L. and Margetts, B.M. (2003) Dietary factors in the pathogenesis of asthma and chronic obstructive pulmonary disease. *Current Allergy and Asthma Reports* **3**, 130–36.

DEFRA (2000) Consumption of selected household foods, 1942 to 1996 Available at: http://www.defra.gov.uk/statistics/foodfarm/food/familyfood/nationalfoodsurvey/ (Accessed 25th July 2011).

DEFRA (2010) UK household purchased quantities of food and drink. Available at: http://www. defra.gov.uk/statistics/foodfarm/food/familyfood/datasets/ (Accessed 25th July 2011).

DEFRA (2011) Family food 2009.Available at: http://www.defra.gov.uk/statistics/files/defra-stats-foodfarm-food-familyfood-2009-110525.pdf) (Accessed 25th July 2011).

Department of Health (1998) *Nutritional Aspects of the Development of Cancer. Report on Health and Social Subjects No. 48.* London: HMSO.

Department of Health (2011) National Diet and Nutrition Survey: headline results from Years 1 and 2 (combined) of the Rolling Programme, 2008/9—2009/10. Available at: http://www.dh.gov.uk/en/Publicationsandstatistics/Publications/PublicationsStatistics/DH_128166 (Accessed 21st July 2011).

Djousse, L., Arnett, D.K., Coon, H., Province, M.A., Moore, L.L. and Ellison, R.C. (2004) Fruit and vegetable consumption and LDL cholesterol: the National Heart, Lung, and Blood Institute Family Heart Study. *American Journal of Clinical Nutrition* **79**, 213–17.

Donovan, J.L. (2004) Flavonoids and the risk of cardiovascular disease in women. *American Journal of Clinical Nutrition* **79**, 522–4.

Eaton, S.B. and Konner, M. (1985) Palaeolithic nutrition: a consideration of its nature and current implications. *New England Journal of Medicine* **312**, 283–9.

EFSA (2011a) EFSA Journal, Scientific Opinion on the substantiation of health claims related to walnuts and maintenance of normal blood LDL-cholesterol concentrations (ID 1156, 1158) and improvement of endothelium-dependent vasodilation (ID 1155, 1157) pursuant to Article 13(1) of Regulation (EC) No 1924/2006. Available at: http://www.efsa.europa.eu/en/efsajournal/pub/2074.htm (Accessed 21 July 2011).

EFSA (2011b) Panel on Dietetic Products, Nutrition and Allergies (NDA) (2011) Scientific Opinion on the substantiation of health claims related to beta-glucans from oats and barley and maintenance of normal blood LDL-cholesterol concentrations (ID 1236, 1299), increase in satiety leading to a reduction in energy intake (ID 851, 852), reduction of post-prandial glycaemic responses (ID 821, 824), and "digestive function" (ID 850) pursuant to Article 13(1) of Regulation (EC) No 1924/2006. *EFSA Journal* **9**, 2207.

EFSA (2011c) European Union Register of nutrition and health claims made on food – Authorized health claims. Available at: http://ec.europa.eu/food/food/labellingnutrition/claims/community_register/authorised_health_claims_en.htm#art135 (Accessed 21 July 2011).

Fletcher, A.E. (2009) Nutrition and the eye in ageing. In: *Nutrition and Healthy Ageing. Report of a British Nutrition Foundation Task Force.* (eds S. Stanner and J. Buttriss). OxfordBlackwell: Blackwell.

Flight, I. and Clifton, P. (2006) Cereal grains and legumes in the prevention of coronary heart disease and stroke: a review of the literature. *European Journal of Clinical Nutrition* **60**, 1145–159.

Ford, E.S. and Mokdad, A.H. (2001) Fruit and vegetable consumption and diabetes mellitus incidence among U.S. adults. *Preventative Medicine* **32**, 33–9.

Fraser, G.E. (1999) Associations between diet and cancer, ischaemic heart disease, and all-cause mortality in non-Hispanic, white California Seventh-day Adventists. *American Journal of Clinical Nutrition* **70**, 532S–538S.

Fung, T.T., Hu, F.B., Pereira, M.A., Liu, S., Stampfer, M.J., Colditz, G.A. and Willet, W.C. (2002) Whole grain intake and the risk of type 2 diabetes: a prospective study in men. *American Journal of Clinical Nutrition* **76**, 535–40.

Gillette-Guyonnet, S., Abellan van Kan, G., Andrieu, S., Barberger-Gateau, P., Berr, C., Bonnefoy, M., Dartigues, JF., De Groot, L., Ferry, M., Galan, P., Hercberg, S., Jeandel, C., Morris, M.C., Nourhashemi, F., Payette, H., Poulain, J.P., Portet, F., Roussel, A.M., Ritz, P., Rolland,Y. and Vellas, B. (2007) IANA Task Force on nutrition and cognitive decline with ageing. *Journal of Nutrition, Health and Aging* **11**, 132–52.

Giovannucci, E., Stampfer, M.J., Colditz, G.A., Colditz, G.A., Hunter, D.J., Fuchs, C., Rosner, B.A., Speizer, F.E and Willett, W.C. (1998) Multivitamin use, folate, and colon cancer in women in the Nurses' Health Study. *Annals of Internal Medicine* **129**, 517–24.

Goldberg, J., Flowerdew, G., Smith., E., Brody, J.A. and Tso, M.O.M. (1998) Factors associated with age-related macular degeneration: an analysis of data from the first National Health and Nutrition Examination Survey. *American Journal of Epidemiology* **128**, 700–10.

Grace, P.B., Taylor, J.I., Low, Y.L., Luben, R.N., Mulligan, A.A., Botting, N.P., Dowsett, M., Welch, A.A., Khaw, K.T., Wareham, N.J. and Bingham, S.H. (2004) Phytoestrogen concentrations in serum and spot urine as biomarkers for dietary phytoestrogen intake and their relation to breast cancer risk in European prospective investigation of cancer and nutrition – Norfolk. *Cancer Epidemiology Biomarkers and Prevention* **13**, 698–708.

Gregory, J., Foster, K., Tyler, H. and Wiseman, M. (1990) *The Dietary and Nutritional Survey of British Adults.* London: HMSO.

Gregory, J., Lowe, S., Bates, C.J., Prentice, A., Jackson, L.V., Smithers, G., Wenlock, R. and Farron, M. (2000) *National Diet and Nutrition Survey, Young People Aged 4 to 18 Years. Volume 1: Report of the Diet and Nutrition Survey.* London: The Stationary Office.

Hamidi, M., Boucher, B.A., Cheung, A.M., Beyene, J. and Shah, P.S. (2011) Fruit and vegetable intake and bone health in women aged 45 years and over: a systematic review. *Osteoporosis International* **22**, 1681–93.

Harland, J.I. and Garton, L.E. (2008) Whole-grain intake as a marker of healthy body weight and adiposity. *Public Health Nutrition* **11**, 554–63.

Harnack, L., Walters, S.A.H. and Jacobs, D.R. (2003) Dietary intake and food sources of whole grains among US children and adolescents. Data from the 1994–1996 Continuing Survey of Food Intakes by individuals. *JADA* **103**, 1015–19.

He, F.J., Nowson, C.A. and MacGregor, G.A. (2006) Fruit and vegetable consumption and stroke: meta-analysis of cohort studies. *Lancet* **367**, 320–6.

He, F.J., Nowson, C.A., Lucas, M. and MacGregor, G.A. (2007) Increased consumption of fruit and vegetables is related to a reduced risk of coronary heart disease: meta-analysis of cohort studies. *Journal of Human Hypertension* **21**, 717–28.

He, M., van Dam, R.M., Rimm, E., Hu, F.B. and Qi, L. (2010) Whole-grain, cereal fiber, bran, and germ intake and the risks of all-cause and cardiovascular disease–specific mortality among women with type 2 diabetes mellitus. *Circulation* **121**, 2162–8.

Heart Outcomes Prevention Evaluation (HOPE) Study Investigators (2000) Effects of an angiotensin converting enzyme inhibitor, ramipril, on cardiovascular events in high-risk patients. *New England Journal of Medicine* **342**, 145–53.

Heiss, C., Schroeter, H., Balzer, J., Kleinbongard, P., Matern, S., Sies, H. and Kelm, M. (2006) Endothelial function, nitric oxide, and cocoa flavanols. *Journal of Cardiovascular Pharmacology* **47**, S128–35.

Henderson, L., Gregory, J. and Swan, G. (2002) *The National Diet and Nutrition Survey; Adults Aged 19 to 64 Years. Volume 1: Types and Quantities of Foods Consumed.* London: The Stationary Office.

Hertog, M.G.L., Feskins, E.J.M., Hollman, P.C.H., Katan, M.B. and Kromhout, D. (1994) Dietary antioxidant flavonoids and cancer risk in the Zutphen Elderly Study. *Nutrition and Cancer* **22**, 175–84

Hertog, M.G., Kromhout, D., Aravanis, C., Blackburn, R., Buzina, R., Fidanza, F., Giamaoli, S., Jansen, A., Menotti, A. and Nedeljkovic, S. (1995) Flavonoid intake and long-term risk of coronary heart disease and cancer in the Seven Countries Study. *Archives of Internal Medicine* **155**, 381–86.

Hodgson, J.M. (2006) Effects of teas and tea flavonoids on endothelial functionand blood pressure: a brief review. *Clinical and Experimental Pharmacology and Physiology* **33**, 838.

Hodgson, J.M., Puddey, I.B., Beilin, L.J., Mori, T.A., Burke, V., Croft, K.D. and Rogers, P.B. (1999) Effects of isoflavonoids on blood pressure in subjects with high–normal ambulatory blood pressure levels: a randomized control trial. *American Journal of Hypertension* **12**, 47–53.

Hollman, P.C. and Katan, M.B. (1999) Health effects and bioavailability of dietary flavonols. *Free Radical Research* **31**, S75–80.

Holt, R.R., Axtis-Goretta, L.-C., Momma, T.Y. and Keen, C.L. (2006) Dietary flavonols and platelet reactivity. *Journal of Cardiovascular Pharmacology* **47**, S187–96.

Hu, F.B. (2003) Plant-based foods and prevention of cardiovascular disease: an overview. *American Journal of Clinical Nutrition* **78**, 544S–551S.

Hu, F.B., Rimm, E.B., Stampfer, M.J., Ascherio, A, Spiegelman, D. and Willett, W.C. (2000) Prospective study of major dietary patterns and risk of coronary heart disease in men. *American Journal of Clinical Nutrition* **72**, 912–21.

Hung, H.-C., Joshipura, K.J., Jiang, R., Hu, F.B., Hunter., D, Smith-Warner, S.A, Colditz, G.A., Rosner, B, Spiegelman, D. and Willett, W.C. (2004) Fruit and vegetable intake and risk of major chronic disease. *Journal of the National Cancer Institute* **96**, 1577–84.

Huxley, R.R. and Neil, H.A.W. (2003) The relation between dietary flavonol intake and coronary heart disease mortality: a meta-analysis of prospective studies. *European Journal of Clinical Nutrition* **57**, 904–8.

Jackson, M. (2003) Potential mechanisms of action of bioactive substances found in foods. In: *Plants: Diet and Health. Report of a British Nutrition Foundation Task Force* (ed. G. Goldberg). Oxford: Blackwell Sciences.

Jacobs, D.R., Meyer, K.A., Kushi, L.H. and Folsom, A.R. (1999) Is whole grain intake associated with reduced total and cause-specific death rates in older women? The Iowa Women's Health Study. *American Journal of Public Health* **89**, 322–9.

Jacobs, D.R., Meyer, H.E. and Solvoll, K. (2001) Reduced mortality among wholegrain bread eaters in men and women in the Norwegian County Study. *European Journal of Clinical Nutrition* **55**, 137–43.

Jenab, M., Ferrari, P., Slimani, N., Norat, T., Casagrande, C., Overad, K., Olsen, A., Stripp, C., Tjonneland, A., Boutron-Ruault, M.C., Clavel-Chapelon, F., Kesse, E., Nieters, A., Bergmann, M., Boeing, H., Naska, A., Trichopoulou, A., Palli, D., Krogh, V., Celentano, E., Tumino, R,. Sacerdote, C., Bueno-de-Mesquita, H.B., Ocke, M.C., Peeters, P.H., Engeset, D., Quiros, J.R., Gonzalez, C.A., Martinez, C., Chirlaque, M.D., Ardanaz, E., Dorronsoro, M., Wallstrom, P., Palmqvist, R., Van Guelpen, B., Bingham, S., San Joaquin, M.A., Saracci, R., Kaaks, R. and Riboli, E. (2004) Association of nut and seed intake with colorectal cancer risk in the European Prospective Investigation into Cancer and Nutrition. Cancer *Epidemiology Biomarkers Preview* **13**, 1595–603.

Jensen, M.K., Hoh-Banerjee, P., Hu, F.B., Franz, M., Sampson, L., Gronbaek, M. and Rimm, E.B. (2004) Intakes of whole grains, bran, and germ and the risk of coronary heart disease in men. *American Journal of Clinical Nutrition* **80**, 1492–6.

Johns, T. and Ezyaguirre, P.B. (2006) Linking biodiversity, diet and health in policy and practice. Proceedings of the Nutrition Society **65**, 182–9.

Joshipura, K.J., Ascherio, A., Manson, J.E, Stampfer, M.J., Rimm, E.B., Speizer, F.E, Hennekens, C.H., Spiegelman, D. and Willett, W.C. (1999) Fruit and vegetable intake in relation to risk of ischaemic stroke. *Journal of the American Medical Association* **282**, 1233–9.

Kang, J., Ascherio, A. and Goldstein, F. (2005) Fruit and vegetable consumption and cognitive function. *Annals of Neurology* **57**, 713–20.

Kay, C.D., Kris-Etherton, P.M. and West, S.G. (2006) Effects of antioxidant-rich foods on vascular reactivity: review of the clinical evidence. *Current Atherosclerosis Reports* **8**, 510–22.

Keinan-Boker, L., van Der Schouw, Y.T., Grobbee, D.E. and Peters, P.H. (2004) Dietary phytoestrogens and breast cancer risk. *American Journal of Clinical Nutrition* **79**, 282–8.

Key, T.J., Allen, N., Appleby, P., Overvad, K., Tjønneland, A., Miller, A., Boeing, H., Karalis, D., Psaltopoulou, T., Berrino, F., Palli, D., Panico, S., Tumino, R., Vineis, P., Bueno-de-Mesquita, H.B, Kiemeney, L., Peeters, P.H., Martinez, C., Dorronsoro, M., Gonzalez, C.A., Chirlaque, M.D., Quiros, J.R., Ardanaz, E., Berglund, G., Egevad, L., Hallmans, G., Stattin, P., Bingham, S., Day, N., Gann, P., Kaaks, R., Ferrari, P. and Riboli, E. (2004) Fruits and vegetables and prostate cancer: no association among 1104 cases in a prospective study of 130544 men in the European Prospective Investigation into Cancer and Nutrition (EPIC). *International Journal of Cancer* **109**, 119–24.

Key, T.J., Fraser, G.E., Thorogood, M., Appleby, P.N., Beral, V., Reeves, G., Burr, M.L., Chang-Claude, J. and Frentzel-Beyme, R. (1998) Mortality in vegetarians and non-vegetarians: a collaborative analysis of 8300 deaths among 76,000 men and women in five prospective studies. *Public Health Nutrition* **1**, 33–41.

Key, T.J.A., Thorogood, M., Appleby, P.N. and Burr, M.L. (1996) Dietary habits and mortality in 11000 vegetarians and health conscious people: results of a 17 year follow-up. *British Medical Journal* **313**, 775–9.

Khaw, K.T. and Barrett-Connor, E. (1987) Dietary fiber and reduced ischemic heart disease mortality rates in men and women: a 12-year prospective study. *American Journal of Epidemiology* **126**, 1093–102.

Khaw, K.T., Bingham, S., Welch, A., Luben, R., Wareham, N., Oakes, S. and Day, N. (2001) Relation between plasma ascorbic acid and mortality in men and women in EPIC-Norfolk prospective study. European Prospective Investigation into Cancer and Nutrition. *Lancet* **357**, 657–63.

Kim, Y.I. (2006) Does a high folate intake increase the risk of breast cancer? *Nutrition Reviews* **64**, 468–75.

Koushik, A., Hunter, D.J., Spiegelman, D., Anderson, K.E., Buring, JE., Freudenheim, J.L., Goldbohm, R.A., Hankinson, S.E., Larsson, S.C., Leitzmann, M., Marshall, J.R., McCullough, M.L., Miller, A.B., Rodriguez, C., Rohan, T.E., Ross, J.A., Schatzkin, A., Schouten, L.J., Willett, W.C., Wolk, A., Zhang, S.M. and Smith-Warner, S.A. (2006) Intake of the major carotenoids and the risk of epithelial ovarian cancer in a pooled analysis of 10 cohort studies. *International Journal of Cancer* **119**, 2148–54.

Knekt, P., Isotupa, S., Rissanen, H., Heliovaara, M., Jarvinen, R., Hakkinen, S., Aromaa, A. and Reunanen, A. (2000) Quercetin intake and incidence of cerebrovascular disease. *European Journal of Clinical Nutrition* **54**, 415–17.

Knekt, P., Jarvinen, R., Reunanen, A. and Maatela, J. (1996) Flavonoid intake and coronary mortality in Finland: a cohort study. *British Medical Journal* **312**, 478–81.

Krinsky, N.I. and Johnson, E.J. (2005) Carotenoid actions and their relation to health and disease. *Molecular Aspects of Medicine* **26**, 459–516.

Kris-Etherton, P.M., Zhao, G., Binkoski, A.E., Coval, S.M. and Etherton, T.D. (2001) The effects of nuts on coronary heart disease risk. *Nutrition Reviews* **59**, 103–11.

Lagiou, P., Samoli, E., Lagiou., A., Tzonou, A., Kalandidi, A., Peterson, J., Dwyer, J. and Trichopoulos, D. (2004) Intake of specific flavonoid classes and coronary heart disease – a case-control study in Greece. *European Journal of Clinical Nutrition* **58**, 1643–8.

Lampe, J.W. (1999) Health effects of vegetables and fruit: assessing mechanisms of action in human experimental studies. *American Journal of Clinical Nutrition* **70** (Suppl), 475S–490S.

Lang, R., Thane, C.W., Bolton-Smith, C. and Jebb, S.A. (2003) Consumption of wholegrain foods by British adults: findings from further analysis of two national dietary surveys. *Public Health Nutrition* **6**, 479–84.

Lanham-New, S. and Loveridge, N. (2007) Bones and ageing. In: *Nutrition and Healthy Ageing. Report of a British Nutrition Foundation Task Force* (eds S. Stanner and J. Buttriss). Oxford: Blackwell.

Law, M.R. and Morris, J.K. (1998) By how much does fruit and vegetable consumption reduce the risk of ischaemic heart disease? *European Journal of Clinical Nutrition* **52**, 549–56.

Lean, M.E., Noroozi, M., Kelly, I., Burns, J., Talwar, D., Sattar, N. and Crozier, A. (1999) Dietary flavonols protect diabetic human lymphocytes against oxidative damage to DNA. *Diabetes* **48**, 176–81.

Leppala, J.M., Virtamo, J., Fogelholm, R., Albanes, D., Taylor, P.R. and Heinonen, O.P. (2000) Vitamin E and beta carotene supplementation in high risk for stroke: a subgroup analysis of the Alpha-Tocopherol, Beta-Carotene Cancer Prevention Study. *Archives of Neurology* **57**, 1503–9.

Lin, P.H., Ginty, F., Appel, L.J., Aickin, M., Bohannon, A., Barnero, P., Barclay, D. and Svetkey, L.P. (2003) The DASH diet and sodium reduction improve markers of bone turnover and calcium metabolism in adults. *Journal of Nutrition* **133**, 3130–36.

Liu, S., Manson, J.E., Lee, I.M., Cole, S.R., Hennekens, C.H., Willett, W.C. and Buring, J.E. (2000a) Fruit and vegetable intake and risk of cardiovascular disease: the Women's Health Study. *American Journal of Clinical Nutrition* **72**, 922–8.

Liu, S., Manson, J., Stampfer, M.J., Rexrode, K.M., Hi, F.B., Rimm, E.B and Willett, W.C. (2000b) Whole grain consumption and risk of ischaemic stroke in women: a prospective study. *Journal of the American Medical Association* **284**, 1534–40.

Liu, S., Stampfer, M.J., Hu, F.B., Giovannucci, E., Mason, J.E., Hennekens, C.H. and Willett, W.C. (1999) Whole-grain consumption and risk of coronary heart disease: results from the Nurse's Health Study. *American Journal of Clinical Nutrition* **70**, 412–19.

de Lorgeril, M., Salen, P., Martin, J.L., Monjaud, I., Delaye, J. and Mamelle, N. (1999) Mediterranean diet, traditional risk factors, and the rate of cardiovascular complications after myocardial infarction: final report of the Lyon Diet Heart Study. *Circulation* **99**, 779–85.

Loria, C.M., Klag, M.J., Caulfield, L.E. and Whelton, P.K. (2000) Vitamin C status and mortality in US adults. *American Journal of Clinical Nutrition* **72**, 139–45.

Lunn, J. and Buttriss, J. (2007) Carbohydrates and dietary fibre. *Nutrition Bulletin* **32**, 21–64.

Lynn, A., Collins, A., Fuller, Z., Hillman, K and Ratcliffe, B (2006) Cruciferous vegetables and colorectal cancer. Proceedings of the Nutrition Society 65, 135–144.

MAFF (1955) *National Food Survey 1954. Annual Report on Food Expenditure, Consumption and Nutrient Intakes.* London: The Stationery Office.

MAFF (1960) *National Food Survey 1959. Annual Report on Food Expenditure, Consumption and Nutrient Intakes.* London: The Stationery Office.

MAFF (1965) *National Food Survey 1964. Annual Report on Food Expenditure, Consumption and Nutrient Intakes.* London: The Stationery Office.

MAFF (1970) *National Food Survey 1969. Annual Report on Food Expenditure, Consumption and Nutrient Intakes.* London: The Stationery Office.

MAFF (1975) *National Food Survey 1974. Annual Report on Food Expenditure, Consumption and Nutrient Intakes.* London: The Stationery Office.

MAFF (1980) *National Food Survey 1979. Annual Report on Food Expenditure, Consumption and Nutrient Intakes.* London: The Stationery Office.

MAFF (1985) *National Food Survey 1984. Annual Report on Food Expenditure, Consumption and Nutrient Intakes.* London: The Stationery Office.

MAFF (1990) *National Food Survey 1989. Annual Report on Food Expenditure, Consumption and Nutrient Intakes.* London: The Stationery Office.

MAFF (1995) *National Food Survey 1994. Annual Report on Food Expenditure, Consumption and Nutrient Intakes.* London: The Stationery Office.

MAFF (2000) *National Food Survey 1999. Annual Report on Food Expenditure, Consumption and Nutrient Intakes.* London: The Stationery Office.

Mannisto, S., Smith-Warner, S.A., Spiegelman, D., Albanes, D., Anderson, K., van den Brandt, P.A., Cerhan, J.R,, Colditz, G., Feskanich, D., Freudenheim, J.L., Giovannucci, E., Goldbohm, R.A., Graham, S., Miller, A.B., Rohan, T.E., Virtamo, J., Willett, W.C. and Hunter, D.J. (2004) Dietary carotenoids and risk of lung cancer in a pooled analysis of seven cohort studies. *Cancer Epidemiology Biomarkers and Prevention* **13**, 40–48.

Marchioli, R. (1999) Antioxidant vitamins and prevention of cardiovascular disease: laboratory, epidemiological and clinical trial data. *Pharmacology Research* **40**, 227–38.

Margetts, B. and Buttriss, J. (2003) Epidemiology linking consumption of plant foods and their constituents with health. In: *Plants: Diet and Health. Report of a British Nutrition Foundation Task Force* (ed. G. Goldberg). Oxford: Blackwell.

Mathers, J.C. (2006) Plant foods for human health: research challenges. *Proceedings of the Nutrition Society* **65**, 198–203.

Mellen, P.B., Walsh, T.F. and Herrington, D.M. (2008) Whole grain intake and cardiovascular disease: a meta-analysis. *Nutrition Metabolism and Cardiovasular Disease* **18**, 283–90.

Mennen, L.I., Sapinho, D., de Bree, A., Arnault, N., Bertrais, S., Galan, P. and Hercberg, S. (2004) Consumption of foods rich in flavonoids is related to a decreased risk in apparently healthy French women. *Journal of Nutrition* **134**, 923–6.

Miedema, I., Feskens, E., Heederik, D. and Kromhout, D. (1993) Dietary determinants of long-term incidence of chronic non-specific lung diseases. *American Journal of Epidemoilogy* **138**, 37–45.

Miller, A.B., Altenburg, H.P and Bueno-de-Mesquita, B. (2004) Fruits and vegetables and lung cancer: findings from the European Prospective Investigation into Cancer and Nutrition. *International Journal of Cancer* **108**, 269–76.

Montonen, J., Knekt, P., Jarvinen, R., Aromaa, A. and Reunanen, A. (2003) Whole-grain and fibre intake and the incidence of type 2 diabetes. *American Journal of Clinical Nutrition* **77**, 622–9.

Morris, C.D. and Carson, S. (2003) Routine vitamin supplementation to prevent cardiovascular disease: a summary of the evidence for the U.S. Preventative Services Task Force. *Annals of Internal Medicine* **139**, 56–70.

Morris, M.C., Evans, D.A., Tangney, C.C., Bienias, J.L. and Willson, R.S. (2006) Associations of vegetable and fruit consumption with age-related cognitive decline. *Neurology* **67**, 1370–76.

National Academy of Sciences (2000) *Food and Nutrition Board: Dietary Reference Intakes for Vitamin C, Vitamin E, Selenium and Carotenoids.* Washington, DC: National Academy Press.

Ness, A.R. and Powles, J.W. (1997) Fruit and vegetables, and cardiovascular disease: a review. *International Journal of Epidemiology* **26**, 1–13.

Ness, A.R. and Powles, J.W. (1999) The role of diet, fruit and vegetables and antioxidants in the aetiology of stroke. *Journal of Cardiovascular Risk* **4**, 229–34.

Nestle, M. (1999) Animal v. plant foods in human diet and health: is the historical record unequivocal? *Proceedings of the Nutrition Society* **58**, 211–18.

Nooyens, A.C.J., Bas Bueno-de-Mesquita, H., van Boxtel, M.P.J., van Gelder, B.M., Verhagen, H. and Monique Verschuren, W.M. (2011) Fruit and vegetable intake and cognitive decline in middle-aged men and women: the Doetinchem Cohort Study. *British Journal of Nutrition* **11**, 1–10.

Obarzanek, E., Sacks, F.M., Vollmer, W.M., Bray, G.A., Miller, E.R., Lin, P.H., Karanja, N.M., Most-Winderhauser, M.M., Moore, T.J,. Swain, J.F., Bales, C.W. and Proschan, M.A. (2001) Effects on blood lipids of a blood pressure lowering diet: the Dietary Approaches to Stop Hypertension (DASH) Trial. *American Journal of Clinical Nutrition* **74**, 80–89.

Patel, B.D., Welch, A.A., Bingham, S.A., Luben, R.N., Day, N.E., Khaw, K.T., Lomas, D.A. and Wareham, N.J. (2006) Dietary antioxidants and asthma in adults. *Thorax* **61**, 388–93.

Paul, A.A. (1977) Changes in food composition – effects of some newer methods of production and processing. *Nutrition Bulletin* **4**, 173–86.

Pereira, M.A., O'Reilly, E., Augustsson, K., Fraser, G.E., Goldbourt, U., Heirmann, B.L., Hallmans, G., Knekt, P., Liu, S., Pietinen, P., Spiegelman, D., Stevens, J., Virtamo, J., Willett, W.C. and Ascherio, A. (2004) Dietary fiber and risk of coronary heart disease: a pooled analysis of cohort studies. *Archives of Internal Medicine* **164**, 370–76.

Pietinen, P., Rimm, E.B., Korhonen, P., Hartman, A.M., Willett, W.C., Albarnes, D. and Virtamo, J. (1996) Intake of dietary fibre and risk of coronary heart disease in a cohort of Finnish men. The Alpha-Tocopherol, Beta-carotene Cancer Prevention Study. *Circulation* **94**, 2720–27.

Plassman, B.L., Williams, J.W. and Burke, J.R. (2010) Systematic review: factors associated with risk for and possible prevention of cognitive decline in later life. *Annals of Internal Medicine* **153**, 182–93.

Riboli, E. and Norat, T. (2003) Epidemiologic evidence of the protective effect of fruit and vegetables on cancer risk. *American Journal of Clinical Nutrition* 78 (suppl), 559S–569S.

Riemersma, R.A., Oliver, M., Elton, R.A., Alfthan, G., Vartiainen, E., Salo, M., Rubba, P., Mancini, M., Georgi, H. and Vuilleumier, J.P. (1990) Plasma antioxidants and coronary heart disease: vitamins C and E, and selenium. *European Journal of Clinical Nutrition* **44**, 143–50.

Rimm, E.B., Ascherio, A., Giovannucci, E., Spiefelman, D., Stampfer, M.J. and Willett, W.C. (1996) Vegetable, fruit, and cereal fiber intake and risk of coronary heart disease among men. *Journal of the American Medical Association* **275**, 447–51.

Romieu, I. and Trenga, C. (2001) Diet and obstructive lung diseases. *Epidemiology Reviews* **23**, 268–87.

Sacks, F.M., Lichtenstein, A., Van Horn, L., Harris, W., Kris-Etherton, P. and Winston, M. (2006) Soya protein, isoflavones and cardiovascular health. *Arteriosclerosis, Thrombosis, and Vascular Biology* **26**, 1689–92.

Sacks, F.M., Svetky, L.P., Vollmer, W.M., Appel, L.J., Bray, G.A., Harsha, D., Obarzane, E., Conlin, P.R., Miller, E.R., Simons-Morton, D.G., Karanja, N. and Lin, P.H. (2001) Effects on blood pressure of reduced dietary sodium and the Dietary Approaches to Stop Hypertension (DASH) diet. DASH-Sodium Collaborative Research Group. *New England Journal of Medicine* **344**, 3–10.

Salonen, J.T., Alfthan, G., Huttunen, J.K., Pikkarainen, J. and Puska, P. (1982) Association between cardiovascular death and myocardial infarctio and serum selenium in a matched-pair longitudinal study. *Lancet* **ii**, 175–9.

Sanjoaquin, M.A., Allen, N., Couto, E., Roddam, A.W. and Key, T.J. (2005) Folate intake and colorectal cancer risk: a meta-analytical approach. *International Journal of Cancer* **113**, 825–8.

Schulz, M., Lahmann, P.H. and Boeing, H. (2005) Fruit and vegetables consumption and risk of epithelial ovarian cancer: the European Prospective Investigation into cancer and nutrition. *Cancer Epidemiology Biomarkers and Prevention* **14**, 2531–5.

Schunemann, H.J., Grant, B.J., Freaudenheim, J.L., Muit, P., Browne, R.W., Drake, J.A., Klocke, R.A. and Trevisan, M. (2001) The relation of serum levels of antioxidant vitamins C and E, retinol and carotenoids with pulmonary function in the general population. *American Journal of Respiratory and Critical Care Medicine* **163**, 1246–55.

Scientific Advisory Committee on Nutrition (SACN) (2006) *Folate and Disease Prevention*. London: The Stationery Office.

Seal, C.J. (2006) Whole grains and CVD risk. *Proceedings of the Nutrition Society* **65**, 24–34.

Seal, C.J., Jones, A.R. and Whitney, A.D. (2006) Whole grains uncovered. *Nutrition Bulletin* **31**, 129.

Sellers, T.A., Kushi, L.H., Cerhan, J.R., Vierkant, A., Gapstur, A., Vachon, C.M., Olson, J.E., Therneau, T.M. and Folsom, A.R. (2001) Dietary folate intake, alcohol, and risk of breast cancer in a prospective study of postmenopausal women. *Epidemiology* **12**, 420–28.

Selmi, C., Mao, T.K., Keen, C.L., Schimtz, H. and Gershwin, E. (2006) The anti-inflammatory properties of cocoa flavanols. *Journal of Cardiovascular Pharmacology* **47**, S163–71.

Seow, A., Yuan, J.M. and Sun, C.L. (2002) Dietary isothiocyanates, glutathione-S-transferase polymorphisms and colorectal cancer risk in the Singapore Chinese Health Study. *Carcinogenesis* **23**, 2055–61.

Sesso, H.D., Gaziano, J.M., Liu, S. and Buring, J.E. (2003) Flavonoid intake and risk of cardiovascular disease in women. *American Journal of Clinical Nutrition* **77**, 1400–8.

Shaheen, SO., Jameson, KA., Syddal, HE., Aigie Sayer, A., Dennison, EM., Cooper, C and Robinson, SM: Hertfordshire Cohort Study Group (2010) The relationship of dietary patterns with adult lung function and COPD. Eur Respir J. 36,277–284.

Shaheen, S.O., Sterne, J.A., Thompson, R.L., Songhurst, C.E., Margetts, B.M. and Burney, P.G. (2001) Dietary antioxidants and asthma in adults: population-based case-control study. *American Journal of Respiratory Critical Care Medicine* **164**, 1823–8.

Singh, R.B., Rastogi, R., Niaz, M.A., Ghosh, S., Singh, R. and Gupta, S. (1992) Effects of fat modified and fruit and vegetable enriched diets on blood lipids in the Indian Diet Heart Study. *American Journal of Cardiology* **70**, 869–874.

Smith-Warner, S.A., Spiegelman, D., Yaun, S.-S., Albanes, D., Beeson, W.L., van den Brandt, P.A., Feskanich, D., Folsom, A.R., Fraser, G.E., Freudenheim, J.L., Giovannucci, E., Goldbohm, RA., Graham, S., Kushi, LH., Miller, AB., Pietinen, P., Rohan, T.E., Speizer, F.E., Willett, W.C. and Hunter, D.J. (2003) Fruits, vegetables and lung cancer: a pooled analysis of cohort studies. *International Journal of Cancer* **107**, 1001–11.

Southgate, D.A.T. (2000) Cereals and cereal products. In: *Human Nutrition and Dietetics* (eds Garrow, J.S., James, W.P.T. and Ralph, A.) pp. 333–47. London: Churchill Livingstone.

Speller, S. (2000) Merging the National Food Survey. *Nutrition Bulletin* **25**, 147–9.

Spencer, J.P. (2010a) The impact of fruit flavonoids on memory and cognition. *British Journal of Nutrition* **104** (Suppl 3), S40–47.

Spencer, J.P. (2010b) Beyond antioxidants: the cellular and molecular interactions of flavonoids and how these underpin their actions on the brain. *Proceedings of the Nutrition Society* **69**, 244–60.

Stanner, S.A., Hughes, J., Kelly, C.N.M. and Buttriss, J. (2004) A review of the epidemiological evidence for the 'antioxidant hypothesis'. *Public Health Nutrition* **7**, 407–22.

Steffen, L.M., Jacobs, D.R., Jr, Stevens, J., Shahar, E., Carithers, T. and Folsom, A.R. (2003) Associations of whole-grain, refined-grain, and fruit and vegetable consumption with risks of all-cause mortality and incident coronary artery disease and ischemic stroke: the Atherosclerosis Risk in Communities (ARIC) Study. *American Journal of Clinical Nutrition* **78**, 383–90.

Stephens, N.G., Parsons, A., Schofield, P.M., Kelly, F., Cheeseman, K. and Mitchinson, M.J. (1996) Randomised controlled trial of vitamin E in patients with coronary disease: Cambridge Heart Antioxidant Study (CHAOS). *Lancet* **347**, 781–6.

Strandhagen, E., Hansson, P.O., Bosaeus, I., Isakkson, B. and Eriksson, H. (2000) High fruit intake may reduce mortality among middle-aged and elderly men. The Study of Men Born in 1913. *European Journal of Clinical Nutrition* **54**, 337–41.

Tavani, A. and La Vecchia, C. (1999) Beta-carotene and risk of coronary heart disease. A review of observational and intervention studies. *Biomedical Pharmacotherapy* **53**, 409–16.

Tavani, A., Spertini, L., Bosetti, C., Parpinel, M., Gnagarella, P., Bravi, F., Peterson, J., Dwyer, J., Lagiou, P., Negri, E. and La Vecchia, C. (2006) Intake of specific flavonoids and risk of acute myocardial infarction in Italy. *Public Health Nutrition* **9**, 369–74.

Thane, C.W., Jones, A.R., Stephen, A.M., Seal, C.J. and Jebb, S.A. (2005) Wholegrain intake by British young people aged 4–18 years. *British Journal of Nutrition* **94**, 825–31.

Tighe, P., Duthie, G., Vaughan, N., Brittenden, J., Simpson, W.G., Duthie, S., Mutch, W., Wahle, K., Horgan, G. and Thies, F. (2010) Effect of increased consumption of whole-grain foods on blood pressure and other cardiovascular risk markers in healthy middle-aged persons: a randomized controlled trial. *American Journal of Clinical Nutrition* **92**, 733–40.

Toussaint_Samat, M. (1992) *History of Food*. Oxford: Blackwell.

Trenga, C.A., Koeing, J.Q. and Williams, P.V. (2001) Dietary antioxidants and ozone-induced bronchial hyper-responsiveness in adults with asthma. *Archives of Environmental Health* **56**, 242–9.

Truswell, A.S. (2002) Cereal grains and coronary heart disease. *European Journal of Clinical Nutrition* **56**, 1–14.

United States Department of Agriculture (USDA) (2011) Choose my plate. Available at: http://www.choosemyplate.gov/ (Accessed 21st July 2011).

Van Gils, C.H., Peeters, P.H.M. and Bueno-de-Mesquita, H.B. (2005) Consumption of vegetables and fruits and risk of breast cancer. *Journal of the American Medical Association* **293**, 183–93.

van't Veer, P., Jansen, M.C., Klerk, M. and Kok, F.J. (2000) Fruits and vegetables in the prevention of cancer and cardiovascular disease. *Public Health Nutrition* **3**, 103–7.

Vivekananthan, D.P., Penn, M.S., Sapp, S.K., Hsu, A. and Topol, E.J. (2003) Use of antioxidant vitamins for the prevention of cardiovascular disease: meta-analysis of randomised trials. *Lancet* **361**, 2017–23.

WHO (2002) *The World Health Report 2002: Reducing Risks, Promoting Healthy Life.* Geneva: World Health Organization.

WHO/FAO (2005) *Fruit and Vegetables for Health.* Report of a Joint FAO/WHO workshop, 1–3 September 2004, Kobe, Japan. Geneva: World Health Organization.

Williamson, C.S. and Buttriss, J.L. (2007) EuroFIR Congress 2006: Food Information Databank Systems – everything you ever wanted to know. *Trends in Food Science and Technology* **18**, 398–406.

WCRF (1997) *Food, Nutrition and the Prevention of Cancer: a Global Perspective.* Washington DC: American Institute for Cancer Research.

WCRF and American Institute for Cancer Research (2007) *Food, Nutrition, Physical Activity and the Prevention of Cancer: a Global Perspective.* Washington DC: American Institute for Cancer Research.

WCRF and American Institute for Cancer Research (2010) Continuous Update Project: colorectal cancer report 2010, summary. Available at: http://www.wcrf.org/cancer_research/cup/index.php

Yochum, L., Kushi, L.H., Meyer, K. and Folsom, A.R. (1999) Dietary flavonoid intake and risk of cardiovascular disease in postmenopausal women. *American Journal of Epidemiology* **149**, 943–9.

Chapter 2

Carbohydrates and lipids

Andrew Salter and Gregory Tucker

Introduction

The macronutrient content of plant-based foods is very variable. Apart from leguminous seeds, these crops tend to be quite low in protein but can often represent rich sources of carbohydrates and lipids. Tubers or roots tend to be rich in carbohydrates whilst seed can be either oil or carbohydrate rich. Table 2.1 lists the composition of some common plant crops.

Sugars in plants are all ultimately derived from photosynthesis as the products of the Calvin or C_3 cycle in the chloroplasts of photosynthetic tissues, primarily leaves. Sugars are removed from the Calvin cycle in the form of fructose-6-phosphate and converted to either sucrose, for transportation around the plant, or for temporary storage within the leaf as starch. Several non-photosynthetic organs, such as tubers and seeds, convert the sucrose into starch for long-term storage in amyloplasts. It is this that forms the major source of dietary carbohydrate. The other major 'sink' for sugars in the plant is the cell walls. These are much more complex structures than starch and are mainly indigestible when forming part of the human diet. They are nonetheless nutritionally significant since they represent the bulk of the fibre in our diets. There are other less prevalent carbohydrates found in plants such as the oligosaccharides, e.g. inulin. However, although these are found in a more restricted distribution and amount they can be nutritionally significant.

In human nutrition the term dietary lipid primarily refers to compounds, largely triacylglycerols (TAG), containing fatty acids. These can be derived from both animal and plant material. In evolutionary terms, most dietary fatty acids will have been consumed as triacylglycerol associated with animal tissue. However, as our ability to manipulate plants through selective breeding has developed, plants, particularly seed oils, have become an increasingly important source of dietary fatty acids. This has had a marked influence on the type of fatty acids consumed, moving from saturated fatty acid (SFA) enriched animal tissues to plant oils rich in monounsaturated (MUFA) and polyunsaturated (PUFA) fatty acids.

Sterols are secondary alcohols belonging to the polyisoprenoid and terpenoid families. In human nutrition the sterol of primary importance is cholesterol which is derived

Phytonutrients, First Edition. Edited by Andrew Salter, Helen Wiseman and Gregory Tucker.
© 2012 Blackwell Publishing Ltd. Published 2012 by Blackwell Publishing Ltd.

Table 2.1 Composition of some major plant commodities[a]

Commodity	Protein	Fat	Carbohydrate
Apple	0.4	0.1	11.8
Banana	1.2	0.3	23.2
Olive	0.9	11.0	Tr
Pea	3.6	0.2	4.2
Soy bean (dried)	35.9	18.6	15.8
Potato	2.1	0.2	17.2
Rice (brown)	6.7	2.8	81.3
Wheat flour (brown)	12.6	2.0	68.5
Cornflour	0.6	0.7	92.0

[a]All values are quoted as g/100g
Source: McCance and Widdowson (2008).

from the tissues of animals and is found in particularly high levels in eggs. While plants do not make cholesterol they do produce a range of other sterols. These have become of particular interest as they have been found to block the absorption of cholesterol in the intestine thereby reducing plasma cholesterol. A range of plant sterol enriched 'functional' foods are now available and sold on the basis of protecting from cardiovascular disease (CVD).

Major carbohydrates

Chemically, carbohydrates are aliphatic polyhydroxy compounds with a carbonyl group and have the empirical formula $(CH_2O)n$. There are three main chemical classes of carbohydrate:

(1) Sugars: these include monosaccharides, disaccharides and polyols. This group includes the major plant storage disaccharide sucrose and the monosaccharides glucose and fructose which are prevalent in many fruit.
(2) Oligosaccharides: these are sugar polymers which have a degree of polymerisation between three and nine and include malto-oligosaccharides and other oligosaccharides. In plants these include raffinose, inulin and stachyose.
(3) Polysaccharides: compounds with a degree of polymerisation >9. In nutrition this group includes starch as well as the dietary fibre complex primarily associated with the carbohydrate polymers found in the plant cell wall. Fruit and vegetables are the main source of dietary fibre in human diets. The majority of plant cell walls in fruit and vegetables are primary plant cell walls from dicotyledonous plants. Some of the non-graminaceous monocotyledons that are important in the human diet such as onions have cell walls similar to dicotyledonous primary plant cell walls. Graminaceous monocotyledons have a slightly different chemical profile.

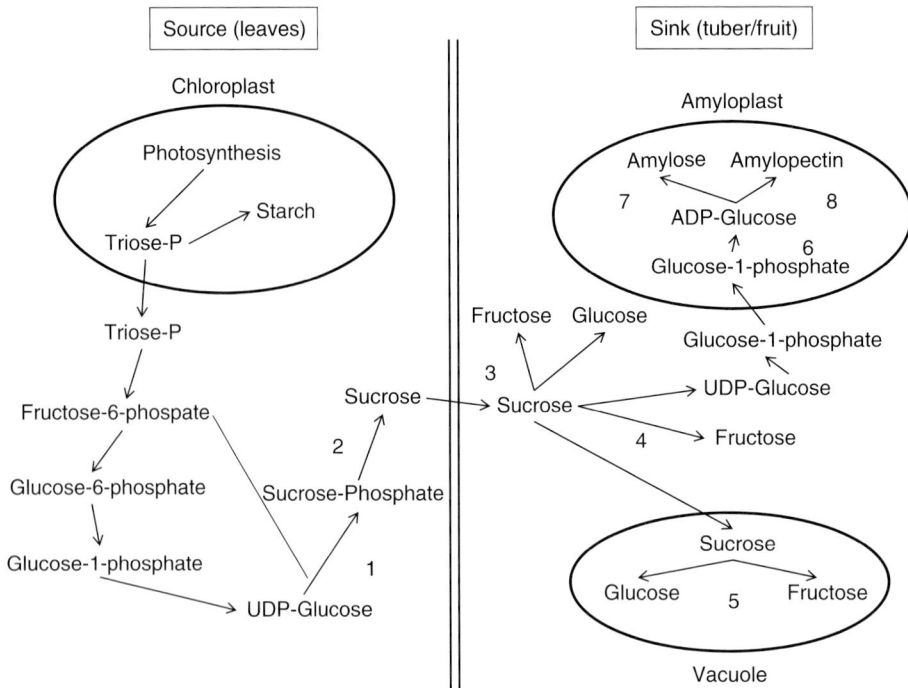

Figure 2.1 Sucrose and starch biosynthesis.

Sugars

The major monosaccharides found in plant foods are glucose and fructose. These are particularly prevalent in fruit where they form a major component, along with organic acids and aromatics, in determining the fruit flavour. Other monosaccharides occur in much smaller concentrations and are normally present as either phosphate or nucleotide diphosphate (NDP) linked glycosides which act as the intermediates in the biosynthesis of polymers. Sucrose is the major disaccharide sugar found in plants. It represents the major transport form for sugars in the plant and is also a major storage form in tissues such as a ripe banana, sugar cane, sugar beet and carrot. Sucrose consists of a β-D-fructofuranose residue linked through its C2 (anomeric carbon) to the anomeric C1 carbon of an α-D-glucopyranose. This linkage serves to protect the reducing groups of both the glucose and fructose and as such makes sucrose a non-reducing sugar. This may have benefits for the plant in that this means that the sucrose is relatively inert and will not react with other components during transport and storage within the plant.

The biosynthesis of sucrose occurs in the cytosol of the cell and is shown in Figure 2.1. Triose-phosphates, from the pool of intermediates in the photosynthetic C_3 cycle, are exported from the chloroplast to the cytosol and converted into fructose-6-phosphate. This fructose-6-phosphate is then converted to glucose-6-phosphate and then into glucose-1-phosphate. The final three intermediates in this pathway represent the major intermediates in the hexose phosphate pool of the plant cell and are inter-converted by the enzymes glucose-6-phosphate isomerase (fructose-6-phosphate to glucose-6-phospahte) and phosphoglucomutase (glucose-6-phosphate to glucose-1-phosphate), respectively. The glucose-1-phosphate then reacts with UTP in a reaction catalysed by UDP-glucose pyrophosphorylase to generate UDP-glucose. This UDP-glucose subsequently reacts with a second fructose-6-phosphate to form sucrose-phosphate in a reaction catalysed by sucrose phosphate synthase. This is an allosteric enzyme, being activated by glucose-6-phosphate, and as such probably represents the main regulatory step for sucrose synthesis. Finally the phosphate group is removed by the enzyme sucrose phosphatase. This final step has a large negative free energy change and at this point the pathway becomes essentially irreversible.

Sucrose is exported from the photosynthetic tissues, transported throughout the plant and eventually delivered to storage organs such as seeds and tubers. It can then either be stored directly or broken down to glucose and fructose by the action of invertase, or to glucose and glucose-1-phosphate by the action of sucrose synthase. In either case the hexoses released can then be imported into the amyloplast (a modified plastid) of the storage organ and used for the synthesis of starch for long-term storage. The advantage of starch as a storage polymer over glucose or sucrose, lies in the reduction of osmotic stress. Storage of a similar level of these soluble metabolites would impose too great an osmotic stress on the cell.

Polysaccharides

Starch

Starch is the major form of storage carbohydrate in plants and as such represents a very significant dietary source of energy. Indeed in 2003 it was estimated that 1000 million tons of starch was produced (The Food and Agriculture Organisation of the United Nations http://www.fao.org). Starch is produced in most crops, but the major dietary sources are cereals such as maize and wheat, other seed endosperm such as rice, and tubers such as potato, carrot and cassava. Since many of these are staples, starch represents the major calorie supplier for a significant proportion of the world's population. Starch is also extracted from these sources and used in a variety of industrial processes, many of which also contribute to our diet. Thus, starch is often used as a thickener and sweetener in commodities such as confectionary.

Starch consists entirely of glucose but is nonetheless a considerably complicated structure which varies between species and indeed within the organs of individual plants. There are two major types of starch polymer, namely amylose and amylopectin. Amylose consists of a linear chain of $\alpha(1-4)$ linked glucose which varies in length but which can contain several hundred sugar residues. Amylopectin also consists primarily of $\alpha(1-4)$ linked glucose but this is a highly branched molecule. The branching is due to $\alpha(1-6)$ linkages which represent about 5% of the total bonds within the polymer. The average length of the $\alpha(1-4)$ linked glucose chains is 20–25 glucose residues but this can be very variable and individual regions can be between 6 or several hundred glucose residues in length. The final size of the polymer can also be variable ranging between around 10 000 and 100 000 glucose residues in total. Neighbouring unbranched chains of between 10 and 15 residues long can pack together to give the amylopectin a semi-crystalline structure (Zeeman et al. 2007).

Starch is essentially insoluble, and is laid down in the plastid (chloroplast or amyloplast) in the form of a starch granule. The detailed structure of the granule is beyond the scope of this chapter but this has been reviewed elsewhere (Jobling 2004; Zeeman et al. 2007). It is thought that the amylopectin is synthesised at the surface of the growing granule to form a scaffold-like structure which is then subsequently 'in-filled' by the synthesis and deposition of amylose within the granule itself. The granules are thus made up of a series of 'growth rings' representing periods of active deposition. Starch granules vary in size, shape and internal structure between organs and species (Jobling 2004). Those in the chloroplasts of leaf tissue tend to be smaller whilst those in storage tissues (amyloplasts) are larger. The relative proportion of amylose to amylopectin is also variable, but generally amylopectin accounts for about 70–80% of the granule.

Starch is a primary product of photosynthesis and can be stored in the leafy tissue of plants. In some species, e.g. soybean (Upmeyer and Koller 1973), starch is the major storage sugar in the leaf, whilst in others, such as spinach (Stitt et al. 1983), sucrose may accumulate as well. This storage though is often transitory with the starch representing a source of carbohydrate to be mobilised during the night. Starch is also synthesised in storage organs (seeds and tubers) normally from imported sucrose as described earlier. This starch is laid down in a modified plastid termed the amyloplast and it is this that represents the major dietary source of this carbohydrate. There are many similarities between the biosynthetic pathways for starch synthesis in these two types of organ but there are also several differences. The majority of research has been carried out on the biosynthetic pathway in storage tissues, and as these represent the major sources of dietary starch, we will concentrate on these tissues. The mechanism underlying the diurnal synthesis and degradation of starch in the photosynthetic leafy type tissues has been recently reviewed by Zeeman et al. (2007).

The biosynthetic pathway for starch is shown in Figure 2.1. As with sucrose, the hexose sugars are obtained from the Calvin cycle and converted into glucose-1-phosphate. This then reacts with ATP in a reaction catalysed by ADP-glucose pyrophosphorylase to form ADP-glucose. This reaction is very similar to that at the start of sucrose biosynthesis, however ADP-glucose is almost exclusively used by the plant for the synthesis of starch whereas UDP-glucose, as well as being a precursor for sucrose synthesis, is also used in the biosynthesis of cell wall polymers (see later section 'Biosynthesis of cell wall polymers'). This simple differentiation has pronounced effects on how these two pathways can be regulated. The location of the ADP-pyrophosphorylase activity within the plant cell is not entirely clear. In leaf tissue this enzyme is found exclusively in the chloroplast where it uses fructose-6-phosphate directly from the Calvin cycle (Zeeman et al. 2007). The enzyme is also localised within the amyloplasts of storage tissues such as maize and potato (Beckles et al. 2001). In this instance the sucrose is broken down to glucose-6-phosphate in the cytosol and this must be transported into the amyloplast. However, it is also evident that in cereals at least, there is an isoform of the ADP glucose pyrophosphorylase located within the cytosol of the seed endosperm cells (Denyer et al. 1996). If this isoform is prevented from acting by genetic modification, then the level of starch in the seed is dramatically reduced, indicating that this is a significant source of the ADP-glucose to be incorporated into starch. Thus, in this instance it is the ADP-glucose that is imported into the amyloplast and a transporter on the plastid membrane to carry out this transportation has been identified.

The ADP-glucose is used to extend pre-existing $\alpha(1–4)$ linked glucose chains by an enzyme called starch synthase. There are several forms of this enzyme located within the amyloplast including granule bound starch synthase (GBSS) which, as its name implies, is exclusively associated with the growing starch granule. If the activity of this enzyme is prevented, either through genetic modification, or in natural mutants such as the waxy mutant of pea, then it has been found that the starch granules are composed entirely of amylopectin. This implies that the GBSS is used by the plant for the synthesis of amylose. The suggestion is that the starch granule 'grows' by having successive shells in which it is the amylopectin that is synthesised first and which then forms a 'scaffold'-like structure. The GBSS becomes incorporated into this 'scaffold' and synthesises amylose to 'fill in' the gaps in the granular structure. This however, is likely to be a very simplistic view. The other starch synthase isoforms SSI and SSII are soluble and located within the stroma of the plastid. These are responsible, along with the two remaining enzymes in the pathway, for the synthesis of the amylopectin. These other two enzymes are starch branching enzyme (SBE) and starch debranching enzyme (SDE). Both occur as isoforms within the amyloplast. The production of amylopectin thus occurs in the following manner: the starch synthase(s) produce linear $\alpha(1–4)$ linked glucose polymers which are then acted on by the SBE which introduces the $\alpha(1–6)$ branch points by catalysing a transglycosylation reaction in which an $\alpha(1–4)$ linkage is broken and the resultant residual 'chain' linked to another glucose reside at a fixed distance along the chain. This can be anything between 8 and 20 residues and it is thought that specific isoforms of the SBE may generate discrete distances between the branching points. In order for the amylopectin to be incorporated into the growing starch granule it is necessary for the polymers to be able to interact to produce a semi-crystalline state. It is thought that the amylopectin, as generated by the SBE, may be unable to do this and that in order to crystallise it may require slight modifications to its three-dimensional structure. These modifications are thought to be brought about by the action of the SDE, possibly in collaboration with other starch synthases and SBE isoforms. However, this final step in the biosynthesis of starch is not well understood and is currently quite speculative. The starch granule is laid down in a number of growth rings each representing a period of rapid photosynthetic activity. The final structure of the granule can be very variable between organs and species (Jobling 2004) and can influence the digestibility of the starch. For example, the synthesis of starch granules in many cereal seeds occurs in two phases, large granules being laid down during the early stages of development and smaller granules later on (Shewry and Morell 2001).

The other aspect of granule formation that is still under examination is the initiation of synthesis. Granule size and number are both thought to be under genetic control (Jane et al. 1994) which is thought to be regulated through control of the initiation process. Starch synthesis in plants is thought to have evolved from the ability of bacteria to synthesis glycogen (Ball and Morell 2003).

In mammals and yeast, glycogen synthesis is primed by a self-glycosylating protein called glycogenin (Alonso et al. 1995). Proteins with homology to glycogenin have been identified in plants but their role, if any, in the synthesis of starch is unclear.

The control of starch synthesis is brought about primarily at the level of ADP-glucose pyrophosphorylase. This is in contrast to the control of sucrose metabolism where the precursor UDP-glucose is required for several other biochemical pathways. ADP-glucose pyrophosphorylase is a hetero-tetramer. It has two identical small sub-units which are responsible for the catalytic activity of the enzyme. In addition, there are two identical large subunits which are thought to play a regulatory role. ADP-glucose pyrophosphory-lase is an allosteric enzyme that is strongly inhibited by phosphate and, in photosynthetic tissues at least, activated by triose phosphates (Preiss 1988). There is also evidence that the ADP-glucose pyrophospharylase may also be regulated by redox conditions within the plastid (Fu et al. 1998). Cysteine residues within the C-terminal domains of the small subunit are subject to redox reactions. In the dark these are oxidised to form disulphide bridges between the two subunits, resulting in an inactivation of the enzyme. Under light conditions the ferridoxin/thioredoxin system in the stroma of the chloroplasts is able to reduce these disulphide bridges, thus activating the enzyme. Such control basically ensures that photosynthetic precursors and starch synthesis are correctly coordinated in a diurnal fashion.

There seem to be a minimal set of 14 core genes responsible for the enzymes involved in starch synthesis across a wide range of organisms. These include two genes encoding ADP-glucose pyrophoshorylase, five for starch synthases, three for starch branching enzymes and four for starch debranching enzymes (Morell and Myers 2005). The homology between these genes across species has meant that genes involved in starch biosynthesis have been identified in a number of plants. This has enabled the manipulation of starch *in planta* to enhance its nutritional or food value (Jobling 2004). Such applications include the production of high amylose starches, which have high gelling strengths that make them useful in the confectionary industry. High amylose starches can also be processed into resistant starch that may have nutritional benefits. High amylase in cereals arises through a natural mutation in the gene encoding the SBE. However, a similar phenotype has been produced in potato tuber by the use of antisense genetic engineering (Schwall et al. 2000). At the other extreme, amylase-free or waxy starches can also have commercial benefits. These include ease of gelatinisation and resistance to freeze–thaw cycles. Again this has been achieved by the identification of mutants in the gene encoding GBSS termed waxy mutants. Waxy mutants of maize and barley have been known for many years and a similar wheat line has been bred. Again, as with the high amylase starch, this trait can also be introduced into other species, such as potato, by using antisense technology (Jobling et al. 2002).

Cell wall polymers

The plant cell wall is another major source of plant-derived dietary carbohydrates. The wall is a complex structure consisting of about 90% polysaccharides and 10% structural protein. The polysaccharides are generally grouped into cellulose, hemicelluloses and pectins. The components of the cell wall are important from a dietary point of view as they form the major source of fibre. Also the physical structure and integrity of the cell wall may impact on the digestibility of plant products and hence affect the availability of other phytonutrients.

The precise structure of the wall is beyond the scope of this review but has been described previously (Carpita and Gibeaut 1993; Carpita and McCann 2000; O'Neill and York 2003; Cosgrove 2005; Somerville et al. 2004). There are two types of cell wall found in plants. Type 1 is common in dicotolydenous plants and this includes most fruit and vegetables. Type 2 cell walls are found in monocots and these include the major cereal crops. The two types of wall both contain cellulose which can account for around 30% of the total wall mass. Cellulose is composed of β1–4 linked glucose residues which form linear polymers that can vary between 5000 and 25 000 residues long. In the plant cell wall these polymers are aggregated together to form crystalline structures called fibrils. Each fibril consists of approximately 36 cellulose polymers, laid down in parallel and held together by hydrogen bonding (Carpita and Gibeaut 1993).

These fibrils interact with a range of hemicellulosic polymers (Ebringerova et al. 2005). Xyloglucans represent the major hemicellulose found in dicotyledonous plants. This polymer consists of a backbone of β1–4 linked glucose residues with the majority of these residues associated with a xylose 'side group'. The distribution of the xylose 'sidegroups' can be variable but the most common motif can be represented by XXXG in which G represents an unsubstituted glucose in the backbone and X a glucose substituted with a xylose. Further substitution of the xylose residues, with galactose and fucose, occurs and this again can be variable. Xyloglucans represent only a minor component of type 2 walls which contain much higher levels of xylans, arabinoxylans, galactomannans and mixed linkage glucans. Arabinoxylans represent major hemicelluloses in starchy endosperm crops and can account for 0.15% of the rice grain and up to 13% of wholegrain flour from barley and 30% of wheat bran (Ebringerova and Hromadkova 1999). This polymer has a linear backbone of xylose residues part-substituted with arabinose on either the O-2 or O-3 positions (Ebringerova and Heinze 2000; Rao and Muralikrishna 2001). Some of these arabinose residues are further esterified to ferulic or coumaric acids. The structure of the polymers is again variable and this can impact on their physical properties, some arabinoxylans being water soluble and others insoluble. Galactomannans are found in the storage tissues of some seeds, in particular guar, locust bean and carob. These represent major sources of gums that are extracted and used commercially in many food products (Reid and Edwards 1995). These polymers are generally composed of an α(1–4)-linked mannan backbone substituted with galactose. Again the structure is variable with degrees of substitution ranging from 30% to 96% and this again can impact on the physical properties of the polymers, with highly substituted forms being more water soluble. The mixed linkage glycans, or β-glycans, consist of a backbone of glucose residues linked together by combinations of β (1–4) and β (1–3) bonds. These polymers are found in cereals such as oat and barley where they can account for up to 3–5% of the dry weight (Wood 2004).

Hemicelluloses, in general, are thought to be able to hydrogen bond with the surface of the cellulose fibril and in some cases may even penetrate the fibril and disrupt its microcrystalline structure (Cosgrove 2005). Hemicellulose may also span the gap between fibrils and generate a cellulose/hemicellulose framework serving to anchor the fibril into the wall (Hayashi et al. 1994). The matrix between the cellulose fibrils in type 1 cell walls is composed primarily of pectin and structural protein. The pectin consists of three major components: homogalacturonan, rhamnogalacturonan I and rhamnogalacturonan II (Thakur et al. 1997; Schols and Voragen 2002; Vincken et al. 2003; Cosgrove 2005).

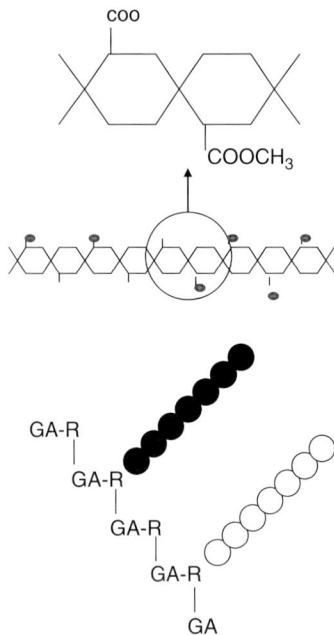

Figure 2.2   Structure of pectin.

Homogalacturonan consists of long chains of α (1–4) linked galacturonic acid residues. These can exist as either the free acid or possibly the methyl esterified at the C6 position (Figure 2.2). Additionally the residues may also be acetylated or in certain polymers may be linked to xylose to form xylogalacturonan. Rhamnogalacturonan 1 consists of an alternating rhamose/galacturonic acid backbone which may be several hundred residues long. The rhamnose residues can be further decorated by side chains of galactose and arabinose residues (Figure 2.2). The structure and distribution of these side chains can vary considerably between polymers. In contrast, the third pectin polymer – rhamnogalactronan-II – seems to be highly conserved between plants but represents only a small proportion of the total pectin in the wall. Pectin can account for up to 30% of a typical type 1 wall but whilst there is some pectin found within some monocotyledons, e.g. onions and banana fruit, they tend to form a much smaller proportion in type 2 walls. In this case the matrix consists largely of hemicellulosic polymers.

Biosynthesis of cell wall polymers

Whilst the cell wall consists of a range of complex polysaccharides, these are composed of only nine major monomeric sugars: glucose, arabinose, xylose, galactose, galacturonic acid, glucuronic acid, rhamnose, mannose and fucose. These are all ultimately derived from glucose produced in photosynthesis. Basically the sugars are all present in the cytosol as nucleotide diphosphate derivative building blocks, similar to those used for the synthesis of starch and sucrose. However, these are normally present at such low levels as to be nutritionally insignificant. The biosynthetic mechanisms for the cell wall polymers are less well characterised than those for starch. This is primarily due to the relative complexity of the polymers involved and because the enzymes involved tend to be membrane bound and as such often lose their catalytic ability upon disruption of the cell. The advent of molecular biology has, however, enhanced this area of cell wall biosynthesis and many potential genes encoding enzymes involved in the synthesis of these polymers have been described (Lerouxel et al. 2006). It is clear that a significant proportion of the genome of a plant may be devoted to the production of enzymes involved in carbohydrate metabolism in some form or other. The initial analysis of the *Arabidopsis* genome sequence resulted in a total of 730 open reading frames being annotated as involved in cell wall biochemistry (Henrissat et al. 2001). Of these, 170 genes alone seem to be related to the turnover/degradation of pectin. Biochemical evidence has confirmed that some of these genes actually encode enzymes involved in the synthesis or degradation of cell wall polymers. A useful database of the large number of enzymes involved in carbohydrate metabolism can be found on the website – carbohydrate active enzymes (http://www.cazy.org). This site categorises these enzymes into families according to their mode of action. As of January 2001these categories includes the glycosyl hydrolases (GH) group with 122 families, the glycosyl transferase (GT) group with 92 families and the polysaccharide lyase (PL) and esterase (PE) groups with 22 and 16 families respectively. The enzymes associated with the GH families are thought to be primarily involved in the degradation of polysaccharides, whilst those in the GT families are more likely to be implicated in biosynthesis.

Cellulose biosynthesis has been reviewed (Appenzeller et al. 2004; Lerouxel et al. 2006; Somerville 2006). This takes place within the plasma membrane and the cellulose polymers are thus produced directly into the wall (Doblin et al. 2003). If the cell membrane is subjected to freeze-fracture and staining then discrete hexameric rosette structures, about 20–30 nm in diameter, can be visualised (Doblin et al. 2002). These are the 'cellulose synthase complexes'. Each rosette consists of six subunits and each of these consists of six cellulose synthase enzymes. These use UDP-glucose generated in the cytoplasm, possibly directly from the breakdown of sucrose, to synthesise a cellulose polymer. Thus, the combined action of the rosette results in the simultaneous production of 36 cellulose polymers which are thought to form a fibril about 3 nm in diameter (Sommerville 2006). The cellulose synthase structure is very complex and the details are only just becoming available. The catalytic activity of the rosettes is associated with the products of the CESA family of genes. These are large (1000 amino acids) proteins that contain eight predicted trans-membrane domains and are indeed integral to the membrane. Ten CESA genes have been identified in *Arabidopsis* and 11 in rice (Keegstra and Walton 2000). It is clear that each subunit of the rosette structure contains six synthase proteins but that they are not identical, indeed in the primary wall there seem to be two of each of three different CESA products. In *Arabidopsis* these are the CESA1, 3 and 6 gene products (Robert et al. 2004). The situation is similar in the synthesis of secondary walls in *Arabidopsis,* but a different subset of the CESA genes (CESA 4, 7 and 8) are involved (Taylor et al. 2004). It is also clear that the CESA products are not the only enzymes required for the correct functioning of the cellulose synthase complex. Mutations in several other genes impact on cellulose biosynthesis. These include KORRIGAN which encodes a β-1–4-glucanase activity (Lane et al. 2001). The role of this enzyme is unclear but it may act to modify the chain lengths of the cellulose polymers. Other genes implicated in cellulose biosynthesis are CYT-1, which seems to be involved in the synthesis of GPD-mannose (Lukowitz et al. 2001), PEANUT which encodes a glycosylphosphoinositol membrane anchor (Gillmor et al. 2005), KOBITOL (Pagent et al. 2002) and COBRA, which is involved in fibril organisation (Roudier et al. 2005). The precise role of these other gene products is not clear.

The other major cell wall polymers – hemicelluloses and pectin – are both synthesised in the Golgi and secreted to the cell wall by directed trafficking. Much less is known about the genetics and biochemistry of these processes. A general pattern is emerging that cellulose synthase-like (CSL) gene products, are probably responsible for the synthesis of the backbone and that a series of glycosyl tranferases (GT) then add the various decorations to this backbone. For example, CSL genes encoding mannan synthase activity have been described (Liepman et al. 2005) and these may be implicated in hemicelluloses synthesis. The synthesis of the backbone of the major dicotyledonous hemicelluloses – xyloglucan – presumably requires a β-glucan synthase. Cocuron et al. (2007) have identified a potential candidate for this activity. Xyloglucan synthesis also requires the action of several glycosyltransferases to add the structural decorations to the β-glucan backbone. Several mutants have been identified in *Arabidopsis* that impact on the structure of xyloglucan. Two of these, *mur2* and *mur3*, have been shown to encode for fucosyl (Vanzin et al. 2002) and galactosyl (Madson et al. 2003) transferase activities, respectively. These were both identified by a reduction in fucose in the xyloglucan of the mutant plants. The *mur3* gene product is responsible for the addition of the galactosyl residue in the third position of the XXXG motif. Since this is the galactose that carries the fucose substitution, this accounts for the lack of fucose phenotype in this mutant. More recently two xylosyltransferase genes have also been implicated in xyloglucan synthesis (Cavalier et al. 2008). The pectin polymers are presumably synthesised by similar mechanisms but since these have more complex and diverse structures, this is likely to be more complex (Mohnen 2002; Bacic 2006). Several dwarfing mutants have been identified which seem to disrupt the synthesis of pectin. These have been termed QUASIMODO1 (Bouton et al. 2002), which encodes a putative membrane bound glycosyltransferase and QUASIMODO2, which seems to encode a putative methyltransferase (Mouille et al. 2007). More specifically, Sterling et al. (2006) described a homogalacturonan galactosyltransferase (GAUT1) activity that may be implicated in the synthesis of the pectin backbone.

Once these polymers have been synthesised in the Golgi, they are then secreted into the cell wall. How they are incorporated into the final three-dimensional structure of the wall or interact with the cellulose fibrils that are synthesised directly into the wall is not really understood.

Cell wall turnover

The primary cell wall is a dynamic structure and undergoes significant turnover to accommodate growth and development of the cell and tissue. This involves a large number of enzymes that are capable of modifying or degrading the various cell wall polymers. The majority, though not all, of these enzymes act as hydrolases (Brummell and Harpster 2001; Fry 2004). The cellulose fibril, being in a highly organised crystalline state, is relatively inert with respect to these degradative enzymes, thus it is the hemicellulose and pectin fractions that undergo the major modifications.

The modification of the pectin is perhaps the most extensive and well studied (Tucker and Seymour 2002). There are a wide range of enzymes that can modify pectin in the cell wall, the major ones being pectinesterase, polygalacturonase and galactanase. Pectinesterase removes the methyl group from the C6 of a galacturonic acid to generate a carboxylic acid moiety. This action can be random, as with the enzyme from many fungal sources, or in the plant itself may result in a block of de-esterified galacturonic acids. These regions of de-esterified pectin can chelate calcium ions and form what is known as an 'egg-box' structure, as first described by Grant et al. (1973). This serves to strengthen the cell wall and is used in the manufacture of jams (Thakur et al. 1997). The extent of this structure can also be important nutritionally as it may dictate to some extent the level of calcium retained within a plant tissue. Polygalacturonase cleaves the bond between two adjacent galacturonic acids thus resulting in the depolymerisation of the pectin backbone and potentially increasing its solubility. The enzyme requires that the galacturonic acids in the active site be in the form of the free acids. Thus there is some potential for synergism between polygalacturonase and pectinesterase with the latter forming sites of action for the former. Many plants contain a related enzyme activity – pectin or pectate lyase (Dominquez Puigjaner et al. 1997) – which can also act to depolymerise the pectin, but does so through a β-elimination reaction that does not always require the presence of de-esterified galacturonic acids at the site of cleavage.

Plants also contain exo-galactanase enzyme activities (Carey et al. 1995), for which one potential role is to modify the galactan side chains found within the rhamnogalacturonan 1. These are particularly prevalent in ripening fruit in which the pectin undergoes a significant loss of neutral sugars. In addition to galactanases there are also arabinosidases present in many plant tissues. These pectin modifying enzymes are often produced in high levels but their activity within the wall is tightly regulated. Thus in the tomato fruit it has been estimated that there is sufficient pectinesterase activity to completely de-esterify the pectin within a matter of minutes. This clearly does not occur in the intact fruit but upon any processing that involves disruption of the tissue, such as the production of tomato pastes, these enzymes can result in extensive modification to their target polymer. It is partly for this reason that tomatoes are heated during processing in order to degrade these enzymes.

The hemicelluloses also undergo modification, the three major enzyme activities being endo-glucanase, xyloglucan endotransglycosylase (XET) and expansin. The endo-glucanase potentially acts by breaking β1–4 linked bonds. Whilst these could reside within a cellulose polymer, the more likely substrate is the backbone of the hemicellulose xyloglucan, although precise modes of action of these enzymes are unclear. The XET can function to modify the xyloglucan by breaking a β1–4 linked bond and then reforming this by addition to either an adjacent polymer or to a short oligosaccharide (Nishitani and Tominaga 1992). This enzyme is sometimes bi-functional and can act simply as a xyloglucan hydrolase. Expansin is unique among the proteins described here as it is not a hydrolase, and does not actually catalyse a chemical reaction at all. The mode of action of expansin is that the protein can intercede between the surface of the cellulose fibril and the hemicelluloses, breaking the hydrogen bond that holds these polymers together and thus allowing slippage of the fibril in relation to the hemicelluloses (McQueen-Mason et al. 1992).

Nutritional benefits of plant carbohydrates

The diet contains a very wide range of carbohydrates, either naturally occurring or as additions made during the processing of the food. These can be loosely divided into 'available'(those that are absorbed in the small intestine) or 'resistant' (those that are poorly absorbed and/or metabolised) (Englyst et al. 2007). The available carbohydrates are thus available for metabolism whilst the 'resistant' have become associated with the term dietary fibre, although the precise definition of dietary fibre, as we shall see, is under some debate. It is not always the case that these 'resistant' carbohydrates cannot be metabolised in the gut since many can be fermented by the microflora of the colon into short-chain fatty acids, which in turn may have nutritional or health promoting benefits.

Our early, hunter-gatherer ancestors consumed relatively low amounts of plant-derived 'available' carbohydrate. Their meat-rich diet was supplemented with fructose from fruit but little plant-derived starch was consumed (Tappy and Lê 2010). This changed dramatically with the advent of agriculture and the production of starch-rich crops. It was not until the eighteenth century that international trade and the development of technologies for large-scale extraction from plant material led to sucrose becoming a significant component of our diet (Tappy and Lê 2010). While originally used as a sweetener for beverages such as tea and coffee, sucrose is now a major component of 'processed' foods and drinks and represents a major energy source. The 2008–2009 National Diet Nutrition Survey (2010) indicated that adults in the United Kingdom were obtaining approximately 26% and 20% of food energy from starch and non-milk extrinsic sugar (primarily sucrose), respectively. While dietary starch is generally considered beneficial to health, considerable concern exists concerning high intakes of fructose from sucrose (and other sources such as fructose-rich corn syrup). Epidemiological evidence suggests that high intakes, particularly in the form of sweetened drinks, may be associated with obesity, insulin resistance, diabetes, non-alcoholic fatty liver disease and increased cardiovascular risk (Tappy and Lê 2010).

By contrast the consumption of dietary fibre is thought to protect from many of these diseases. A high intake of foods rich in fibre, such as wholegrain cereals, has been associated with a reduction in the incidence of CVD (Flight and Clifton 2006; Seal 2006), although the specific contribution of the fibre to this protective effect remains to be firmly established. Similarly, high intakes of dietary fibre have also been associated with reduced risks of some cancers (Gonzalez and Riboli 2010) and diabetes (Lindstrom et al. 2006). The mode of action of the fibre in each case has not been fully elucidated, however this is likely to vary depending on the physiological response being investigated.

Major sources of dietary fibre within the diet and recommended intakes

In adult humans, the main source of dietary fibre comes from primary plant cell walls. Most of these are derived from the dicotyledonous primary cell walls of fruit and vegetables. Wholegrains are another rich source of fibre and these provide us with a range of hemicelluloses such as β1–4-glucans. However, the proportions of the various polymers vary depending on our diet. Humans tend to eat very few secondary cell walls and specifically avoid eating the most woody secondary cell walls.

In the UK there has been a recommendation for the intake of non-starch polysaccharides (NSP) as it was felt to be more definable than giving a recommendation for the intake of dietary fibre. The NSP fraction makes up about 90% of the total dietary fibre. The recommended UK dietary reference value (DRV) for NSP for an adult was set in a COMA report in 1991 at 18 g/day (DoH 1991). The minimum intake is 12 g of NSP/day with an average intake of 18 g recommended and an individual maximum of 24 g/day not to exceed 32 g/day. The reasoning is that levels below 12 g/day clearly cause problems with constipation – the only recognised problem associated with a deficiency of dietary fibre. The thinking behind the limitation on intake is the concern that high phytate in the diet may bind minerals. However, there has been no clear evidence that a diet high in plant cell wall material will cause a mineral deficiency. Pectins do bind divalent ions, such as calcium; however, they are completely fermented in the colon and the ions are absorbed there.

Definition and measurement of dietary fibre

The definition of 'dietary fibre' has been the subject of some debate. Burkitt and Trowell (1977) defined dietary fibre as 'that portion of food which is derived from the cellular wall of plants which is digested very poorly by human beings'. An alternative definition that has been suggested is 'Any dietary component that reaches the colon without being absorbed in a healthy human gut' (Ha et al. 2000). The first definition restricts 'fibre' to those polymers originally associated with the plant cell wall – primarily the pectins, hemicelluloses and cellulose fractions. Using this physiological definition, plant cell wall components which are not carbohydrates such as cutin, lignins, tannins and waxes are part of the fibre concept. This definition also includes material that may be digestible but arrives at the colon packaged within an undigested particle. Having a definitive definition is important for two main reasons. First, the need to be able to associate any physiological response to a defined chemical constituent in the diet, and secondly to be able to accurately measure the said component and thus provide useful nutritional information on any food label. In this respect the definition of 'dietary fibre' (if this term must be used) as relating to plant cell wall polymers is perhaps more applicable.

In the past in nutrition, carbohydrate was measured by difference. It was what was left after the protein, fat, ash and moisture content of the food had been determined. This was not very accurate as a number of non-carbohydrate compounds such as lignin, tannins, waxes and some Maillard products are also included in this measure.

If a chemical definition of fibre as being the non-starch polysaccharides and lignin arising from the plant cell wall is used then this can be more accurately assessed, and analytical methods to determine these dietary carbohydrates have been developed (Englyst et al. 2007). This does, however, tend to omit 'resistant' starch and those oligosaccharides that also resist digestion. The potential importance of these in the diet needs to be further assessed. Resistant starch in particular is often considered as fibre and has several functional advances as a food additive and may be nutritionally beneficial (Fuentes-Zaragoza et al. 2010).

Much of the nutrition literature differentiates dietary fibre into 'soluble' and 'insoluble' fibre. The soluble fraction tends to be enriched in pectin polymers from the cell wall. However, this pectin represents only a small proportion of the total pectin within a plant cell wall, yet all pectin became classified as soluble. Similarly a small part of the hemicellulose fraction is solubilised whilst most hemicellulose fractions are classified as insoluble. This classification has little to do with the chemistry, function or position of the polymers within the plant cell wall but it has been used extensively in the nutrition literature to describe the health effects of dietary fibre.

Physiological effects of dietary fibre

Burkitt and Trowell (1977) brought to prominence the idea that dietary fibre could be important in the diet, linking a decreased intake of fibre in the West with an increased incidence of chronic diseases such as cancer, coronary heart disease and diabetes mellitus. Dietary fibre is not a new concept though, with Hippocrates first mentioning that coarse plant foods could relieve constipation. If consumption of fibre does have positive physiological effects it is essential to determine how these are mediated and which polysaccharides may be most important. This, however, is very difficult for several reasons. The plant cell wall is an extremely complex matrix consisting of several distinct polymers. Moreover, the nature of this wall will vary between cells in a tissue, between tissues in a plant and between plant species. This makes any attempt at defining the precise chemical composition of 'dietary fibre' very difficult. Researchers have tried to overcome this particular problem by investigating the effect of individual polymers. Thus Jenkins et al. (1978) examined the potential of wheat bran and several individual polymers for their ability to modify postprandial hyperglycaemia. The physiological significance of such an approach may be questioned in terms of doses applied and whether the response to an individual polymer is the same as that to the polymer when presented as part of the cell wall matrix. The plant cell wall will have an effect on digestion and absorption as a single, complex matrix. The make-up of the plant cell wall matrix will also influence the behaviour of the polymers during digestion and absorption. This again will be unique to each plant type and will also be influenced by the stage of maturity. The fact that much of our plant food is cooked prior to consumption may also impact on the nature and function of the dietary fibre (McDougall et al 1996).

There has been a lot of emphasis on the protective effects of wholegrains. Meta-analysis has shown that a high intake of wholegrains protects against a multitude of diseases, more so than a high intake of fruit and vegetables. However when individual parts of the wholegrain are tested for the physiological response, the protection is not so great. It is postulated that other phytonutrients present in the grain, such as vitamin E, provide the protective effect (Slavin 2003).

Despite these limitations there have been several suggestion put forward as to how dietary fibre may elicit beneficial physiological responses. These mechanisms are likely to vary dependent upon the position in the gastrointestinal tract and the physiological response involved. One potential mechanism is through the increased viscosity of the digestate. This may delay glucose and lipid uptake resulting in the food exhibiting a lower glycaemic index. This may be important for the regulation of glucose responses in patients with non-insulin-dependent diabetes. Dietary fibre also serves to increase faecal mass, soften stool consistency and decreases gastrointestinal transit time. These properties may aid in the relief of constipation. The latter may also serve to chelate potential carcinogens and decrease the exposure time to potential toxins within the gut. Finally, much of the dietary fibre can be fermented by the colonic microflora and the resultant short-chain fatty acids (SCFA) can be absorbed and may have beneficial effects (Topping and Clifton 2001).

Epidemiological studies have indicated that diets high in dietary fibre, along with other nutritional and lifestyle factors, can be associated with reduced risk of developing type 2 diabetes (Lindstrom et al. 2006). This could be linked to the impact on the glycaemic index of the food (Wolever et al. 1992). If a diet high in 'insoluble' fibre was eaten, triglyceride levels increased. The glycaemic index, defined as the area under the 2-h blood glucose response curve (AUC) following the ingestion of a fixed portion of carbohydrate (usually 50 g) relative to pure glucose, was proposed as a way of determining if a food would help with the control of blood sugar levels (reference). The theory behind this is that the more slowly a food releases sugar into the bloodstream, the more likely it is that a constant blood sugar level will be maintained, eliminating swings. One theory is that the gradual breakdown of cells within the food results in the slow leeching of sugars and may restrict access of digestive enzymes such as amylase to the starch. It has been observed for instance that some starch is encapsulated in this way and reaches the large intestine intact. This would explain some of the differences in glycaemic index between foods.

Epidemiological Studies also suggest that diets rich in water-soluble fibre are associated with decreased risk of CVD (Theuwissen and Mensink 2008, Flight and Clifton 2006; Seal 2006). However, such diets are frequently rich in wholegrain foods which contain many potentially beneficial nutrients, including antioxidants (such as vitamin E) and polyphenolics, along with fibre. There is good evidence from well-controlled intervention studies suggesting that water-soluble fibre from a variety of sources will effectively lower serum LDL cholesterol concentrations. It has been calculated that for every gram of water-soluble fibre added to the diet, LDL will decrease by 0.029 mmol/L (Theuwissen and Mensink 2008).

The mechanism whereby soluble fibre reduces plasma cholesterol remains to be fully established. One suggestion is that it may interfere with the absorption of bile acids in the gut, thus increasing faecal excretion and stimulating the conversion of cholesterol to bile acids in the liver. This could be through direct binding of fibre to bile acids or formation of a thick unstirred water layer within the intestine which hinders absorption of bile acids and lipids (Theuwissen and Mensink 2008). Other alternative mechanisms suggested include the direct effects of SCFAs, produced as a result of fermentation of soluble fibre in the colon, on hepatic lipogenesis and/or improved insulin sensitivity as a result of slowed glucose absorption from the intestine (Theuwissen and Mensink 2008).

Consumption of wholegrain cereal also seems to provide protection against various cancers (Slavin 2003). Again, the mechanism is unclear and may reside in bioactive compound(s) other than fibre. More specifically it has been suggested that a high fibre diet may be protective against certain forms of cancer, in particular colon cancer (Bingham et al. 2003; Gonzalez and Riboli 2010); however, several earlier studies failed to identify such an effect.

It has been suggested that such anamolies may be the result of differences in efficacy of different sources of fibre and/or nutrient–gene interactions within specific populations.

Suggested potential mechanisms for this protection include the fact that many polysaccharides, e.g. pectin, can act as biological response modifiers and augment the immune response (Leung et al. 2006). Additionally some extracted dietary fibres, through binding and complexing, could modulate the toxicity of various carcinogens. Finally the fermentation products in the colon may serve to protect from colonic cancer.

Lipids

Lipids tend to be defined on the basis of their physical properties rather than any common chemical structure. They can be defined as compounds that are insoluble in water and are instead extractable by non-polar organic solvents. This definition encompasses a wide range of molecular structures including some very complex waxes that are, for instance, constituents of the plant cuticle. The lipid content of plant food is very variable. Vegetative tissue tends to contain between 5% and 10% lipid on a dry weight basis (Ohlrogge and Browse 1995) whilst oilseeds can contain up to 60% dry weight lipid (Wallis and Browse 2010). The four major seed oil crops are soya, oil palm, rape and sunflower which between them account for 70–75% of global trade (Murphy 1996). The types of lipid in these crops can also be very varied. However, the most abundant lipids are those that are derived from the fatty acid and glycerolipid biosynthetic pathways and it is these that are perhaps the most nutritionally significant. These include the 'complex' lipids such as phosphatidylcoline, which are normally found within the membranes of the plant cell, and the more nutritionally important triacylglycerols, which constitute the major lipids in oilseeds.

Fatty acids consist of a hydrocarbon chain with a terminal carboxylic acid group. Because of their method of synthesis, most plant and animal fatty acids consist of an even number of carbons. The carbon chain can be saturated or contain one or more double bonds. Animals and plants produce unsaturated fatty acids containing double bonds in the *cis* conformation (with hydrogen atoms on opposite sides of the double bond). However, bacterial (such as in the rumen of cattle and sheep) and chemical hydrogenation can result in the formation of *trans* double bonds. The production of partially hydrogenated vegetable oils, as replacements for animal fat, led to a considerable increase in consumption of *trans* fatty acids in the second half of the twentieth century. Growing concern about their potential health effects has led to a marked reduction, and even elimination, of such fats from foods in many countries. Fatty acid nomenclature is based on the number of carbon atoms and the number and position of double bonds within the chain. The carbon atoms are numbered from the carboxylic acid residue and the site of the double bond is identified by the number of the first carbon involved in the bond. Hence, linoleic (octadecadienoic) acid, an 18-carbon fatty acid with two *cis* double bonds, one between the 9 and 10 carbons and the other between the 12 and 13 carbons may be referred to as $C18:2^{cis, cis \Delta 9, \Delta 12}$. However, fatty acids are also frequently referred to in terms of the 'metabolic family' to which they belong. Animals are unable to insert double bonds between an existing double bond and the methyl end of the fatty acid chain. Thus, while linoleic acid may be further elongated and desaturated, the first double bond from the methyl end will always be

Table 2.2 Some common plant fatty acids

Common name	Systematic name	Stucture	Family	Common plant sources
Lauric	*n*-Dodecanoic	C12:0	–	Coconut oil
Myristic	*n*-Tetradecanoic	C14:0	–	Coconut oil
Palmitic	*n*-Hexadecanoic	C16:0	–	Palm oil
Stearic	*n*-Octadecanoic	C18:0	–	Cocoa butter
Oleic	*Cis*-9-octadecenoic	C18:1$^{cis\Delta9}$	Omega-9	Olive oil Rapeseed oil
Linoleic acid	*Cis,cis*-9,12-octadecadienoic	C18:2$^{cis,cis\Delta9,\Delta12}$	Omega-6	Sunflower oil Safflower oil Corn oil Soya oil
Alpha-linolenic	All-*cis*-9,12,15-octadecatrienoic	C18:3$^{cis,cis,cis\Delta9,\Delta12,\Delta15}$	Omega-3	Flaxseed oil
Gamma-linolenic	All-*cis*-6,9,12-octadecatrienoic	C18:3$^{cis,cis,cis\Delta6,\Delta9,\Delta12}$	Omega-6	Evening primrose oil

between the sixth and seventh carbon atoms, leading to such fatty acids being described as members of the omega-6, or n-6, family. By contrast fatty acids derived from alpha-linolenic acid represent those of the omega-3, or n-3, family. Table 2.2 lists some of the more common dietary fatty acids together with their structures and common occurrences in plant oils.

Free fatty acids are very rare in plant tissues; the majority are attached to glycerol to form glycerolipids. This review will firstly describe the common pathway for the synthesis of glycerolipids; however, the situation in plants in much more complex.

Synthesis of fatty acids in plants

All plant tissues have the capacity to synthesise fatty acids. It is beyond the scope of this chapter to cover this biosynthesis in detail but there have been several reviews published (Browse and Sommerville 1991; Ohlrogge and Browse 1995; Wallis and Browse 2010). In animals, fatty acid synthesis occurs within the cytosol, but in plants it is localised within the plastid. As in all other organisms, acetyl-CoA is the precursor for fatty acid synthesis in plants, and the first step is the conversion of this acetyl-CoA into malonyl-CoA by acetyl coenzyme A carboxylase (ACCase). Plants are complicated because they usually have at least two ACCase isoforms, one located within the plastid and the other being cytosolic. The plastid isoform is often referred to as the prokaryotic type, as it consists of separate subunits similar to the situation in bacteria. However, unlike the bacterial enzymes, the subunits in plants often assemble into 700KD complexes (Sasaki et al. 1993). The second type of ACCase is located in the cytosol and the three components of the reaction are all catalysed by a large multifunctional single peptide. This is the situation in dicots and probably also in monocots, however the Gramineae family of plants would seem to have just the multifunctional forms but still with plastid and cytosolic localisations (Konishi and Sasaki 1994). In either case it seems that malonyl-CoA, as synthesised by the isoform in the plastid, is used exclusively for the synthesis of fatty acids. The cytosolic activity is presumably required to provide malonyl-CoA for the biosynthesis of other compounds such as the flavonoids.

The malonyl CoA formed is then fed into the chain elongation activity of the fatty acid synthase complex (FAS). FAS found in the plastids of plants seems to be structurally similar to that found in *Escherichia coli,* as it is composed of easily dissociable multi-subunits rather than the multifunctional protein found in animal species. The FAS carries out repeated cycles of four reactions catalysed by 3-ketoacetyl-ACP synthase, 3-keto-ACP reductase, 3-hydroxacyl-ACP dehydratase and enoyl-ACP reductase that, by sequentially adding two carbon units to the growing acyl chain, can produce a range of fatty acids normally containing an even number of carbon atoms. These are attached to an acyl carrier protein (ACP). The first enzyme in this cycle – 3-keto-ACP synthase (KAS) – is known to exist in plants in at least three isoforms. KASIII is thought to be involved in the initial condensation of the first malonyl-CoA and acetyl-CoA to produce the four carbon unit. KASI is the major isoform involved in the extension of the acyl chain up to 16 units, at which point it can either be released from the FAS complex as a free fatty acid, by the action of oleoyl-ACP thioesterase, or used directly for the synthesis of glycerolipids in the plastid by the action of acyl transferase (see the next section 'Synthesis of glycerolipids in plants'). However, many of the acyl chains are further extended to form stearic acid and then desaturated to oleic acid. The addition of the two extra carbon atoms is thought to be mediated by KASII and this again can be released from the FAS. However, plants also contain a soluble stearoyl, ACP desaturase, within the stromal compartment of the plastid. This enzyme is unusual because the majority of desaturases are membrane bound. The stearoyl-ACP desaturase is capable of inserting a *cis* double bond at the 9-position of the C18:0, whilst still attached to the ACP, to produce oleic acid (C18:1). This fatty acid can then be released from the ACP, again through the action of either oleoyl-ACP thioesterase or acyl transferase. The stearoyl-ACP desaturase is normally very effective, so in most plant cells the predominant fatty acids produced within the plastid are C16:0 and C18:1. Sometimes, however, especially in oil producing seeds (one of the most extreme examples being cocoa beans), a significant amount of C18:0 is also released from the plastid. Also a few plants are able to desaturate C16:0-ACP and generate C16:1. In some plant tissues (e.g. coconut) shorter chain saturated fatty acids may be released.

Synthesis of glycerolipids in plants

In plants, as in all other organisms, there is very limited accumulation of free fatty acids. Once formed, the fatty acids are predominantly incorporated into glycerolipids for inclusion into membranes, or more significantly from a nutritional point of view, into triacylglycerols (TAG) within storage organs such as seeds and fruit. While a proportion of newly synthesised fatty acids may be used for glycerolipid synthesis within the plastid itself, the majority are exported into the cytosol, complexed with CoA and then used for glycerolipid assembly at the endoplasmic reticulum (ER). These two glycerolipid pathways (plastid and ER) are very similar but give quite different end products.

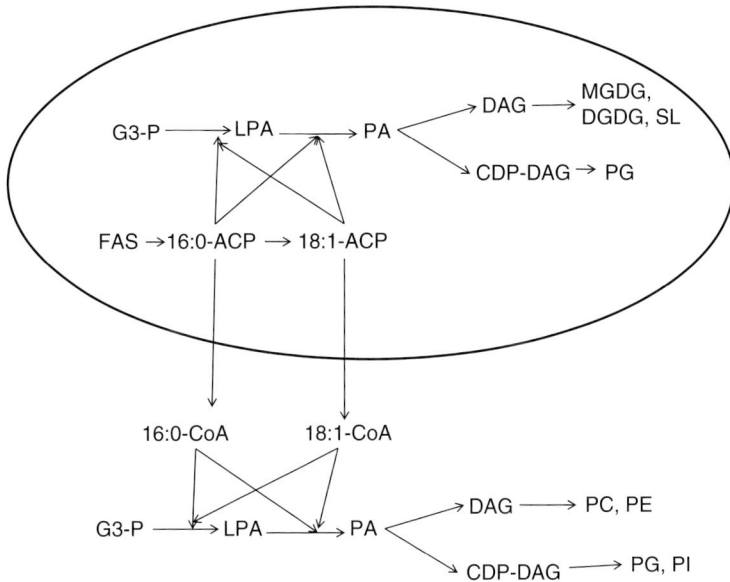

Figure 2.3   Outline of biosynthesis of glycerolipids.

The general pathway is illustrated in Figure 2.3. The glycerol 3-phosphate backbone is formed by the reduction of dihydroxyacetone phosphate. Fatty acids are then added sequentially to positions 1 and 2 of the glycerol by the transfer of the acyl group from either an acyl-ACP (plastid) or acyl-CoA (cytosol), to produce lysophosphatidic acid (LPA) and phosphatidic acid (PA), respectively. The major difference between the two pathways (plastid and cytosolic) is in the nature of the fatty acids that are placed in the 1 and 2 positions of the glycerol backbone, and this in turn is dictated by the relative isoforms of glycerol-3-phosphate acyl transferase enzymes involved. In the plastid position 2 of the glycerol is predominantly occupied by 16:0, whilst both 16C and 18C fatty acids occur at position 1. This is a form of glycerolipid found in cyanobacteria and as such this pathway is referred to as the prokaryotic pathway. In contrast, the cytosolic pathway is referred to as the eukaryotic pathway since the products have 18C predominantly at position 2, again with a mixture of 16C and 18C at position 1, a eukaryotic form of glycerolipid.

The phosphatidic acid (PA) is further converted to diacylglycerol (DAG) or CDP-DAG prior to forming a range of complex glycolipids such a phosphatidylcholine (PC), phosphatidylinositol (PI) and phosphatidyl ethanolamine (PE). These are used primarily to form the membranes within the plant cell and are quite conservative in the nature of the fatty acids that are incorporated, these being primarily either 16C or 18C.

The products of the prokaryotic pathway serve as precursors for a wide range of relatively specialised lipids for inclusion in the plastid membranes. These are listed on Figure 2.3 but are of little nutritional significance. The products of the eukaryotic pathway, which as discussed resides primarily in the ER, are precursors for the membranes in

```
                        DAG
                      ↗     ↖
        PA ⟶ PC-18:1 ⟶ PC-18:2 ⟶ PC-18:3
        ↑                  ↓         ↓              ⟶ TAG
        LPA              18:2      18:3
        ↑↖
        G3-P          ┌──────────┐
                      │ Acyl-Pool │ ←
                      └──────────┘    20:1, 22:1
                         ↑          ⟶
                      ╱  │  ╲       18:1
                     ╱   │   ╲  ↗
        ═══════════════════════════════════════════
                   ╱     │     ╲
                16:0   18:0   18:1         Plastid
                         FAS
```

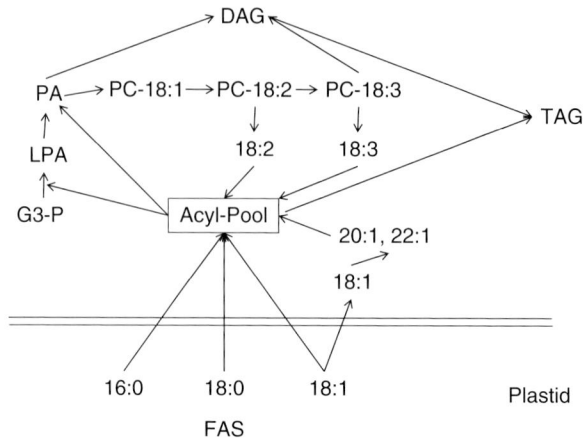

Figure 2.4 Outline biosynthesis of triacylglycerols.

the rest of the cell organelles and plasma membrane. In addition these are also the precursors for the synthesis of the TAGs which are the major form of lipid store.

The TAG synthesis pathway is outlined in Figure 2.4 and has been the subject of several reviews (Browse and Sommerville 1991; Voelker and Kinney 2001). This is a complex pathway with essentially two major routes. This occurs primarily in the ER of oil produc- ing tissues. The cytoplasmic acyl-CoA pool is populated by 16:0, 18:0 and 18:1 exported from the plastid. This is complimented in some tissues by the products of the elongation of 18:1 into 20:1 and possibly 22:1. In addition 18:2 and 18:3 are provided by release from PC. The immediate precursor for TAG synthesis is DAG. This can be generated either through PA via the Kennedy pathway or by a direct reversal of the formation of PC. In either case the DAG is acetylated in the third position by the enzyme diacylglycerol acyl- transferase (DAGAT).

The lipids in most plant tissues are stored as oil bodies (Huang 1996) formed by a bud- ding process from the ER. They are spherical bodies of approximately 1 μm in diameter and consist of a matrix of TAG surrounded by phospholipids. The oil bodies in storage organs such as seeds are extremely stable and do not aggregate. This stability is due to the presence of coating proteins called oleosins. These are small, 15–26KD amphiphilic pro- teins which serve to coat, and stabilise, the surface of the oil bodies. These oleosins can represent a considerable proportion of the protein content (up to 8%) and as such can be nutritionally significant (Tzen et al. 1993).

The major fatty acids found in seed oils are 16:0, 18.0, 18:1, 18:2 and 18:3. These are also the major fatty acids found in membranes. However, it has been estimated that in excess of 300 different fatty acids can be produced by plants. These other fatty acids are rarely associated with membrane lipids but rather accumulate (often to high levels) in the TAG fractions. Some plants have the capacity to produce lipids with chains longer than 18C. The brassica family, which includes oilseed rape, along with several other species is capable of elongating 18:1-CoA to 20:1 or 22:1 which can then enter the cyto- solic fatty acid pool for inclusion into PA or DAG. On the other hand, palm or coconut oil is very high in the short-chain saturated fatty acids 10:0, 12:0 and 14:0 (Browse and Somerville 1991).

In all plant tissues the major glycolipids are synthesised using 16:0 and 18:1. In the eukaryotic pathway, the PC thus formed serves as the substrate for further rounds of desaturation. First by the action of a $\Delta12$ desaturase to form linoleic acid (LA, C18:$2^{\Delta9,\Delta12}$), then secondly by a $\Delta15$ desaturase to form α-linolenic acid (ALA, C18:$3^{\Delta9,\Delta12,\Delta15}$). These can then be released from the PC to join the cytosolic fatty acid pool for the *de novo* synthesis of PA and DAG prior to being incorporated into TAG, or the PC itself can be converted directly to DAG.

Some plants, such as borage, also contain a $\Delta6$ desaturase which can convert linoleic acid (LA, C18:2$\Delta9$,12) into γ-linolenic acid (γ-LnA, C18:3$\Delta6$,9,12) or α-linolenic acid (α-LnA, C18:3$\Delta9$,12,15) into octadecatetraenoic acid (C18:4 $\Delta6$,9,12,15).

Quantitatively and nutritionally the most important plant polyunsaturated fatty acids are LA and ALA. The enzymes responsible for these further desaturations can be found either within the plastid or on the ER. In general, they are located in the chloroplast of photosynthetically active cells whereas the microsomal pathway predominates in non-green tissues and developing seeds. Selective breeding, and more recently genetic manipulation, have been highly successful in altering the relative activity of these desaturases to alter the fatty acid composition of the lipids produced. This is particularly evident in the development of seed oil crops (see next section).

Modification of plant lipids

Naturally occurring oilseed oil is not always optimal in terms of nutritional value. A good example of this is the composition of traditional oilseed rape cultivars which contain around 45% of the nutritionally undesirable erucic acid (C22:1) in addition to palmitic acid (5%), stearic acid (1%), oleic acid (15%), linoleic acid (14%) and α-linolenic acid (9%) (Ackman, 1990). In the 1950s attempts to produce low erucic acid varieties were initiated. The approach taken was to exploit mutations resulting in cultivars with naturally low levels of erucic acid. These were first identified in the German *B. napus* forage cultivar, Liho, in 1959. These low erucic acid plants were used in breeding programmes and by 1974, 95% of the rapeseed grown in Canada contained low erucic acid (Eskin et al. 1996).The use of natural, or induced, mutants to modify rapeseed oil has been applied in many other cases to generate high erucic acid, low linolenic acid, high oleic acid and low saturated fatty acid varieties, often primarily for industrial purposes (see Scarth and Tang 2006 for a review).

The use of natural variation and mutants is very effective but does have limitations in the nature and extent of the seed oil modifications that can be achieved. Thus, when the ability to genetically modify plants became available it was perhaps not surprising, given their commercial value and relative ease of transformation, that oilseed crops, in particular soya and oilseed rape, became major targets for this new technology (Murphy 1996; Scarth and Tang 2006). Commercial exploitation of the modification of these crops, as with several others, was targeted primarily at herbicide or pest resistance. However, in the case of oilseeds the quality of the oil was also a target for manipulation. One of the first commercial applications was in the generation of rape seed with high lauric acid (C12:0) content. This was achieved by the expression of a lauroyl-ACP thioesterase from the California Bay plant, in oilseed rape (Voelker et al. 1992). This resulted in the premature termination of the FAS reaction at C12. Normal oilseed rape oil contains less than 0.1% of lauric acid whilst oil from the transgenic plants accumulated up to 40% of this fatty acid. The oil was targeted at the soap and detergent industries and obviously had no nutritional significance. A second major application was in the generation of high stearic acid cultivars (Knutzon et al. 1992) by the expression of an antisense construct against stearate desaturase. This resulted in the accumulation of stearic acid to around 40% of the total fatty acids. Again this was not nutritionally motivated but was useful for the generation of oils able to produce solid fats and also to reduce the rancidity of the oil.

The most nutritionally significant fatty acids are the linoleic and α-linolenic acids, since humans are unable to synthesis these two essential fatty acids. All plants can synthesis these two fatty acids. In contrast the ability to synthesis γ-linolenic acid (GLA) and octadecatetraenoic acid (ODA, commonly called stearidonic acid) is restricted to a limited number of higher plants. Whilst these are not essential fatty acids, it has been suggested that increased consumption is beneficial. Thus the accumulation of these fatty acids in food crops has become a major target for the genetic modification of oilseeds. The capacity to synthesis GLA and ODA, in plants such as borage, resides in their unique expression of a Δ6 desaturase enzyme. The transfer of a gene encoding this enzyme to commercial oilseed crops was thus an obvious target for early genetic modification. The first demonstration of this was reported by Reddy and Thomas in 1996. Since then this technology has been used to generate soya oil (Sato et al. 2004) and oilseed rape (Huang et al. 2004) with up to 50% or 40% GLA, respectively. More recently there has been considerable interest in producing crops enriched in ODA. This is because it has been suggested that it may be more readily converted in to longer chain omga-3 PUFA, than its precursor ALA, in humans (Whelan 2009). Through conventional breeding of crops naturally rich in ODA, such as *Echium*, and genetic manipulation of more conventional crops, such as oilseed rape, oils specifically enriched in ODA have been produced. The latter has been achieved through introduction of Δ6 and Δ12 desaturases from the fungus *Mortierella alpine* (Ursin 2003).

Other fatty acids that are not essential but are nonetheless thought to be beneficial if enhanced in the diet include the long-chain polyunsaturated fatty acids (LC-PUFA), arachidonic acid (AA, 20:4 Δ5,8,11,14), eicosapentoenoic acid (EPA, 20:5 Δ5,8,11,14,17) and docosahexaenoic acid (DHA, 22:6 Δ4,7,10,13,16,19). Higher plants do not have the capacity to synthesise these LC-PUFAs. However, this ability is found in various organisms such as mosses, algae and bacteria. Major dietary sources of these fatty acids are in meat (AA) or in fish oil (EPA/DHA) where it has accumulated because of the consumption of marine algae by the fish. Mosses, algae and bacteria have a range of pathways available for the synthesis of the LC-PUFAs. There is an anaerobic pathway but this is unlikely to lend itself to transfer to higher plants. In contrast the more heavily studied aerobic pathway has been used successfully to transfer the ability to synthesise LC-PUFAs in higher plants. There have been several reviews of this complex technology over the past few years (Singh et al. 2005; Graham et al. 2007; Truksa et al. 2009; Venegas-Caleron et al. 2010). The aerobic route for biosynthesis can follow either of two pathways and

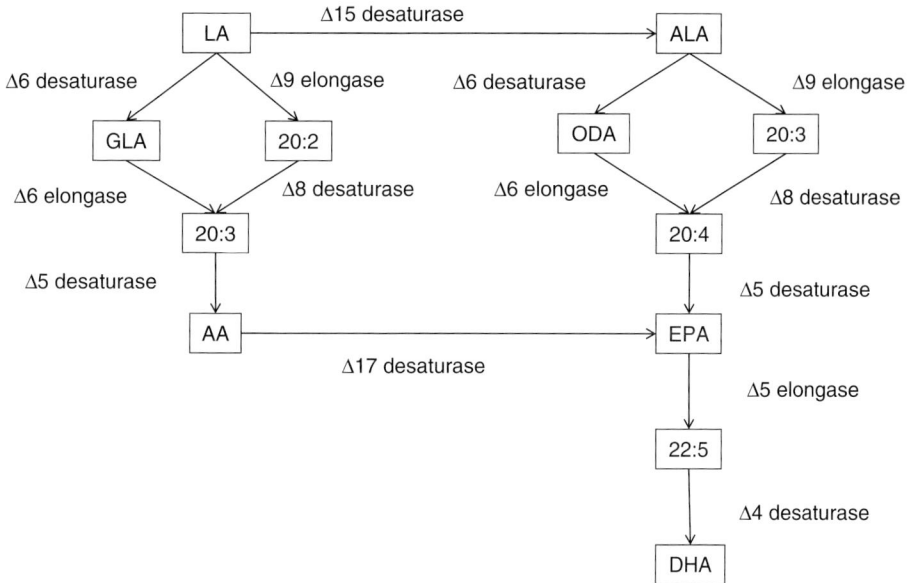

Figure 2.5   Aerobic pathways for the production of LC-PUFAs.

these are outlined in Figure 2.5. The precursors in either pathway are LA and ALA. In general, LA is the precursor of AA, and ALA the precursor of EPA and DHA. The first step of the 'classical' or Δ6 pathway involves the conversion of LA to GLA or ALA to ODA by the action of a Δ6 desaturase (as described earlier). These are then recognised by a specific Δ6 elongase enzyme and converted to 20:3 and 20:4, respectively. Subsequent action of a Δ5 desaturase generates AA and EPA and elongation of the latter by a specific Δ5 elongase followed by a further Δ4 desaturase results in the production of DHA. Some organisms also exhibit an alternate 'Δ8' pathway in which LA and ALA are firstly elongated by a specific Δ9 elongase enzyme followed by a Δ8 desaturase reaction to generate the 20:3 and 20:4 intermediates as before. These then follow the classical pathway for the generation of AA, EPA and DHA. Some species possess a Δ17 desaturase activity which can convert AA to EPA.

Since all plants can synthesis LA and ALA, the ability to produce LC-PUFAs can be achieved in several different ways by the introduction of a series of suitable genes to catalyse the appropriate steps shown in Figure 2.5. This was first demonstrated in *Arabidopsis* leaves (Qi et al. 2004) by the use of the Δ8 pathway. This was achieved by the expression of Δ9 elongase, Δ8 desaturase and Δ5 desaturase enzymes and resulted in the accumulation of around 7% AA and 3% EPA in the total lipid. Interestingly, they found that LC-PUFAs accounted for about 40% of the acyl-CoA pool in these transgenic plants. An alternative approach using the Δ6 pathway was first described by Abbadi et al. (2004) in tobacco and linseed oil. This group introduced genes encoding for Δ6 desaturase, Δ6 elongase and Δ5 desaturase enzymes and found high levels of

GLA and ODA in the seed oils but less than 1% of AA, EPA or DHA. These results served to illustrate the complexity of using genetic modification to manipulate lipid synthesis and highlighted some potential bottlenecks involved in the adoption of this technology. Thus, for the $\Delta 8$ pathway the accumulation of non-native fatty acids in the acyl-CoA pool of the transgenic plants could be interpreted as an inability of the native enzymes to incorporate these fatty acids into glycerolipids. Similarly, the accumulation of GLA and ODA using the $\Delta 6$ approach could be interpreted as an inability to transfer non-native fatty acids from their site of synthesis on PC into the acyl-CoA pool for further modification and synthesis of TAG. These bottlenecks are being overcome by the heterologous expression of elongases and desaturases (Venegan-Caleron et al. 2010) and more recent transgenic plants have the capacity to produce up to 25% AA and 15% EPA. DHA expression to date has not been so successful with only around 1.5% in transgenics.

Given the very wide range of fatty acids that can be produced in higher plants, the potential for the production of 'designer oils' is immense. Many of these will be targeted at commercial uses rather than for nutritional improvement. One potential advance that may be made in the future, however, is the production of conjugated fatty acids. The nutritional target here would probably be conjugated linolenic acid (CLA), which has been suggested to have a range of potential health benefits (Bhattacharya et al. 2006). Although this fatty acid has yet to be produced in transgenic oilseeds, another conjugated fatty acid – calendic acid – has been synthesised at high levels (20–25%) in soy oil by the introduction of a gene from marigold (Cahoon et al. 2001).

Fatty acid composition of plant foods

All plant tissue will contain some lipid, but the specific amounts and the fatty acid composition will depend on the species of plant, the environmental conditions in which it was grown and, even more importantly, the part of the plant being consumed. In general photosynthetic tissues contain relatively small amounts of lipid. The lipid content of cereals and grains varies from about 3–4% in wheat, rice and barley to in excess of 6% in oats and corn. The latter represents a major source of refined oil in many parts of the world. In general, the mesocarp or pulp of fruits also contains low amounts of lipid, although there are notable exceptions including avocado, palm and olive. Fruit seeds and nuts tend to be high in lipid, and oil extracted from these sources represents an important commercial source of plant lipid. Oilseeds are defined as crops or seeds grown specifically for their oil content and it is their development that has dramatically altered the fatty acid composition of the human diet in many parts of the world. A more detailed discussion of the fatty acid composition of some of these plant foods follows.

Vegetables

A vegetable can be described as an edible plant or part of a plant other than a sweet fruit or seed. In general they may contain 0.1–1% of lipid on a fresh weight basis. As can be

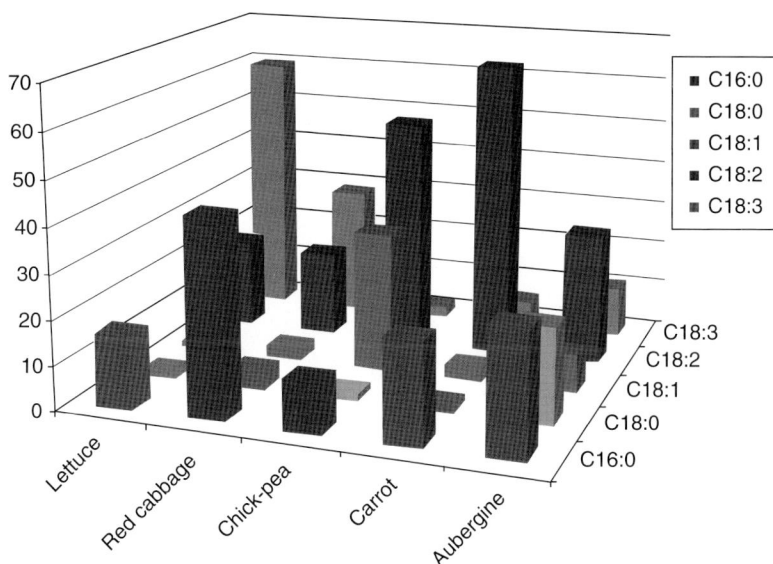

Figure 2.6 Fatty acid composition of some common vegetables (data from Vidrih et al. 2009).

seen from Figure 2.6 their fatty acid composition can vary dramatically depending on the specific tissue being consumed.

Cereals

Cereals, grains or cereal grains, are grasses cultivated for the edible components of their fruit seeds. As with most plants the fatty acids that predominate are palmitic, stearic, oleic, linoleic and linolenic acids. Of the cereal oils, corn oil is commercially the most important and tends to be rich in oleic (19–50) and linoleic (34–62%) acids.

Fruit

As noted above, most fruits have relatively low lipid contents. Of the exceptions, saturated fatty acid-rich palm fruits and oleic acid-rich olive constitute major oil crops (see following). Figure 2.7 gives examples of the widely differing fatty acid compositions of other some fruits.

Oil seeds

For the purpose of this discussion, oilseeds can be described as varieties of oil-rich seeds, nuts, fruits and cereals that are used in vegetable oils and fats for cooking, food manufacture, soap making, specialised lubricating oils and cosmetics. The primary sources of vegetable oils are: coconut, corn, cotton seed, oil palm, olive, peanut (groundnut or arachis oil), safflower, soybean, sunflower seed, and rape seed. As discussed earlier, these crops have been subject to considerable genetic alternation to produce high yields

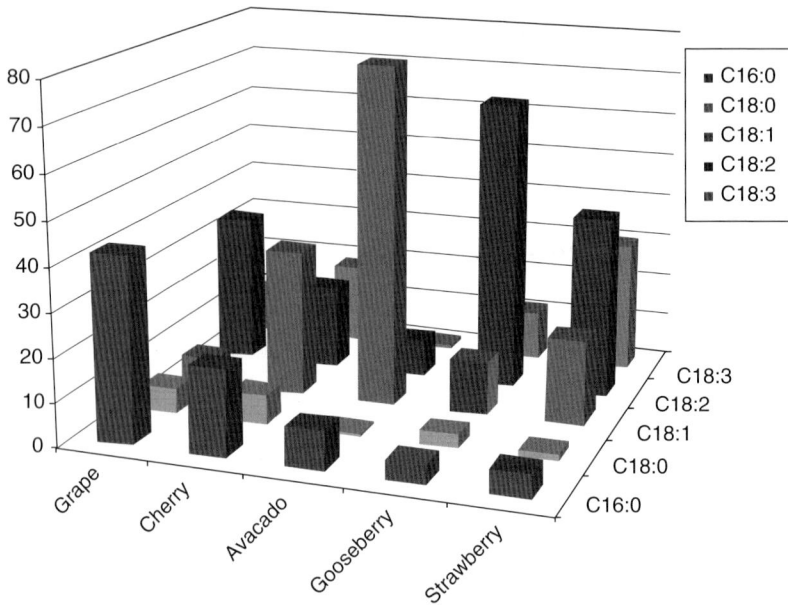

Figure 2.7   Fatty acid composition of some common fruits (data from Kamel and Kakuda 1992).

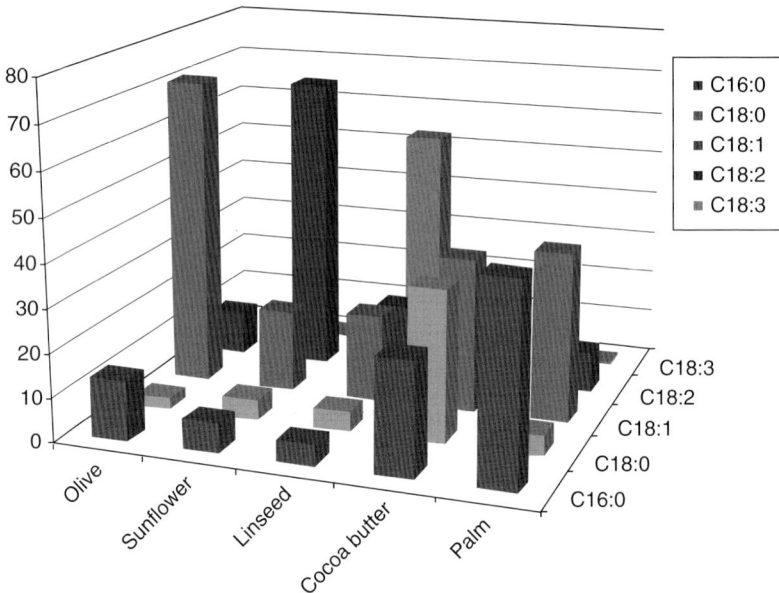

Figure 2.8   Fatty acid composition of some common plant oils (data taken from White 1992).

of oil of specific fatty acid composition. Figure 2.8 shows some of the most diverse examples from highly saturated palm oil and cocoa butter to oleic acid-rich olive oil and polyunsaturated fatty acid-rich sunflower oil (predominantly linoleic acid) and linseed oil (predominantly α-linolenic acid).

Dietary lipids and human health

Our hunter-gatherer ancestors probably derived a significant proportion of their food energy from lipids of animal origin. With a move toward the cultivation of crops this probably declined substantially, but then rose again with the domestication of farm animals. One of the biggest changes will have been in the large-scale production of ruminant milk and its introduction as a major component of the human diet. By the middle of the twentieth century, a growing recognition of the potential link between saturated fatty acid (SFA) intake, plasma cholesterol and CVD led to world-wide public health campaigns which frequently advocated replacing animal fats with plant oils. Data from the 2008–2009 National Diet Nutrition Survey (2010) suggest that total fat now contributes approximately 36% of food energy, of which about 40% is directly derived from meat and milk. The average intake of SFAs has declined from a peak of about 20% in the 1970s to 13.6 in the most recent survey.

The shift from diets rich in SFAs to those containing increased amounts of MUFA and/or PUFA has generally been viewed as beneficial, particularly with respect to plasma cholesterol and the associated risk of CVD. A recent meta-analysis has confirmed the benefits of replacing SFAs with omega-6 PUFA in terms of cardiovascular events (Mozaffarian et al. 2010). However, some concern has been expressed over the proportions on omega-6 and omega-3 PUFA currently consumed. As discussed, many plant oils are relatively rich in omega-6 PUFA (primarily linoleic) and relatively poor in omega-3 PUFA (primarily ALA). Considerable evidence exists to suggest that longer chain omega-3 fatty acids such as EPA (C20:5) and DHA (C22:6) can be protective against a variety of diseases, including CVD, because of their conversion to less inflammatory eicosanoids than those derived from omega-6 PUFA (Simopoulos 2008). These can be consumed directly within the diet through consumption of marine fish and mammals and, to a lesser extent, terrestrial mammals. Alternatively, they can be synthesised from shorter precursors, primarily as ALA. However, fatty acids of both the omega-3 and omega-6 pathways compete for enzymes involved in elongation and desaturation to produce the long-chain PUFA. It has been suggested that the high ratio of omega-6 to omega -3 fatty acids associated with many 'modern' diets may predispose individuals to a more pro-inflammatory state and increase the risk of a range of chronic diseases including CVD, cancer, and inflammatory and autoimmune diseases. This has led to calls to try and redress the ratio of these two fatty acid classes in our diet (Simopoulos 2008) and hence an interest in manipulating plant species to produce more omega-3 fatty acids (see earlier). However, the limited ability of humans to convert ALA to EPA and/or DHA, suggests that dietary intakes of the longer chain PUFA may be more crucial (Harris 2006) and hence the interest in genetically manipulating plants to produce these fatty acids. This has also led to an interest in producing crops enriched in omega-3 C18:4 (ODA; see earlier section 'Modification of plant lipids') as this could bypass the first Δ6-desaturation which may be rate limiting in the production of EPA in mammals (Whelan 2009).

The mechanisms by which dietary fatty acids influence CVD risk remain to be fully elucidated. However, as indicated above PUFA act as precursors of eicosanoids which exert effects on a whole range of physiological functions, with those derived from omega-3 PUFA specifically being anti-inflammatory and anti-thrombotic (Adkins &

Kelley 2010). Fatty acids may also act by modulating the activity of the transcription factors and the nuclear hormone receptors involved in regulating the expression of genes for the various proteins involved in lipid and lipoprotein metabolism (Salter and Tarling 2007). For example, fatty acid derivatives (particularly those from omega-3 PUFA) may act as ligands for the peroxisome proliferator activated receptor-alpha (PPAR-alpha). PPAR-alpha plays a major role in regulating genes for enzymes involved in fatty acid oxidation. Increased fatty acid oxidation may, at least in part, be responsible for the TAG-lowering effects of omega-3 PUFA. PUFA are also known to inhibit the activity of sterol regulatory binding protein 1c (SREBP1c). This transcription factor plays a major role in regulating the expression of lipogenic enzymes. It has been suggested that this is the result of inhibiting the association of another nuclear hormone receptor, the liver X receptor (LXR), with its oxysterol ligands. LXR directly activates the expression of SREBP1c (Salter and Tarling 2007). Dietary saturated fatty acids seems to reduce the expression of LDL receptors in the liver, thereby slowing the removal of these particles from the circulation. By contrast, omega-6 PUFA may increase LDL turnover, though the mechanisms underlying these effects remain to be fully elucidated (Vallim & Salter 2010).

Dietary lipids may also play an important role in the pathogenesis of other diseases including cancer and diabetes. A recent critical review indicated that high total fat intakes may be associated with a range of different cancers, though this may be partly the result of the association of such diets with obesity (Gerber 2009). Relationships between specific cancers and individual fatty acid classes were much harder to confirm, though evidence of protective effects of long-chain omega-3 PUFA were suggested. Diets rich in SFAs have been suggested to induce insulin resistance, metabolic syndrome and ultimately type 2 diabetes, although this may again be related to the obesogenic nature of such diets. By contrast, growing evidence suggests that long-chain omega-3 PUFA may alleviate insulin resistance (Melanson 2009).

Phytosterols

Sterols are isoprenoid-derived molecules that occur in all eukaryotic species. In mammals the major sterol is cholesterol (Figure 2.9). Due to its hydrophobicity and solubility in organic solvents, and its close association with other lipids within lipoproteins, cell membranes and other cellular compartments, cholesterol is often referred to as a lipid. In contrast to mammals, higher plants are unable to synthesise cholesterol but do produce a wide range other sterols, usually predominately sitosterol (Benveniste 2004), which differs only in the nature of the side chain (Figure 2.9). Until recently, it was generally accepted that the differences between plants and animals begins at the cyclisation step at the level of 2,3-oxidosqualene (Figure 2.10). In mammals, through the action of lanosterol synthase (LAS), lanosterol is produced and then converted to cholesterol. In higher plants it was believed that 2,3-oxidosqualene was converted to cycloartenol, by the action of cycloartenol synthase (CAS), prior to the production of phytosterols (such as sitosterol and camposterol). However, more recent evidence suggests that plants do possess LAS and a small proportion of phytosterols may be synthesised via lanosterol (Ohyama et al.

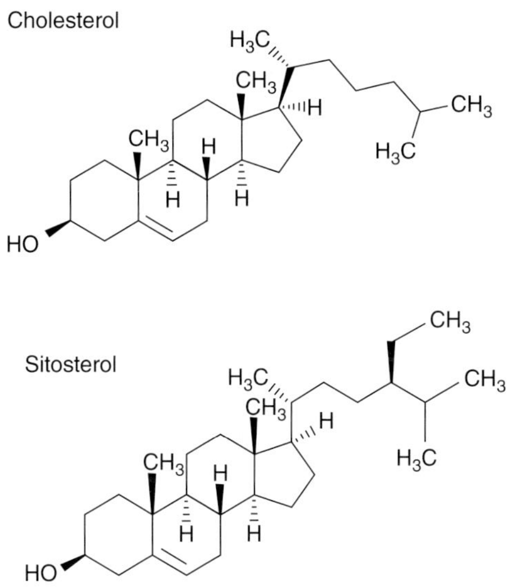

Cholesterol

Sitosterol

Figure 2.9   Structures of cholesterol and sitosterol.

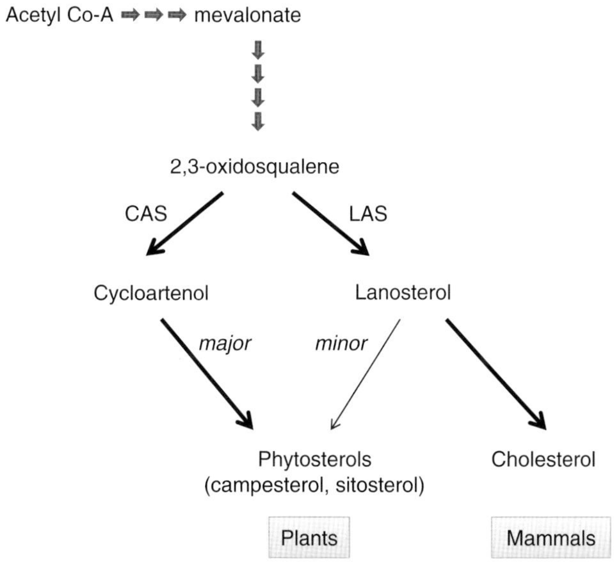

Acetyl Co-A ⇒ ⇒ ⇒ mevalonate

2,3-oxidosqualene

CAS   LAS

Cycloartenol   Lanosterol

major   *minor*

Phytosterols   Cholesterol
(campesterol, sitosterol)

Plants   Mammals

Figure 2.10   Synthesis of sterols in higher plants and mammals.

2009). Saturated forms of phytosterols – phytostanols – are also produced. These compounds, which are not abundant in nature, are saturated at the carbon-5.

It has been estimated that human intake of phytosterols from natural sources is within the range of 250–300 mg/day, an intake which is a similar order of magnitude to that of cholesterol itself (Gibney et al. 2008). In general, phytosterols (0.4–3.5%) and phytostanols (0.02–0.3%) are poorly absorbed by humans. However, in the rare autosomal disorder sitosterolaemia, plasma levels have been seen to rise by as much as 100-fold (Salen et al. 1999). This is associated with the accumulation of phytosterols in the tissues and severe atherosclerosis. Sitosterolaemia has been shown to be a result of mutations in the ABCG5 and ABCG8 transporters, which are believed to be involved in transporting phytosterol out of the intestinal epithelial cells back into the intestinal lumen (Calpe-Berdiel et al. 2009).

Interest in phytosterols and phytostanols has increased dramatically with the finding that supplementation of the diet with these compounds can significantly reduce plasma cholesterol. It has been estimated that intakes of 2 g/day can reduce plasma levels of the atherogenic low density lipoprotein cholesterol by 6–10% (Devaraj and Jialal, 2006). The primary mode of action seems to be through blocking cholesterol absorption (Calpe-Berdiel et al. 2009). There is now a range of 'functional' foods (primarily spreads and dairy-based drinks) that are supplemented with either phytosterols or phytostanols, which are marketed on the basis of their cholesterol-lowering properties.

References

Abbadi, A., Domergue, F., Bauer, J., Napier, J.A., Welti, R., Zahringer, U., Cirpus, P. and Heinz, E. (2004) Biosynthesis of very-long-chain polyunsaturated fatty acids in transgenic oilseeds:constraints on their accumulation. *Plant Cell* **16**, 2734–48.

Ackman, R.G. (1990) Canola fatty acids – an ideal mixture for health, nutrition, and food use. In: *Canola and Rapeseed: Production, Chemistry, Nutrition and Processing Technology* (ed. Shahidi, F.), pp. 81–98. New York: Van Nostrand Reinhold.

Adkins, Y. and Kelley, D.S. (2010) Mechanisms underlying the cardioprotective effects of omega-3 polyunsaturated fatty acids. *Journal of Nutritional Biochemistry* **21**, 781–92.

Alonso, M.D., Lomako, J., Lomako, W.M. and Whelan, W.J. (1995) A new look at the biogenesis of glycogen *FASEB Journal* **9**, 1126–37.

Appenzeller, L., Doblin, M., Barreiro, R., Wang, H., Niu, X., Kollipara, K., Carrigan, L., Tomes, D., Chapman, M. and Dhugga, K.S. (2004) Cellulose synthesis in maize: isolation and expression analysis of the cellulose synthase (CesA) gene family. *Cellulose* **11**, 287–99.

Bacic, A. (2006) Breaking an impass in pectin biosynthesis. *Proceedings of the National Academy of Sciences USA* **103**, 5639–40.

Ball, S. and Morell, M.K. (2003) From bacterial glycogen to starch: understanding the biogenesis of the starch granule. *Annual Review of Plant Biology* **54**, 207–33.

Beckles, D.M., Smith, A.M. and Après, T. (2001) A cytosolic ADP-glucose pyrophosphorylase is located in a feature of graminaceous endosperms but not of other starch storing organs. *Plant Physiology* **125**, 818–27.

Benveniste, P. (2004) Biosynthesis and accumulation of sterols. *Annual Review of Plant Biology* **55**, 429–57.

Bhattacharya, A., Banu, J., Rahman, M., Causey, J. and Fernandes, G. (2006) Biological effects of conjugated linoleic acids in health and disease. *Journal of Nutritional Biochemistry* **17**, 789–810.

Bingham, S.A., Day, N.E., Luben, R., Ferrari, P., Slimani, N., Norat, T., Clavel-Chapelon, F., Kesse, E., Nieters, A., Boeing, H., Tjonneland, A., Overvad, K., Martinez, K., Dorronsora, M., Gobzalez,

C.A., Key, TJ., Trichopoulou, A., Naska, A., Vineis, P., Tumino, R., Krogh, V., Bueno-de-Mesquita, H.B., Peeters, P.H.M., Berglund, G., Hallmans, G., Lund, E., Skele, G., Kaaks R. and Riboli, E. (2003) Dietary fibre in food and protection against colorectal cancer in the European Prospective Investigation into Cancer and Nutrition (EPIC): an observational study. *Lancet* **361**, 1496–501.

Bouton, S., Leboeuf, E., Mouilee, G., Leydecker, M.-T., Talbotec, J., Granier, F., Lahaye, M., Hofte, H. and Truong, H.-M. (2002) QUASIMODO1 encodes a putative membrane-bound glycosyltransferase required for normal pectin synthesis and cell adheshion in *Arabidopsis*. *Plant Cell* **14**, 2577–90.

Browse, J. and Sommerville, C. (1991) Glycerolipid synthesis: biochemistry and regulation. *Annual Review of Plant Physiology and Molecular Biology* **42**, 467–506.

Brummell, D.A. and Harpster, M.H. (2001) Cell wall metabolism in fruit softening and quality and its manipulation in transgenic plants. *Plant Molecular Biology* **47**, 311–40.

Burkitt, D.P. and Trowell, H.C. (1977) Dietary fibre and western diseases. *Irish Medical Journal* **70**, 272–7.

Cahoon, E.B., Ripp., K.G., Hall, S.E. and Kinney, A.J. (2001) Formation of conjugated $\Delta 8$, $\Delta 10$-double bonds by $\Delta 12$- oleic acid desaturase related enzymes: biosynthetic origin of calendic acid. *Journal of Biological Chemistry* **276**, 2637–43.

Calpe-Berdiel, L., Escolà-Gil, J.C. and Blanco-Vaca, F. (2009) New insights into the molecular actions of plant sterols and stanols in cholesterol metabolism. *Atherosclerosis* **203**, 18–31.

Carey, A., Holt, K., Picard, S., Wilder, R., Tucker, G.A., Bird, C.R., Schuch, W. and Seymour, G.B. (1995) Tomato exo-(1-]4)-beta-d-galactanase – isolation, changes during ripening in normal and mutant tomato fruit, and characterization of a related cDNA clone. *Plant Physiology* **108**, 1099–107.

Carpita, N.C. and Gibeaut, D.M. (1993) Structural models of primary cell walls in flowering plants: consistency of molecular structure with the physical properties of the walls during growth. *Plant Journal* **3**, 1–30.

Carpita, N.C. and McCann, M. (2000) The cell wall. In: *Biochemistry and Molecular Biology of Plants* (eds Buchanan, B.B., Wilhelm, G. and Jones, R.L.), pp. 52–108. American Society of Plant Physiologists.

Cavalier, D.M., Lerouxel, O., Neumetzler, L., Yamauchi, K., Reinecke, A., Freshour, G., Zabotina, O.A., Hahn, M.G., Burgert, I., Pauly, M., Raikhel, N.V. and Keegstra, K. (2008) Disrupting two *Arabidopsis thaliana* xylosyltransferase genes results in plants deficient in xyloglucan, a major primary cell wall component. *Plant Cell* **20**, 1519–37.

Cocuron, J.C., Lerouxel, O., Drakakaki, G., Alonso, A.P., Liepman, A.H., Keegstra, K., Raikhel, N. and Wilkerson, C.G. (2007) A gene from the cellulose synthase-like C family encodes a beta-1, 4 glucan synthase. *Proceedings of the National Academy of Sciences USA* **104**, 8550–55.

Cosgrove, D.J. (2005) Growth of the plant cell wall. Nature Reviews **6**, 850–861.

Denyer, K., Dunlap, F., Thorbjornsen, T., Keeling, P. and Smith, A.M. (1996) The major form of ADP-glucose pyrophosphorylase in maize endosperm is extra-plastidial. *Plant Physiology* **112**, 779–85.

Devaraj, S. and Jialal, I. (2006) The role of dietary supplementation with plant sterols and stanols in the prevention of cardiovascular disease. *Nutrition Reviews* **64**, 348–54.

Doblin, M.S., Vergara, C.E., Read, S.M., Newbigin, E. and Bacic, A. (2003) Plant cell wall biosynthesis: making the bricks. In: *The Plant Cell Wall* (ed. J.K.C. Rose), pp. 183–222. Oxford: Blackwell.

Doblin, M.S., Kurek, I., Jacob-Wilk, D. and Delmer, D.P. (2002) Cellulose biosynthesis in plants; from genes to rosettes. *Plant Cell Physiology* **43**, 1407–20.

DoH (1991) *Dietary reference values of food energy and nutrients for the United Kingdom.* Report on Health and Social Subjects 41. London: Department of Health.

Dominguez Puigjaner, E., Vendrell, M. and Prat, S. (1997) A cDNA clone highly expressed in ripe banana fruit shows homology to pectate lyases. *Plant Physiology* **114**, 1071–6.

Ebringerová, A. and Heinze, T, (2000) Xylan and xylan derivatives – biopolymers with variable properties, 1 – Naturally occurring xylan structures, procedures and properties. *Macromolecular Rapid Communications* **21**, 542–56.

Ebringerová, A. and Hromádková, Z. (1999) Xylans of industrial and biomedical importance. In: *Biotechnology and Genetic Engineering Reviews* (ed. Harding, S.E.), Volume 16, pp. 325–46. England: Intercept.

Ebringerova, A., Hromadkova, Z. and Heinze, T. (2005) Hemicellulose. *Advances in Polymer Sciences* **186**, 1–67.

Englyst, K.N., Liu, S. and Englyst, H.N. (2007) Nutritional characterization and measurement of dietary carbohydrates. *European Journal of Clinical Nutrition* **61**, S19–39.

Eskin, N.A.M., McDonald, B.E., Przybylski, R., Malcolmson, L.J., Scarth, R., Mag, T., Ward, K. and Adolph, D. (1996) Canola oil. In: *Edible Oil and Fat Products: Oil and Oil Seed* (ed. Hui, Y.H.), pp. 1–96. New York: John Wiley & Sons.

Flight, I. and Clifton, P. (2006) Cereal grains and legumes in the prevention of coronary heart disease and stroke: a review of the literature. *European Journal of Clinical Nutrition* **60**, 1145–59.

Fry, S.C. (2004) Primary cell wall metabolism: tracking the careers of wall polymers in living plant cells. *New Phytologist* **161**, 641–75.

Fu, Y., Ballicora, M.A., Leykam, J.F., and Preiss, J. (1998) Mechanism of reductive activation of potato tuber ADP-glucose pyrophosphorylase. *Journal of Biological Chemistry* **273**, 25045–52.

Fuentes-Zaragoza, E., Riquelme-Navarrete, M.J., Sanchez-Zapata, E. and Perez-Alvarez, J.A. (2010) Resistant starch as functional ingredient: a review. *Food Research International* **43**, 931–42.

Gerber, M. (2009) Background review paper on total fat, fatty acid intake and cancers. *Annals of Nutrition and Metabolism* **55**, 140–61.

Gibney, M.J., Hearty, A., Duffy, E., Joyce, J. and O'Connor, C. (2008) Phytosterol-enriched products on the Irish market: examination of intake and consumption patterns. *Public Health Nutrition* **12**, 1–8.

Gillmor, C.S., Lukowitz, W., Brininstool, G., Sedbrook, J.C., Hamann, T., Poindexter, P. and Somerville, C. (2005) Glycosylphosphatidyl inositol-anchored proteins are required for cell wall synthesis and morphogenesis in *Arabidopsis*. *Plant Cell* **17**, 1128–40.

Gonzalez, C.A. and Riboli, E. (2010) Diet and cancer prevention: contributions from the European Prospective Investigation into Cancer and Nutrition (EPIC) study. *European Journal of Cancer* **46**, 2555–62.

Graham, I.A., Larson, T. and Napier, J.A. (2007) Rational metabolic engineering of transgenic plants for the biosynthesis of omega-3 polyunsaturates. *Current Opinions in Biotechnology* **18**, 142–7.

Grant, G.T., Morris, E.R., Rees, D.A., Smith, P.J.C. and Thorn, D. (1973) Biological interactions between polysaccharides and divalent cations: the egg box model. FEBS Letters. 32, 195–198.

Ha, M.-A., Jarvis, M.C. and Mann, J.I. (2000) A definition for dietary fibre. *European Journal of Clinical Nutrition* **54**, 861–4.

Harris, W.S. (2006) The omega-6/omega-3 ratio and cardiovascular disease risk: uses and abuses. *Current Atherosclerosis Reports* **8**, 453–9.

Hayashi, T., Ogawa, K. and Mitsuishi, Y. (1994) Characterisation of the adsorption of xyloglucan to cellulose. *Plant Cell Physiology* **35**, 1199–205.

Henrissat, B., Coutinho, P.M. and Davies, G.J. (2001) A census of carbohydrate-active enzymes in the genome of *Arabidopsis thaliana*. *Plant Molecular Biology* **47**, 55–72.

Huang, A.H.C. (1996) Oleosins and oil bodies in seed and other organs. *Plant Physiology* **110**, 1055–61.

Jane, J.-L., Kasemsuwan, T., Leas, S., Zobel, H. and Robyt, J.F. (1994) Anthology of starch granule morphology by scanning electron microscopy. *Starch-Staarke* **46**, 121–9.

Jenkins, D.J.A., Wolever, T.M.S., Leeds, A.E., Gassuli, M.A., Haisman, P., Dilawari, J., Goff, D.V., Metz, G.L. and Alberti, K.G.M.M. (1978) Dietary fibres, fibre analogues and glucose intolerance: importance of viscosity. *British Medical Journal* **1**, 1392–4.

Jobling, S. (2004) Improving starch for food and industrial applications. *Current Opinions in Plant Biology* **7**, 210–18.

Jobling, S.A., Westcott, R.J., Tayal, A., Jeffcoat, R. and Schwall, G.P. (2002) Production of a freeze–thaw stable potato starch by antisense inhibition of three starch synthase genes. *Nature Biotechnology* **20**, 295–9.

Kamel, B.S. and Kakuda, Y. (1992) Fatty acids in fruit and fruit products. In: *Fatty Acids in Foods and their Health Implications* (ed. C.K. Chow). New York: Marcel Dekker.

Keegstra, K. and Walton, J. (2000) Plant science: β-glucans-brewers bane, dieticians delight. *Science* **311**, 1872–3.

Knutzon, D.S., Thompson, G.A., Radke, S.E., Johnson, W.B., Knauf, V.C. and Kridi, J.C. (1992) Modification of *Brassica* seed oil by antisense expression of a stearoyl-acyl carrier protein desaturase gene. *Proceedings of the National Academy of Sciences USA* **89**, 2624–8.

Konishi, T. and Sasaki, Y. (1994) Compartmentalization of two forms of acetyl-CoA carboxylase in plants and the origin of their tolerance towards herbicide. *Proceedings of the National Academy of Sciences USA* **91**, 3598–601.

Lane, D.R., Wiedemeier, A., Peng, L.C., Hofte, H., Vernhettes, S., Desprez, T., Hocart, C.H., Birch, R.J., Baskin, T.I., Burn, J.E., Arioli, T., Betzner, A.S. and Williamson, R.E. (2001) Temperature-sensitive alleles of RSW2 link the KORRIGAN endo-1, 4-β-glucanase to cellulose synthesis and cytokinesis in *Arabidopsis. Plant Physiology* **126**, 278–88.

Lerouxel, O., Cavalier, D.M., Liepman, A.H. and Keegstra, K. (2006) Biosynthesis of plant cell wall polysaccharides-a complex process. *Current Opinion in Plant Biology* **9**, 621–30.

Lessire, R., Cahoon, E., Chapman, K., Dyer, J., Eastmond, P. and Heinz, E. (2009) Highlights of recent progress in plant lipid research. *Plant Physiology and Biochemistry* **47**, 443–7.

Leung, M.Y.K., Liu, C., Koon, J.C.M. and Fung, K.P. (2006) Polysaccharide biological response modifiers. *Immunology Letters* **105**, 101–14.

Liepman, A., Wilkerson, C. and Keegstra, K. (2005) Expression of cellulose synthase-like (Csl) genes in insect cells reveals that CslA family members encode mannan synthases. *Proceedings of the National Academy of Sciences USA* **102**, 2221–6.

Lindstrom, J., Ilanne-Parikka, P., Peltonen, M., Aunola, S., Eriksson, J.G., Hernia, H., Hornalainen, H., Harkonen, P., Keinanen-Kiukaanniemi, S., Laakso, M., Louheranta, A., Mannelin, M., Paturi, M., Sundvall, J., Valle, T.T., Uusitupa, M. and Tuomilehto, J. (2006) Sustained reduction in the incidence of type 2 diabetes by lifestyle intervention: follow-up of the Finnish diabetes prevention study. *Lancet* **368**, 1673–9.

Lukowitz, W., Nickle, T.C., Meinke, D.W., Last, R.L., Conklin, P.L. and Somerville, C.R. (2001) *Arabidopsis* cyt11 mutants are deficient in a mannose-1-phosphate quanyltransferase and point to a requirement of N-linked glycosylation for cellulose biosynthesis. *Proceedings of the National Academy of Sciences USA* **98**, 2262–7.

McCance, R.A. and Widdowson, E.M. (2008) *The Composition of Foods*, 6th edition. London: Food Standards Agency.

McDougall, G.J., Morrison, I.M., Stewart, D. and Hillman, J.R. (1996) Plant cell walls as dietary fibre: range, structure, processing and function. *Journal of the Science of Food and Agriculture* **70**, 133–50.

Madson, M., Dunand, C., Li, X.L., Vanzin, G.K, Caplan, J., Shoue, D.A., Carpita, N.C. and Reiter, W.D. (2003) The *MUR3* gene of *Arabidopsis thaliana* encodes a xyloglucan galactosyltransferase that is evolutionarily related to animal exostosins. *Plant Cell* **15**, 1662–70.

McQueen-Mason, S., Durachko, D.M. and Cosgrove, D.J. (1992) Two endogenous proteins that induce cell wall expansion in plants. *Plant Cell* **4**, 1425–33.

Melanson, E.L., Astrup, A. and Donahoo, W.T. (2009) The relationship between dietary fat and fatty acid intake and body weight, diabetes, and the metabolic syndrome. *Annals of Nutrition and Metabolism* **55**, 229–43.

Mohnen, D. (2002) Biosynthesis of pectins. In: *Pectins and their Manipulation* (eds Seymour, G.B. and Knox, J.P.), pp. 52–98. Oxford: Blackwell.

Morell, M.K. and Myers, A.M. (2005) Towards the rational design of cereal starches. *Current Opinion in Plant Biology* **8**, 204–10.

Mouille, G., Ralet, M.-C., Cavelier, C., Eland, C., Effroy, D., Hematy, K., McCartney, L., Troung, H.M., Gaudon, V., Thibault, J.-F., Marchant, A. and Hofte, H. (2007) Homogalacturonan synthesis in *Arabidopsis thaliana* requires a Golgi-localised protein with a putative methyltransferase domain. *Plant Journal* **50**, 605–14.

Mozaffarian, D., Micha, R. and Wallace, S. (2010) Effects on coronary heart disease of increasing polyunsaturated fat in place of saturated sat: a systematic review and meta-analysis of randomized controlled trials. *PLoS Medicine* **7**(3), e1000252.

Murphy, D.J. (1996) Engineering oil production in rapeseed and other oil crops. *Trends in Technology* **14**, 206–13.

National Diet Nutrition Survey (2010) Tables – NDNS Headline results from Year 1 of the Rolling Programme (2008/2009). http://www.food.gov.uk/multimedia/pdfs/publication/ndnstables0809.pdf (Accessed 10 January 2011).

Nishitani, K. and Tominaga, T. (1992) Endo-xyloglucan transferase, a novel class of glycosyltransferase that catalyses transfer of a segment of xyloglucan molecule to another xyloglucan molecule. *Journal of Biological Chemistry* **267**, 21058–64.

Ohlrogge, J. and Browse, J. (1995) Lipid biosynthesis. *Plant Cell* **7**, 957–70.

Ohyama, K., Suzuki, M., Kikuchi, J., Saito, K. and Muranaka, T. (2009) Dual biosynthetic pathways to phytosterol via cycloartenol and lanosterol in *Arabidopsis. Proceedings of the National Aacademy of Sciences USA* **106**, 725–730.

O'Neill, M.A. and York, W.S. (2001) *The Plant Cell Wall* (ed. J.K.C. Rose), pp. 1–54. Oxford: Blackwell.

Pagant, S., Bichet, A., Sugimoto, K., Lerouxek, O., Desprez, T., McMann, M., Lerouge, P., Vernhettes, S. and Hofte, H. (2002) KORBITO 1 encodes a novel plasma membrane protein necessary for normal synthesis of cellulose during cell expansion in *Arabidopsis. Plant Cell* **14**, 2001–13.

Preiss, J. (1988) Biosynthesis of starch and its regulation. In: *The Biochemistry of Plants* (ed. Preiss, J.), Volume 14, pp. 181–254. London: Academic Press.

Qi, B., Fraser, T., Mugford, S., Dobsion, G., Sayanova, O, Butler, J., Napier, J.A., Stobart, A.K. and Lazarus, C.M. (2004) Production of very long chain polyunsaturated omega-3 and omega-6 fatty acids in plants. *Nature Biotechnology* **22**, 739–45.

Rao, M.V.S.S.T.S. and Muralikrishna, G. (2001) Non-starch polysaccharides and bound phenolic acids from native and malted finger millet (Ragi, *Eleusine coracana*, Indif-15). *Food Chemistry* **72**, 187–92.

Reddy, A.S. and Thomas, T.L. (1996) Expression of a cyanobacterial Δ6 desaturase gene results in γ-linolenic acid production in transgenic plants. *Nature Biotechnology* **14**, 639–42.

Reid, J.S.G. and Edwards, M.E. (1995) Galactomannans and other cell wall storage polysaccharides in seeds. In: *Food Polysaccharides and their Applications* (ed. A.M. Stephen), p. 155. New York: Marcel Dekker.

Robert, S., Mouille, G. and Hofte, H. (2004) The mechanism and regulation of cellulose synthesis in primary cell walls: lessons from cellulose-deficient *Arabidopsis* mutants. *Cellulose* **11**, 351–64.

Roudier, F., Fernandez, A.G., Fujita, M., Himmelspach, R., Borner, G.H.H., Schindelman, G., Song, S., Baskin, T.I., Dupree, P., Wasteneys, G.O. and Benfey, P.N. (2005) COBRA, an *Arabidopsis* extracellular glycosyl-phosphadyl inositol-anchored protein, specifically controls highly anisotropic expansion through its involvement in cellulose microfibril orientation. *Plant Cell* **17**, 1749–63.

Salen, G., Shefer, S., Nguyen, L.B., Ness, G.C. and Tint, G.S. (1999) Sitosterolaemia. In: *Lipoproteins in Health and Disease* (eds D.J. Betteridge, D.R. Illingworth and J. Shepherd), pp. 815–27. London: Arnold.

Salter, A.M. and Tarling, E.J. (2007) Regulation of gene transcription by fatty acids. *Animal* **1**, 1314–20.

Sasaki, Y., Hakamada, K., Suama, Y., Nagano, Y., Furusawa, I. and Matsuno, R. (1993) Chloroplast-encoded protein as a subunit of acetyl-CoA carboxylase in pea plant. *Journal of Biological Chemistry* **268**, 25118–23.

Sato, S., Xing, A., Schweiger, B., Kinney, A., Graef, G. and Clemente, T. (2004) Production of γ-linolenic acid and stearidonic acid in seed of marker-free transgenic soybean. *Crop Science* **44**, 646–52.

Scarth, R. and Tang, J. (2006) Modification of *Brassica* oil using conventional and transgenic approaches. *Crop Science* **46**, 1225–36.

Schneeman, B.O. (1999) Building scientific consensus: the importance of dietary fibre. *American Journal of Clinical Nutrition* **45**, 129–32.

Schols, H.A. and Voragen, A.G.J. (2002) The chemical structure of pectins. In: *Pectins and their Manipulation* (eds G.B. Seymour and J.P. Knox), pp. 1–29. Oxford: Blackwell.

Schwall, G.P., Safford, R., Westcott, R.J., Jeffcoat, R., Tayal, A., Shi, Y.C., Gidley, M.J. and Jobling, S.A. (2000) Production of very-high-amylose potato starch by inhibition of SBE A and B. *Nature Biotechnology* **18**, 551–4.

Seal, C.J. (2006) Whole grains and CVD risk. *Proceedings of the Nutrition Society* **65**, 24–34.

Shewry, P.R. and Morell, M. (2001) Manipulating cereal endosperm structure, development and composition to improve end-use properties. *Advances in Botanical Research* **34**, 165–236.

Simopoulos, A.P. (2008) The importance of the omega-6/omega-3 fatty acid ratio in cardiovascular disease and other chronic diseases. *Experimental Biology and Medicine* **233**, 674–88.

Singh, S.P., Zhou, X.-R., Liu, Q., Stymne, S. and Green A.G. (2005) Metabolic engineering of new fatty acids in plants. *Current Opinions in Plant Biology* **8**, 197–203.

Slavin, J. (2003) Why whole grains are protective: biological mechanisms. *Proceedings of the Nutrition Society* **62**, 129–34.

Somerville, C. (2006) Cellulose synthesis in higher plants. *Annual Review of Cellular and Developmental Biology* **22**, 53–78.

Somerville, C., Bauer, S., Brininstool, G., Facette, M., Hamann, T., Milne, J., Osborne, E., Paredez, A., Persson, S., Raab, T., Vorwerk, S. and Youngs, H. (2004) Towards a systems approach to understanding plant cell walls. *Science* **306**, 2206–11.

Sterling, J.D., Atmodjo, M.A., Inwood, S.E., Kolli, V.S.K., Quigley, H.F., Hahn, M.G. and Mohhnen, D. (2006) Functional identification of an *Arabidopsis* pectin biosynthetic homogalacturonan galactosyltransferase. *Proceedings of the National Academy of Sciences USA* **103**, 5236–41.

Stitt, M., Gerhardt, R., Kurzel, B. and Heldt, H.W. (1983) A role for fructose2, 6-bisphosphate in the regulation of sucrose synthesis in spinach leaves. *Plant Physiology* **72**, 1139–41.

Tappy, L. and Lê, K.-A. (2010) Metabolic effects of fructose and the worldwide increase in obesity. *Physiological Reviews* **90**, 23–46.

Taylor, N.G., Gardiner, J.C., Whiteman, R. and Turner, S.R. (2004) Cellulose synthesis in *Arabidopsis* secondary cell walls. *Cellulose* **11**, 329–38.

Thakur, B.R., Singh, R.K. and Handa, A.K. (1997) Chemistry and uses of pectin- a review. *Critical Reviews in Food Science and Nutrition* **37**, 47–73.

Theuwissen, E. and Mensink, R.P. (2008) Water-soluble dietary fibers and cardiovascular disease. *Physiology and Behaviour* **94**, 285–92.

Topping, D.L. and Clifton, P.M. (2001) Short-chain fatty acids and human colonic function: roles of resistant starch and nonstarch polysaccharides. *Physiological Reviews* **8**, 1031–64.

Truksa, M., Vrinten, P. and Qui, X. (2009) Metabolic engineering of plants for polyunsaturated fatty acid production. *Molecular Breeding* **23**, 1–11.

Tucker, G.A. and Seymour, G.B. (2002) Modification and degradation of pectins. In: *Pectins and their Manipulation* (eds G.B. Seymour and J.P. Knox), pp. 150–73. Oxford: Blackwell.

Tzen, J.T.C., Lie, G.C., Laurent, P., Ratnayake, C. and Huang, A.H.C. (1993) Lipids, proteins, and structure of seed oil bodies from diverse species. *Plant Physiology* **101**, 267–76.

Upmeyer, D.J. and Koller, H.R. (1973) Diurnal trends in net photosynthetic rate and carbohydrate levels of soyabean leaves. *Plant Physiology* **51**, 871–4.

Ursin, V.M. (2003) Modification of plant lipids for human health: development of functional land-based omega-3 fatty acids. *Journal of Nutrition* **133**, 4271–4.

Vallim, T. and Salter, A.M. (2010) Regulation of hepatic gene expression by saturated fatty acids. *Prostaglandins, Leukotrienes and Essential Fatty Acids* **88**, 2565–75.

Vanzin, G.F., Madson, M., Carpita, N.C., Raikhel, N.V., Keegstra, K. and Reiter, W.D. (2002) The mur2 mutant of *Arabidopsis thaliana* lacks fucosylated xyloglucan because of a lesion in fucosyltransferase AtFUT1. *Proceedings of the National Academy of Sciences USA* **99**, 3340–5.

Venegas-Caleron, M., Sayanova O. and Napier, J.A. (2010) An alternative to fish oils: metabolic engineering of oil-seed crops to produce omega-3 long chain polyunsaturated fatty acids. *Progress in Lipid Research* **49**, 108–19.

Vidrih, R., Filip S. and Hribar, J. (2009) Content of higher fatty acids in green Vegetables. *Czechoslavakian Journal of Food Science* **27**, S125–9

Vincken, J,P., Schols, H.A., Oomen, R.J., McCann, M.C., Ulvskov, P., Voragen, A.G. and Visser, R.G. (2003) If homogalacturonan were a side chain of rhamnogalacturonan I, implications for cell wall architecture. *Plant Physiology* **132**, 1781–9.

Voelker, T. and Kinney, A.J. (2001) Variations in the biosynthesis of seed-storage lipids. *Annual Review of Plant Physiology and Molecular Biology* **52**, 335–64.

Voelker, T.A., Worrell, A.C., Anderson, L., Bleibaum, J., Fan, C., Hawkins, D.J., Radke, S.E. and Davies, H.M. (1992) Fatty acid biosynthesis redirected to medium chain in transgenic oilseed plants. *Science* **257**, 72–74.

Wallis, J.G. and Browse, J. (2010) Lipid biochemists salute the genome. *Plant Journal* **61**, 1092–106.

Whelan, J. (2009) Dietary Stearidonic Acid Is a Long Chain (n-3) Polyunsaturated Fatty Acid with Potential Health Benefits. Journal of Nutrition, 139, 5–10.

White, P.J. (1992) Fatty acids in oilseeds (vegetable oils). In: *Fatty Acids in Foods and their Health Implications* (ed. C.K. Chow). New York: Marcel Dekker.

Wolever, T.M.S., Jenkins, D.J.A., Vuksan, V., Jenkins, A.L., Buckley, G.C., Wong, G.S. and Josse, R.G. (1992) Beneficial effect of a low glycemic index diet in type-2 diabetes. *Diabetic Medicine* **9**, 451–8.

Wood, P.J. (2004) Relationships between solution properties of cereal beta-glucans and physiological effects – a review. *Trends in Food Science and Technology* **15**, 313–20.

Zeeman, S.C., Smith, S.M. and Smith, A.M. (2007) The diurnal metabolism of leaf starch. *Biochemical Journal* **401**, 13–28.

Chapter 3

Carotenoids

Úrsula Flores-Perez and Manuel Rodriguez-Concepcion

Introduction

Carotenoids are isoprenoid pigments synthesised by all photosynthetic organisms (including plants, algae and cyanobacteria) and some bacteria and fungi. Carotenoids synthesised in plant chloroplasts are essential for photoprotection and participate in light harvesting. When chlorophyll is degraded in leaves or missing in non-photosynthetic organs such as roots, flowers and fruits, the distinctive yellow to red colours of carotenoids become visible. Thus, carotenoids provide the autumn colours of many leaves and are responsible for the yellow colour of corn, the orange colour of carrots, pumpkin and oranges, and the red colour of tomato and watermelon. In addition, their oxidative cleavage produces growth regulators such as abscisic acid. Humans cannot synthesise carotenoids *de novo,* but must obtain them through the diet as a source for the production of essential retinoids such as retinol (vitamin A), retinal (the main visual pigment) and retinoic acid (a regulator of gene expression) (Bollag 1996; Handelman 2001; Demmig-Adams and Adams 2002; Johnson 2002). Some animals (shrimp, lobster, trout, salmon, goldfish, flamingoes) also use dietary carotenoids for coloration, which in the case of many birds is used as a signal of mate quality (Blount 2004).

The major value of carotenoids (particularly β-carotene) in human nutrition is their use as vitamin A precursors. Deficient vitamin A intake is one of the most common dietary problems affecting children worldwide, leading to blindness and premature death (West 2003). Additionally, carotenoids have been proposed to confer other health benefits. For instance, an inverse relationship exists between the dietary intake of carotenoid-rich foods and the incidence of some cancers, coronary heart disease, light-induced erythema, cataracts and macular degeneration (Johnson 2002; Fraser and Bramley 2004; Stahl and Sies 2005). The discovery of the health-related properties of carotenoids is spurring their use as nutraceuticals, and it is expected that the future demand for some carotenoids will exceed the levels that can be currently achieved by chemical synthesis or extraction from natural sources.

The main pathway for carotenoid biosynthesis is now known, and some of the identified biosynthetic genes have been successfully used in metabolic engineering approaches

Phytonutrients, First Edition. Edited by Andrew Salter, Helen Wiseman and Gregory Tucker.
© 2012 Blackwell Publishing Ltd. Published 2012 by Blackwell Publishing Ltd.

to overproduce carotenoids of interest in plants, the main source of carotenoids in the human diet. Plant carotenoid biotechnology might contribute not only to producing carotenoid-enriched foods with improved health benefits but also to providing novel sources for the production of natural pigments of industrial interest. For instance, astaxanthin and canthaxanthin are carotenoids produced by marine bacteria and microalgae that are added to the feed of aquaculture-grown salmon, trout, lobster and shrimp to provide the characteristic pink colour that these animals acquire in the wild from their diet. Astaxanthin, lutein and zeaxanthin are also extensively used to enhance the yellow pigmentation of eggs and poultry. Besides other industrial applications of carotenoids such as β-carotene as colourants for human food, the economic value (consumer acceptance) of many fruits, vegetables and flowers can be increased by enhancing their carotenoid-derived colour and flavour. In this review, we summarise the current knowledge on plant carotenoid biosynthesis and function and review the contribution of plant food carotenoids to human nutrition and health. Biochemical, molecular, regulatory and biotechnological aspects of carotenoid biosynthesis have been extensively reviewed elsewhere (Bartley and Scolnik 1995; Britton 1995; Armstrong and Hearst 1996; Demmig-Adams et al. 1996; Cunningham and Gantt 1998; Giuliano et al. 2000; Hirschberg 2001; Sandmann 2001; Bramley 2002; Fraser and Bramley 2004; Botella-Pavía and Rodríguez-Concepción 2006).

Structure, biosynthesis and function of plant carotenoids

Hundreds of carotenoid structures are known to occur in nature. All of them derive from a backbone formed by several isoprene units with a series of conjugated double bonds which, after subsequent modifications such as cyclisations and oxidations, determines their physical and biological properties (Britton 1995). With the exception of a few bacterial carotenoids with 30, 45 or 50 carbon atoms, most carotenoids are 40-carbon isoprenoids (tetraterpenes). The basic 40-carbon polyene chain of plant carotenoids is synthesised from the 5-carbon units isopentenyl diphosphate (IPP) and its isomer dimethylallyl diphosphate (DMAPP), the building blocks of all isoprenoid compounds (Figure 3.1). In plastids, these precursors are synthesised from pyruvate and glyceraldehyde 3-phosphate by the methylerythritol 4-phosphate (MEP) pathway (Lichtenthaler 1999; Eisenreich et al. 2001; Rodríguez-Concepción and Boronat 2002). Although all the MEP pathway enzymes are located in the plastid, they are encoded by the nuclear genome (Rodríguez-Concepción and Boronat 2002). Interestingly, engineered upregulation of some of the MEP pathway genes results in enhanced accumulation of carotenoids, indicating that precursor supply is limiting for carotenoid biosynthesis in plants (Estévez et al. 2001; Mahmoud and Croteau 2001; Botella-Pavía et al. 2004; Carretero-Paulet et al. 2006).

Plant carotenoid biosynthesis takes place in the plastids (Cunningham and Gantt 1998). The sequential and linear addition of three molecules of IPP to one molecule of DMAPP generates the 20-carbon geranylgeranyl diphosphate (GGPP) molecule, which serves as the immediate precursor not only for carotenoids but also for the biosynthesis of gibberellins and the isoprenoid moiety of chlorophylls, phylloquinones, plastoquinones and tocopherols. The first committed step in plant carotenoid biosynthesis is the head-to-head condensation of two GGPP molecules to yield phytoene (Figure 3.1). This reaction, catalysed in a two-step

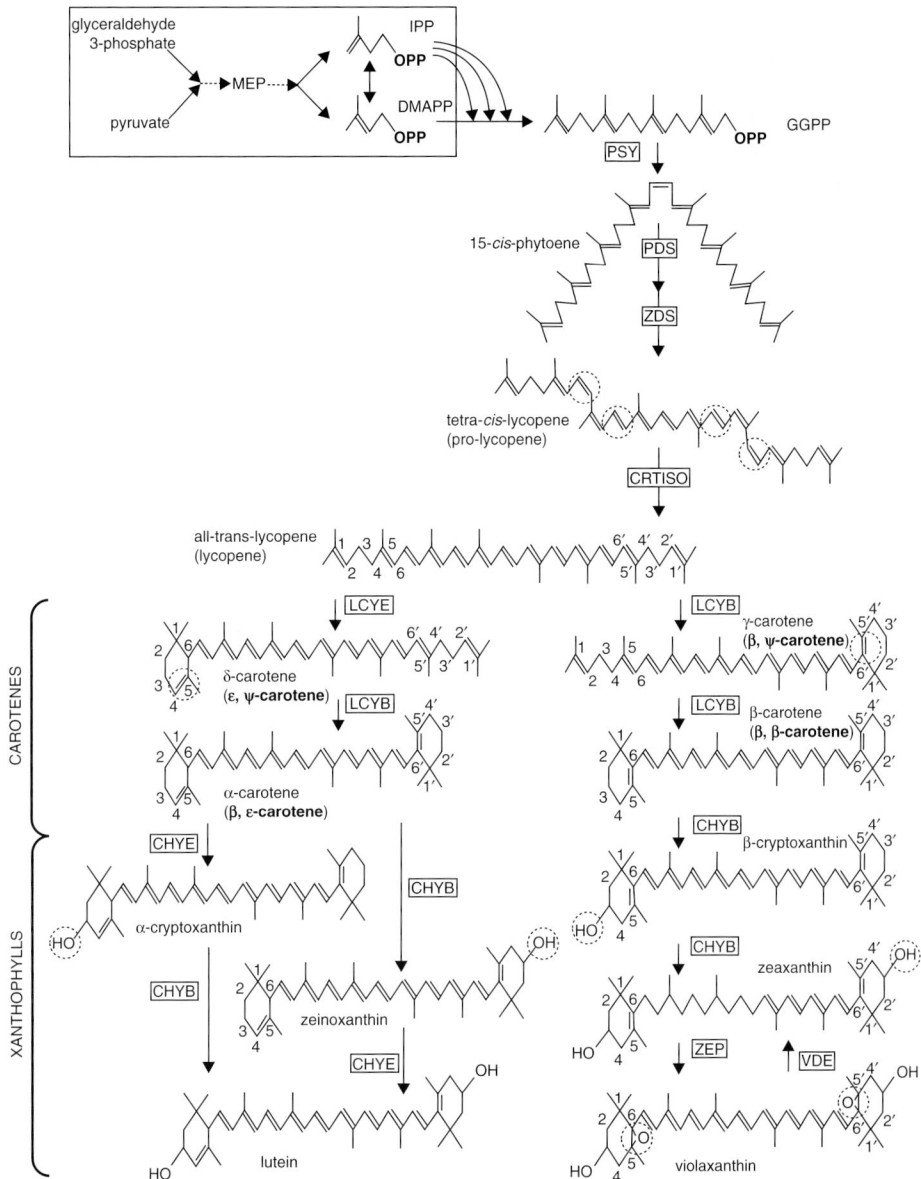

Figure 3.1 Carotenoid biosynthesis pathway in plants. MEP, methylerythritol 4-phosphate; IPP, isopentenyl diphosphate; DMAPP, dimethylallyl diphosphate; GGPP, geranylgeranyl diphosphate. The MEP pathway is boxed. Enzymes of the carotenoid pathway are also boxed: PSY, phytoene synthase; PDS, phytoene desaturase; ZDS, ζ-carotene desaturase; CRTISO, carotenoid isomerase; LCYB, lycopene β-cyclase; LCYE, lycopene ϵ-cyclase; CHYB, carotene β-hydroxylase; CHYE, carotene ϵ-hydroxylase; ZEP, zeaxanthin epoxidase; VDE, violaxanthin deepoxidase.

process by the enzyme phytoene synthase (PSY), has been proposed as the main flux-controlling step of the pathway in plants (Hirschberg 2001; Fraser and Bramley 2004). Colourless phytoene then undergoes a series of four sequential desaturation (dehydrogenation) reactions catalysed by phytoene desaturase (PDS) and ζ–carotene desaturase (ZDS) that increase the conjugated series of double bonds to eventually produce the red-coloured lycopene. In non-photosynthetic tissues, a carotenoid isomerase (CRTISO) activity is additionally required to transform poly-*cis* lycopene (pro-lycopene), the actual product of PDS and ZDS activities, into the all-*trans* isomer (lycopene) found in plant cells (Figure 3.1). Photoisomerisation can substitute the CRTISO activity in chloroplasts (Isaacson et al. 2002; Park et al. 2002).

Cyclisation of one or both ends of the linear lycopene molecule by the related cyclises, lycopene cyclase B (LCYB) and lycopene cyclase E (LCYE), represents a branching point in the plant pathway. One branch leads to the orange-coloured β-carotene, which contains two β-ionone rings, whereas the other branch leads to carotenes with β and/or ε rings (Figure 3.1). With the exception of lettuce lactucaxanthin, carotenoids with two ε rings are not commonly found in plants. Other unusual cyclic end groups are the κ and ψ end groups. The presence of the cyclopentane κ ring in capsanthin and capsorubin, carotenoids that accumulate in ripe pepper fruit, is responsible for their characteristic red colour (Cunningham and Gantt 1998). The enzymatic oxygenation of carotenes results in the production of xanthophylls, which have distinct and complementary functions in photosystem assembly, light harvesting and photoprotection. Carotenoid ε-ring hydroxylase (CHYE) enzymes are cytochrome P450-type monooxygenases that catalyse the hydroxylation of ε rings (Tian et al. 2004), whereas two types of monooxygenases (non-haeme di-iron and P450) have been shown to have β ring hydroxylase (CHYB) activity (Fiore et al. 2006; Kim and DellaPenna 2006). Hydroxylation of the C-3 and C-3′ positions of α-carotene and β-carotene result in the formation of the xanthophylls lutein and zeaxanthin, respectively. The enzyme zeaxanthin epoxidase (ZEP) readily converts zeaxanthin into violaxanthin via antheraxanthin by introducing 5,6-epoxy groups into the 3-hydroxy β rings. In the last step of the chloroplast carotenoid pathway, the allenic xanthophyll neoxanthin is formed from violaxanthin (Cunningham and Gantt 1998).

In chloroplasts, most carotenoids are located together with chlorophylls in functional pigment-binding protein structures embedded in thylakoid membranes (Demmig-Adams et al. 1996). Besides acting as membrane stabilisers, chloroplast carotenoids play two major roles in photosynthesis: light collection and photoprotection. Carotenoids act as accessory light-harvesting pigments that absorb at 450–570 nm (where chlorophyll does not absorb efficiently) and transfer the excitation energy to chlorophyll. But the essential role of carotenoids in green plants is the protection against the highly reactive photooxidative species that are generated as by-products of photosynthesis under strong light (Demmig-Adams et al. 1996). Carotenoids can efficiently quench chlorophyll triplets, preventing the generation of oxygen singlets. The protection of biomembranes against oxidative damage can also be achieved via the modification of the physical properties of the lipid phase of the membranes (Gruszecki and Strzalka 2005). When plants grow under full sunlight and light levels exceed the maximum that can be used productively by the photosynthetic apparatus, carotenoids can also dissipate excess light energy absorbed by the antenna pigments in a process known as thermal dissipation or non-photochemical quenching of chlorophyll fluorescence (Baroli and Niyogi 2000; Muller et al. 2001). Some carotenoid species such as zeaxanthin are more efficient in this process. Under light conditions that do not exceed the photosynthetic capacity of chloroplasts, plants have a remarkably similar carotenoid composition with high levels of lutein (45% of the total), β-carotene (25–30%), violaxanthin (10–15%), and neoxanthin (10–15%) and low levels of zeaxanthin (Demmig-Adams et al. 1996; Baroli and Niyogi 2000). However, under strong (excess) light, violaxanthin is transformed into zeaxanthin by the enzyme violaxanthin de-epoxidase (VDE) to improve photoprotection. Low light conditions result in the transformation of zeaxanthin back into violaxanthin by the activity of ZEP (Figure 3.1). This reversible interconversion of zeaxanthin and violaxanthin is known as the xanthophyll cycle and has a key role in the adaptation of plants to changing light intensities (Demmig-Adams et al. 1996; Baroli and Niyogi 2000; Muller et al. 2001).

In non-photosynthetic organs, the red, orange and yellow colours of carotenoids are not masked by chlorophyll. The yellow colour of the cotyledons of dark-grown seedlings is due to the accumulation of high levels of lutein and violaxanthin in etioplasts, basically associated to a crystalline structure called a prolamellar body (Park et al. 2002). And the accumulation of very high levels of carotenoids in differentiated plastids, the chromoplasts, results in the characteristic colour of carrot roots and some flower petals and ripe fruits. Unlike chloroplasts and etioplasts, the carotenoid composition of chromoplasts varies widely among different plant species and tissues. Chromoplast carotenoids are associated with lipids and proteins in specialised structures with globular, membranous, fibrilar, crystalline and tubular shapes that sequester large amounts of these lipophylic compounds (Bartley and Scolnik 1995; Camara et al. 1995). The main function of carotenoids in flowers and fruits seems to be the attraction of animals for pollination and dispersal of seeds.

Dietary sources and health benefits

Humans, like all animals, do not synthesise carotenoids *de novo* and rely upon their diet as the only source of these essential molecules. Fruits and vegetables are the major source of dietary carotenoids. The most prevalent carotenoids in the human diet are lycopene, α-carotene, β-carotene, β-cryptoxanthin, lutein and zeaxanthin. As a general rule, β-carotene, α-carotene, β-cryptoxanthin and lycopene are found in yellow to red fruits and vegetables, whereas the xanthophylls lutein and zeaxanthin, together with β-carotene, are abundant in dark-green leafy vegetables. However, the carotenoid profile varies widely among different foods (Holden et al. 1999), as shown in Figure 3.2. The carotenoid composition of a given plant food can also show a qualitative and quantitative variability because of factors such as stage of maturity, variety or cultivar, harvesting season, production practices, post-harvest handling, processing and storage (Rodriguez-Amaya 2003). There are also important differences in the type of food people consume as the source of some carotenoids among different countries. For example, carrots are the major source of β-carotene in most European countries whereas spinach is the most important source in Spain (O'Neill et al. 2001). An important exception is lycopene, with most of its dietary intake coming from tomato, ripe fruit and derived products such as juice, soup,

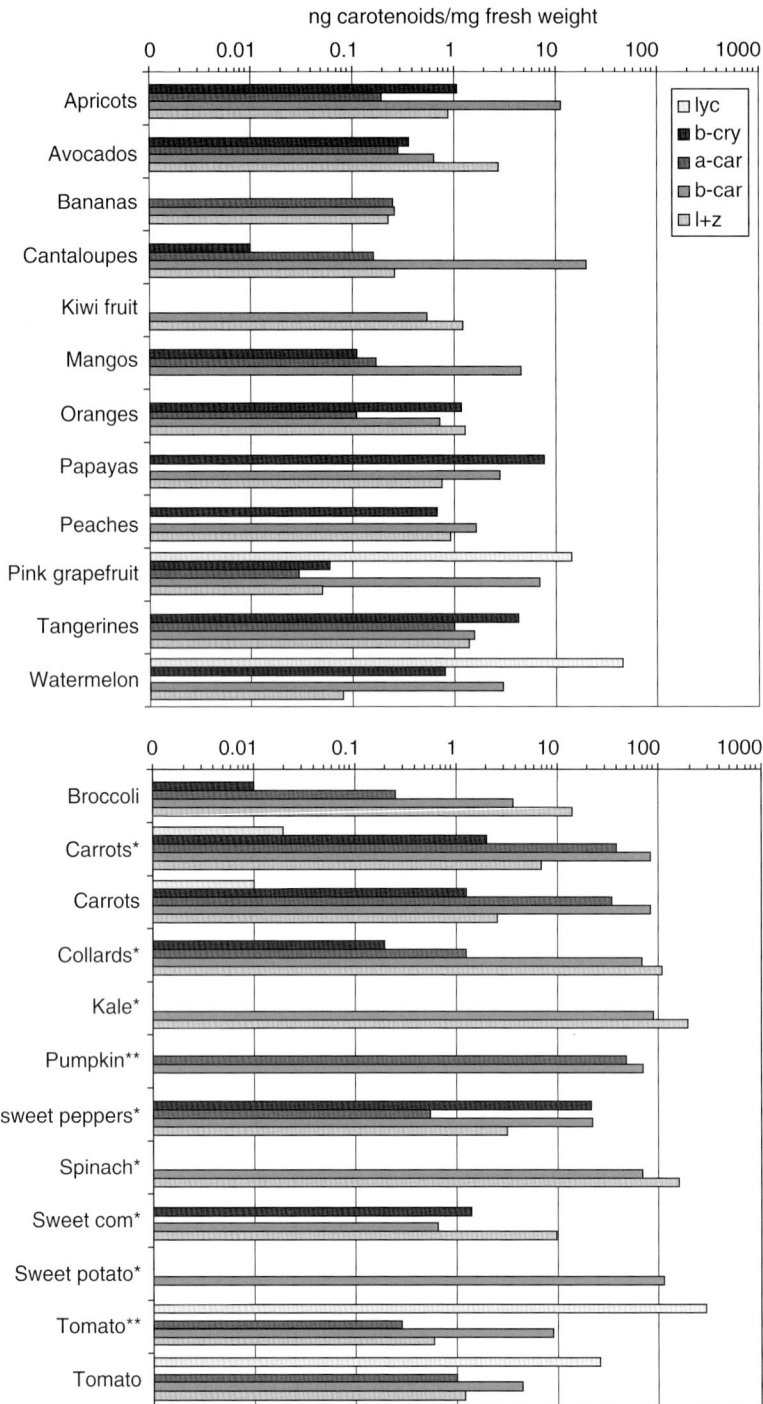

Figure 3.2 Carotenoid levels in fruits and vegetables. Data were collected from the United States Department of Agriculture (USDA) and Nutrition Coordination Center (NCC) Carotenoid Database (Holden et al., 1999) and correspond to raw foods unless indicated with an asterisc (cooked) or two asteriscs (canned). Note that the carotenoid content scale is logarithmic. lyc, lycopene; b-cry, β-cryptoxanthin; a-car, α-carotene; b-car, β-carotene; l+z, lutein and zeaxanthin. See plate section for colour version of this figure.

sauce or ketchup (Clinton 1998; Fraser and Bramley 2004). The main reason is that lycopene is only present in a few products (Holden et al. 1999). Because carotenoids are widely used in animal feed, they can also enter the human food chain in dairy products (β-carotene), eggs, poultry, seafood and fish (xanthophylls).

Dietary carotenoids fulfil essential requirements for human and animal nutrition (Bollag 1996; Rice-Evans et al. 1997; Demmig-Adams and Adams 2002; Johnson 2002). The major value of carotenoids in human nutrition is their use as vitamin A precursors. Provitamin A activity, however, is restricted to carotenoids with β rings, such as β-carotene (the most potent dietary precursor of vitamin A), α-carotene and β-cryptoxanthin (Figure 3.1). It is widely accepted that the incidence of some cancers, UV-induced skin damage (erythema or sunburn), cardiovascular disease (CVD), cataracts and macular degeneration is negatively correlated with the ingestion of carotenoid-rich foods (Handelman 2001; Demmig-Adams and Adams 2002; Johnson 2002; Fraser and Bramley 2004; Stahl and Sies 2005). High carotenoid intake has also been associated with enhanced immune system functions (Hughes 2001) and protection from type 2 diabetes (Ylonen et al. 2003). However, these data cannot be used to establish a requirement for carotenoid intake because it is not clear whether the observed effects are directly mediated by carotenoids or may be due to other substances found in carotenoid-rich food. In fact, a combination of carotenoids (and other phytonutrients) in food products is more effective than dietary supplements of single components (Stahl et al. 2000; Giovannucci et al. 2002; Miller et al. 2002; Wright et al. 2003).

Most of the health benefits associated with a carotenoid-rich diet seem to be derived from the antioxidant properties of these compounds. The conjugated double bond system of the carotenoid backbone results in a high capacity for quenching singlet oxygen and acting as free radical scavengers. The length of the polyene chain in the carotenoid molecule is correlated with its efficiency in quenching singlet oxygen, lycopene being the most effective carotenoid (DiMascio et al. 1989). Molecules such as hydrogen peroxide, singlet oxygen, nitrogen oxides, superoxide anion and other reactive species can also be inactivated by carotenoids (Paiva and Russell 1999). Although important for plants, the relevance of the antioxidant properties of carotenoids to human health is less clear. Besides its antioxidant mechanism of action, dietary carotenoids and the metabolites resulting from their oxidative degradation may achieve their potential biological activity of preventing certain diseases by other mechanisms, including the enhancement of intercellular communication activity via gap junctions (which play a role in the regulation of cell growth, differentiation and apoptosis), stimulation of detoxification enzymes, and anti-inflammatory and immune-related properties (Yeum and Russell 2002; Nagao 2004; Tapiero et al. 2004).

Some dietary carotenoids may have more protective roles than others, and certainly they have different degrees of biological activity and antioxidant capacities. High intake of tomato products rich in lycopene, a potent antioxidant, seems to prevent CVD (Rissanen et al. 2002) and prostate cancer (Giovannucci et al. 2002; Barber 2003). A diet rich in tomatoes can also reduce prostate tissue oxidative damage in patients with cancer, suggesting that lycopene can be used not only for the prevention but also for the treatment of prostate cancer (Chen et al. 2001; Kim et al. 2002). An inverse relationship has been reported between the intake of lycopene-rich food or serum lycopene and the risk of other cancers (Giovannucci 1999). However, additional evidence is required to confirm whether these findings are related specifically to lycopene intake or to other factors associated with tomato-rich diets.

Another potent antioxidant is β-cryptoxanthin, a xanthophyll which also has a mild provitamin A activity (Melendez-Martinez et al. 2004). Dietary β-cryptoxanthin seems to be a preventive agent against risk of some cancers (Yuan et al. 2003; Binns et al. 2004; Mannisto et al. 2004) and rheumatoid arthritis (Pattison et al. 2004). Lutein and zeaxanthin accumulate in the macula of the human eye where, along with their oxidative metabolites, they are collectively known as the macular pigments. These two powerful antioxidants participate in the scavenging of free radicals formed in the photoreceptors, protecting the macula from light-induced damage and age-related macular degeneration (AMD). Both carotenoids absorb UV and blue light and serve to protect the lens from oxidative damage (Krinsky et al. 2003). Macular pigment concentration can be elevated by dietary carotenoids in fruits and vegetables and lutein and zeaxanthin supplements, resulting in a significant reduction in the risk for AMD (Seddon et al. 1994; Mares-Perlman et al. 2002; Snellen et al. 2002; Goodrow et al. 2006). Dietary intake of high levels of these xanthophylls is also associated with a lower risk of cataract (Snodderly 1995; Jacques 1999; Lyle et al. 1999). In addition to ocular benefits, lutein supplementation seems to result in protection of skin from UV-induced damage (Eichler et al. 2002), anticancer activity (Chew et al. 1996) and enhanced immune function (Snodderly 1995). Zeaxanthin, a widely used colourant in the cosmetics and food industries, may also play a critical role in the prevention of cancer (Nishino et al. 2002). Epoxy xanthophylls such as antheraxanthin, violaxanthin and neoxanthin are also dietary carotenoids with antioxidant properties. Neoxanthin has been reported as protective against cancer (Chang et al. 1995; Kotake-Nara et al. 2001). The relationships observed between a high intake of these individual xanthophylls and the reported health benefits, however, are not clear-cut.

Besides the role of β-carotene as provitamin A, a protective effect of this carotenoid against UV-mediated sunburn has been reported (Gollnick et al. 1996; Stahl et al. 2000; Eichler et al. 2002). However, claims that β-carotene is effective as a sunscreen remain to be conclusively proven. Other studies suggest that β-carotene supplementation does not significantly protect against CVD (ATBCCPSG 1994; Brown et al. 1994; Hennekens et al. 1996; Omenn et al. 1996b; Cooper et al. 1999). Its ability to reduce the risk of certain types of cancer is controversial. Trials using β-carotene supplements (such as the pills typically sold in stores) have shown that the risk of lung cancer is actually increased in heavy smokers consuming such supplements, perhaps because under these circumstances β-carotene has pro-oxidant rather than antioxidant activity (ATBCCPSG 1994; Albanes et al. 1996; Omenn et al. 1996a; Pryor et al. 2000). These results illustrate that a diet rich in fruit and vegetables is probably safer and more effective than supplementation with individual carotenoids. Metabolic engineering approaches to enrich crops with nutritionally relevant carotenoids also seem to be more appropriate than supplementing the diet with single components as evidenced by the health benefits provided by carotenoid mixtures and their synergy with other phytonutrients and components of fruits and vegetables (Yeum and Russell 2002; Fraser and Bramley 2004; Botella-Pavía and Rodríguez-Concepción 2006). The feasibility of enhancing the levels of endogenous carotenoids and of producing novel carotenoids in plant systems has been reviewed elsewhere (Hirschberg 2001; Sandmann 2001; Fraser and Bramley 2004; Botella-Pavía and Rodríguez-Concepción 2006).

Programs to improve carotenoid levels in crop plants, however, should also take into account the factors that influence the absorption and metabolism of such carotenoids in the human body for optimal bioavailability.

Absorption and bioavailability of dietary carotenoids

Humans accumulate carotenoids in various tissues including liver (where the highest concentrations of carotenoids are found), adipose, serum, breast milk, adrenal, prostate, macula, kidney, lung, brain and skin (Deming and Erdman 1999). But for dietary carotenoids to be available for storage or metabolism, they must first be released from the ingested food and absorbed intestinally. Mastication, gastric action and digestive enzymes release carotenoids from the food matrix soon after the ingestion of food (Deming and Erdman 1999). Since carotenoids are non-polar lipidic compounds that cannot dissolve in aqueous solutions, they are incorporated in the stomach into mixed micelles consisting of bile acids, free fatty acids, monoglycerides and phospholipids, and absorbed via passive diffusion by the mucosa of the small intestine, mainly in the duodenum (Parker et al. 1999; Yeum and Russell 2002). The amount of carotenoid incorporated into micelles depends on the polarity of the carotenoid and on micellar fatty acid composition and saturation (Deming and Erdman 1999). Non-provitamin A carotenoids (lycopene, lutein, zeaxanthin) can be absorbed intact or undergo oxidative cleavage before absorption from the intestinal lumen. Lutein and zeaxanthin esters (common in fruits and vegetables) are also cleaved in the lumen of the small intestine before their uptake by the mucosa. The oxidative cleavage of provitamin A carotenoids (β-carotene, α-carotene, β-cryptoxanthin) partly converts them to vitamin A in the intestinal mucosa. The absorption of both carotenoids and derived products occurs with their assembly into large lipoprotein particles (chylomicrons) created by enterocytes, the absorptive cells that line the small intestine. Chylomicrons with their packaged carotenoids (and other dietary lipids such as triglycerides, phospholipids and cholesterol) are then released by exocytosis from enterocytes into the lymphatic circulation for delivery to the bloodstream (Deming and Erdman 1999). Levels of chylomicron-associated carotenoids are highest 4–8 h after food ingestion. In the blood, chylomicrons are rapidly degraded by endothelium-associated lipoprotein lipase and the carotenoid-containing remnants are taken up mostly by the liver (Parker et al. 1999). In the liver, carotenoids are stored or secreted back into the bloodstream associated with very low density lipoproteins (VLDL). In the fasting state, however, most plasma carotenoids are associated with low density lipoproteins (LDL) and, to a lesser extent, with high density lipoproteins (HDL). Lycopene and β-carotene are found mostly associated with LDL, whereas lutein and zeaxanthin are more evenly distributed between LDL and HDL fractions. A reason for this distribution might be that lycopene and β-carotene are mainly found in the core of the lipoprotein, whereas the more polar xanthophylls are mainly located on the surface. Therefore, transfer between lipoproteins might be easier for lutein and zeaxanthin, resulting in a more equal balance between LDL and HDL. Although serum concentrations show an enormous variability, HDL and LDL carotenoid levels were found to peak 16–48 h and 24–48 h, respectively, after food ingestion (Yeum and Russell 2002). It is most likely that the liver or the adipose tissue, with a large number of LDL receptors, can accumulate carotenoids passively. By contrast, the variety of carotenoid forms and concentrations detected in different tissues suggests the existence of other factors regulating the uptake and storage of carotenoid in a particular tissue. For instance, lycopene is found in most human tissues but its levels in the adrenals and testes are much higher. Similarly, high levels of two particular carotenoids, lutein and zeaxanthin, are found in the macula of the eye, suggesting that a specific mechanism exists for the preferential deposition of specific carotenoids in those tissues (Yeum and Russell 2002). Because carotenoids are highly lipophilic molecules, the existence of specific binding and transport proteins, such as those described for other lipids, has been proposed. Recent results suggest that lipoprotein-bound carotenoids might be distributed to target tissues by a protein-mediated transport involving class B scavenger receptors (von Lintig et al. 2005). These cell-surface receptors, which play a key role in HDL metabolism in mammals (Rigotti et al. 1997), might be involved in the cellular uptake of carotenoids from the circulating lipoprotein complexes, contributing to body distribution of dietary carotenoids.

Bioavailability, i.e. the proportion of ingested carotenoids that can be either stored or used in normal physiological functions, is influenced by multiple factors affecting their release from the food matrix, uptake, transport and storage (Castenmiller and West 1998; Deming and Erdman 1999; Yeum and Russell 2002; Kopsell and Kopsell 2006). These factors include carotenoid type, the food matrix in which the carotenoid is incorporated, and host-related factors.

Carotenoid type

Differential absorption and/or interactions between carotenoids have been observed in controlled feeding studies (Castenmiller and West 1998; Deming and Erdman 1999; Yeum and Russell 2002; Kopsell and Kopsell 2006). The bioavailability of xanthophylls is relatively higher than that of carotenes. This is probably because non-polar carotenes migrate to the triacylglycerol-rich core of lipid micelles, whereas the more polar nature of xanthophylls facilitates their incorporation into the surface monolayer of the micelles and therefore they can be more easily taken up by the enterocyte and incorporated into chylomicrons (van het Hof et al. 1999; Johnson et al. 2000). Plant food carotenoids are usually in the all-*trans* form, but heating, light or mechanical homogenisation can increase the levels of carotenoid species in *cis* configuration (Rodriguez-Amaya 2003; Kopsell and Kopsell 2006). For lycopene, the *cis* isomer is better absorbed than the all-*trans* form (Stahl and Sies 1992; Boileau et al. 2002). By contrast, the bioavailability of the all-*trans* form of β-carotene seems to be higher than that of the *cis* forms (Castenmiller and West 1998; Yeum and Russell 2002; Kopsell and Kopsell 2006). A substantial proportion of β-carotene and lycopene isomerisation has also been observed between ingestion and appearance in plasma (You et al. 1996; Re et al. 2001).

Food matrix

Food carotenoids are complexed with other components that influence their bioavailability. Several studies have found that carotenoids in uncooked vegetables and fruit are poorly absorbed when compared to the equivalent dose in a pure formulation, basically because they do not need to be released from the plant matrix (Stahl and Sies 1992; de Pee et al. 1995; van het Hof et al. 2000). However, when plant cell walls and carotenoid–protein complexes are disrupted by mechanical homogenisation and/or heat treatment, the levels of serum carotenoids are significantly increased compared with the same unprocessed (raw) food (Stahl and Sies 1992; Gartner et al. 1997; Rock et al. 1998; Castenmiller et al. 1999). In addition, absorption of carotenoids seems to be much more efficient when they are ingested in a meal (Shiau et al. 1994). But perhaps the most important food parameter for optimising carotenoid absorption is the ingestion of dietary fat during the same eating period. Even small amounts of dietary fat (3–5 g) significantly increase the absorption of pure and food carotenoids (Castenmiller and West 1998; Deming and Erdman 1999; Parker et al. 1999; Yeum and Russell 2002; Kopsell and Kopsell 2006). By contrast, the presence of dietary fibre decreases carotenoid bioavailability, which may partly explain why the bioavailability of carotenoids from dark-green leafy vegetables is lower than that of fruit carotenoids (Rock and Swendseid 1992; de Pee et al. 1998; Hoffmann et al. 1999).

Carotenoid metabolism in humans

In the human body, dietary carotenoids with β ring end groups (such as β-carotene, α-carotene, or β-cryptoxanthin; Figure 3.1) act as precursors for the production of vitamin A (retinol) and its derivatives (retinoids). Retinoids are essential for a wide diversity of physiological processes, including vision, embryonic development, reproduction, immune responses, and differentiation and maintenance of various epithelia (Bollag 1996). In animals, 11-*cis*-retinal and closely related compounds act as the chromophores of rhodopsin, a protein found in the rod cells of the eye. Light-induced isomerisation of the chromophore from 11-*cis*-retinal to all-*trans*-retinal results in activation of the photoreceptor molecule and the transduction of light into visual signals. Retinoic acid, another vitamin A derivative, mediates most of the non-visual functions of vitamin A. Retinoic acid binds to nuclear receptors, eventually resulting in the binding of the ligand–receptor complexes to DNA and the regulation of gene expression (Chambon 1996). Vitamin A is transformed into retinoic acid by two rounds of oxidation *via* retinal (Figure 3.3). The reversible transformation of retinol into retinal is catalysed by two classes of retinol dehydrogenase (RDH) enzymes: microsomal members of the short-chain dehydrogenases/reductases family, and cytosolic members of the alcohol dehydrogenase family (Napoli 1999; Duester 2000; Liden et al. 2003). The production of retinoic acid from retinal is catalysed by NAD^+-dependent retinal dehydrogenase (RALDH), a member of the aldehyde dehydrogenase family (Napoli 1999; Duester 2001). Retinal can also be oxidised to retinoic acid by oxygen-dependent aldehyde oxidase (Huang and Ichikawa 1994; Huang et al. 1999).

The committed step in vitamin A formation is the oxidative cleavage at the C-15,C-15′ double bond of β-carotene into two retinal molecules (Figure 3.3) catalysed by the enzyme β-carotene-15,15′-oxygenase (BCO). The sequence of the human BCO was only recently identified and shown to share homology with non-haeme iron monooxygenases involved in the cleavage of carotenoids for the production of apocarotenoids such as abscisic acid in plants (Yan et al. 2001). Because human BCO has been shown to be a

β-carotene

β-ionone

BCO   BCO2

2 × Retinal
(vitamin A
aldehyde)

β-10′-carotenal

RDH

RALDH

Retinol
(vitamin A)

Retinoic acid
(vitamin A acid)

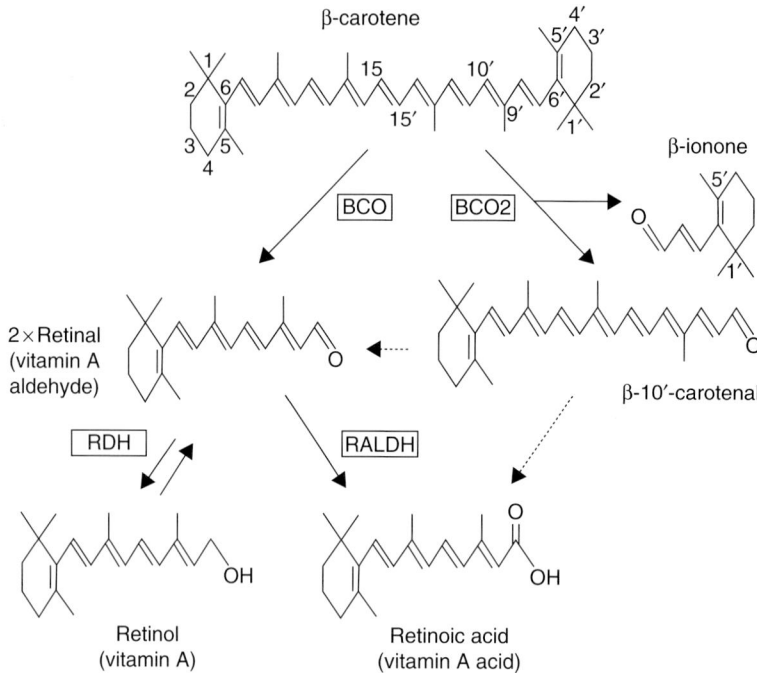

Figure 3.3 Enzymatic carotenoid cleavage in humans. BCO, β-carotene-15,15′-oxygenase
(EC 1.14.99.36); BCO2, β-carotene-9′,10′-oxygenase; RDH, retinol dehydrogenase
(EC 1.1.1.105); RALDH, retinal dehydrogenase (EC 1.2.1.36). Retinal may also be converted
into retinoic acid by retinal/aldehyde oxidase (EC 1.2.3.11).

soluble hydrophylic protein localised in the cytosol (Lindqvist and Andersson 2002), it is
probable that specific binding proteins are required *in vivo* to deliver and to pick up the
highly lipophilic carotenoid substrate and retinal product, respectively. Synthesis of vitamin A from dietary carotenoids takes place mostly in epithelial cells of the intestinal
mucosa. Retinal formed from β-carotene (or other provitamin A carotenoids) is further
converted to retinyl ester and thereafter incorporated into chylomicrons and transported
to the liver for storage (Napoli 1999; Nagao 2004; Harrison 2005). Hepatocytes store
vitamin A as retinyl esters that, when required, can be de-esterified and released into the
bloodstream as retinol to be delivered *via* retinol-binding proteins to target cells and tissues. As described above, provitamin A carotenoids are also stored in the liver.
Interestingly, BCO-encoding transcripts are found in not only in the small intestine and
liver but also in other tissues such as kidney, prostate, testis, ovary, skeletal muscle and the
retinal pigment epithelium of the human eyes (Yan et al. 2001; Lindqvist and Andersson
2002). This expression pattern suggests that retinoid metabolism in at least some cell
types and tissues might depend not only on vitamin A supply via the blood circulation but
also on the availability of provitamin A carotenoids that could be cleaved to retinal by
BCO activity.

A protein sharing homology with BCO, named BCO2, has been shown to be a
β-carotene-9′,10′-oxygenase specifically catalysing the asymmetric cleavage of β-carotene

at the C-9′,C-10′ double bond to produce β-ionone and β-10′-carotenal (Kiefer et al. 2001). As shown in Figure 3.3, β-10′-carotenal (and other β-apocarotenals that might result from the asymmetric cleavage of β-carotene) can be shortened to retinal and to β-apocarotenoid acids that can subsequently be transformed into retinoic acid (von Lintig et al. 2005). The specific role of BCO2 in the vitamin A biosynthetic pathway, however, still remains to be conclusively proven. Since BCO2 can also catalyse the oxidative cleavage of lycopene *in vitro* (Kiefer et al. 2001), a detailed investigation of BCO2 substrate specificity and product fate will be required to understand the physiological functions of this enzyme.

Besides the specific enzymatic cleavage of some carotenoids, the high reactivity of the conjugated double bond system to active oxygen species may result in the oxidation of carotenoids to a number of compounds. A cleavage reaction at the conjugated double bond backbone can result from autoxidation, enzymatic cooxidation, radical-mediated oxidation, or direct reaction with singlet oxygen and free radicals (Yeum and Russell 2002; Nagao 2004). The oxidation products, which might be formed in biological tissues under oxidative stress and also in normal physiological conditions, may then be metabolised and eventually eliminated from the body. A detailed analysis of human plasma showed eight kinds of carotenoid oxidation products that retained the carbon skeleton of their parental carotenoids (Khachik et al. 1997), but the *in vivo* formation of oxidation metabolites of lower molecular weight (other than retinoids) remains to be fully investigated. The reports showing that some apocarotenoids might be biologically active substances potentially affecting human health in not only beneficial but also harmful ways (Yeum and Russell 2002; Nagao 2004; von Lintig et al. 2005) enforce the need for unveiling the *in vivo* pathways for the oxidative metabolism of carotenoids and their relevance for human health.

Meeting the dietary demand and consequences for imbalance

Vitamin A deficiency (VAD) is the most important problem derived from a carotenoid-poor diet. The roles exerted by vitamin A derivatives (retinoids) in human physiology explain why VAD not only causes visual defects but also affects the immune system, leads to infertility, and causes malformations during embryogenesis. In developing countries, VAD is the leading cause of preventable blindness in children, causing xerophthalmia (dry eyes), growth retardation, and increased risk and severity of diseases from such common childhood infections as diarrhoea and measles, leading to premature death (West 2003). As well as young children, VAD most strongly affects pregnant women. VAD is critical during the last trimester when the demand of vitamin A by both the unborn child and the mother is highest. The impact of VAD on mother-to-child HIV transmission needs further investigation.

The high risk of disease and death caused by VAD in more than half of all the world's countries, especially Africa and South-East Asia, can be successfully corrected not only with vitamin A supplementation programmes but also with long-term sustainable solutions such as diet improvement (increasing the use of available carotenoid-rich foods) and food fortification. According to the World Health Organization (WHO) the periodic supply of high-dose vitamin A to VAD-affected children between 6 months and 6 years of age has produced remarkable results, reducing mortality by 23% overall and by up to 50% for those with acute measles. These supplements have averted an estimated 1.25 million deaths since 1998 in 40 countries. Food fortification to maintain vitamin A status in high-risk groups and needy families takes over where supplementation leaves off. As well as the active forms of vitamin A obtained from animal products, which are immediately available to the body, vitamin A can be synthesised from provitamin A carotenoids present in fruits and vegetables. Engineering staple foods to create varieties enriched in provitamin A carotenoids that could be freely distributed in high-risk countries might have a tremendous impact on the fight against VAD. The production of β-carotene in rice represented a very promising first step in this direction (Ye et al. 2000). Although anti-GMO activists campaigned against the so-called 'golden rice' as 'fools' gold' because of the relatively low levels of β-carotene accumulated in the grain, the significantly increased accumulation levels achieved in 'golden rice 2' (31 μg/g fresh weight) could actually be enough to provide most of the vitamin A required by high-risk groups in regions where rice is a staple food (Paine et al. 2005).

VAD is rarely seen in developed countries, where vitamin A and retinoid supplements are mostly used in cosmetic and medical applications applied to the skin (Orafanos et al. 1997). Because vitamin A is required for optimal functioning of epithelial tissues, retinoids are used to treat xerosis (dry skin), keratosis (gooseflesh skin), psoriasis and acne. Vitamin A derivatives are also used as 'anti-ageing' treatments because they increase the rate of skin turnover, resulting in a temporary increase in collagen and giving a more youthful appearance. Research is also being done into the ability of retinoids to treat skin cancers. Vitamin A overdose (hypervitaminosis A) can be harmful or even fatal. Toxicity is typically reported in people consuming either large amounts of liver or, most commonly, excess vitamin A supplements. An excess of vitamin A intake can cause osteoporosis, central nervous system disorders and birth defects (Penniston and Tanumihardjo 2006). These harmful effects have only been reported with vitamin A itself or the ester (animal) forms. High-dose supplementation of provitamin A carotenoids causes no hypervitaminosis in humans, probably because cleavage to vitamin A is tightly regulated (Solomons 2001; von Lintig et al. 2005). However, excess carotenoid intake may lead to hypercarotenaemia, a transient and not dangerous condition that causes yellow to orange discoloration of the skin. Most importantly, as described earlier, supplementation with β-carotene has been reported to increase the incidence of lung cancer in some people, particularly smokers. Overall, dietary intake of all carotenoid-rich fruits and vegetables is highly recommended because of their health-promoting benefits. Supplementation with formulated individual carotenoids such as β-carotene could sometimes be recommended but it may not be efficient for the general population and may even have undesired effects on human health.

Acknowledgements

Work in our laboratory is supported by grants from the Spanish Ministerio de Educación y Ciencia and FEDER (BIO2005-00367), Consejo Superior de Investigaciones Científicas (Intramural 200620/165) and Generalitat de Catalunya (Distinció) to MRC. UFP received a PhD fellowship of the Ministerio de Educación y Ciencia FPU program.

References

Albanes, D., Heinonen, O.P., Taylor, P.R., Virtamo, J., Edwards, B.K., Rautalahti, M., Hartman, A.M., Palmgren, J., Freedman, L.S., Haapakoski, J. et al. (1996) Alpha-tocopherol and beta-carotene supplements and lung cancer incidence in the alpha-tocopherol, beta-carotene cancer prevention study: effects of base-line characteristics and study compliance. *Journal of the National Cancer Institute* **88**, 1560–70.

Armstrong, G.A. and Hearst, J.E. (1996) Carotenoids 2: Genetics and molecular biology of carotenoid pigment biosynthesis. *FASEB Journal* **10**, 228–37.

ATBCCPSG. (1994) The effect of vitamin E and beta carotene on the incidence of lung cancer and other cancers in male smokers. The Alpha Tocopherol Beta Carotene Cancer Prevention Study Group. *New England Journal of Medicine* **330**, 1029–35.

Barber, N. (2003) The tomato: an important part of the urologist's diet? *BJU International* **91**, 307–9.

Baroli, I. and Niyogi, K.K. (2000) Molecular genetics of xanthophyll-dependent photoprotection in green algae and plants. *Philosophical Transactions of the Royal Society of London B Biological Science* **355**, 1385–94.

Bartley, G.E. and Scolnik, P.A. (1995) Plant carotenoids: pigments for photoprotection, visual attraction, and human health. *Plant Cell* **7**, 1027–38.

Binns, C.W., Jian, L.J.L. and Lee, A.H. (2004) The relationship between dietary carotenoids and prostate cancer risk in Southeast Chinese men. *Asia Pacific Journal of Clinical Nutrition* **13**(Suppl.), S117.

Blount, J.D. (2004) Carotenoids and life-history evolution in animals. *Archives of Biochemistry and Physics* **430**, 10–15.

Boileau, T.W., Boileau, A.C. and Erdman, J.W. (2002) Bioavailability of all-trans and cis-isomers of lycopene. *Experimental Biology and Medicine* **227**, 914–19.

Bollag, W. (1996) The retinoid revolution. Overview. *FASEB Journal* **10**, 938–9.

Botella-Pavía, P., Besumbes, O., Phillips, M.A., Carretero-Paulet, L., Boronat, A. and Rodríguez-Concepción, M. (2004) Regulation of carotenoid biosynthesis in plants: evidence for a key role of hydroxymethylbutenyl diphosphate reductase in controlling the supply of plastidial isoprenoid precursors. *Plant Journal* **40**, 188–99.

Botella-Pavía, P. and Rodríguez-Concepción, M. (2006) Carotenoid biotechnology in plants for nutritionally improved foods. *Physiologia Plantarum* **126**, 369–81.

Bramley, P.M. (2002) Regulation of carotenoid formation during tomato fruit ripening and development. *Journal of Experimental Botany* **53**, 2107–13.

Britton, G. (1995) Structure and properties of carotenoids in relation to function. *FASEB Journal* **9**, 1551–8.

Brown, N.F., Anderson, R.C., Caplan, S.L., Foster, D.W. and McGarry, J.D. (1994) Catalytically important domains of rat carnitine palmitoyltransferase II as determined by site-directed mutagenesis and chemical modification. Evidence for a critical histidine residue. *Journal of Biological Chemistry* **269**, 19157–62.

Camara, B., Hugueney, P., Bouvier, F., Kuntz, M. and Moneger, R. (1995) Biochemistry and molecular biology of chromoplast development. *International Review of Cytology* **163**, 175–247.

Carretero-Paulet, L., Cairo, A., Botella-Pavia, P., Besumbes, O., Campos, N., Boronat, A. and Rodriguez-Concepcion, M. (2006) Enhanced flux through the methylerythritol 4-phosphate pathway in Arabidopsis plants overexpressing deoxyxylulose 5-phosphate reductoisomerase. *Plant Molecular Biology* **62**, 683–95.

Castenmiller, J.J.M. and West, C.E. (1998) Bioavailability and bioconversion of carotenoids. *Annual Review of Nutrition* **18**, 19–38.

Castenmiller, J.J., West, C.E., Linssen, J.P., van het Hof, K.H. and Voragen, A.G. (1999) The food matrix of spinach is a limiting factor in determining the bioavalability of beta-carotene and to a lesser extent of lutein in humans. *Journal of Nutrition* **129**, 349–55.

Chambon, P. (1996) A decade of molecular biology of retinoic acid receptors. *FASEB Journal* **9**, 940–54.

Chang, J.M., Chen, W.C., Hong, D. and Lin, J.K. (1995) The inhibition of DMBA-induced carcino-genesis by neoxanthin in hamster buccal pouch. *Nutrtion and Cancer* **24**, 325–33.

Chen, L., Stacewicz-Sapuntzakis, M., Duncan, C., Sharifi, R., Ghosh, L., van Breemen, R., Ashton, D. and Bowen, P. E. (2001) Oxidative DNA damage in prostate cancer patients consuming tomato sauce-based entrees as a whole-food intervention. *Journal of the National Cancer Institute* **93**, 1872–9.

Chew, B.P., Wong, M.M. and Wong, T.S. (1996) Effects of lutein from marigold extract on immunity and growth of mammary tumors in mice. *Anticancer Research* **16**, 3689–94.

Clinton, S.K. (1998) Lycopene: chemistry, biology, and implications for human health and disease. *Nutrition Review* **56**, 35–51.

Cooper, D. A., Eldridge, A. L. and Peters, J. C. (1999) Dietary carotenoids and certain cancers, heart disease, and age-related macular degeneration: a review of recent research. *Nutrition Review* **57**, 201–14.

Cunningham, F.X. and Gantt, E. (1998) Genes and enzymes of carotenoid biosynthesis in plants. *Annual Review of Plant Physiology and Plant Molecular Biology* **49**, 557–83.

de Pee, S., West, C.E., Muhilal, Karyadi, D. and Hautvast, J.G. (1995) Lack of improvement in vitamin A status with increased consumption of dark-green leafy vegetables. *Lancet* **346**, 75–81.

de Pee, S., West, C.E., Permaesih, D., Martuti, S., Muhilal and Hautvast, J.G. (1998) Orange fruit is more effective than are dark-green, leafy vegetables in increasing serum concentrations of retinol and beta-carotene in schoolchildren in Indonesia. *American Journal of Clinical Nutrition* **68**, 1058–67.

Deming, D.M. and Erdman, J.W. (1999) Mammalian carotenoid absorption and metabolism. *Pure and Applied Chemistry* **71**, 2213–23.

Demmig-Adams, B. and Adams, W.W. (2002) Antioxidants in photosynthesis and human nutrition. *Science* **298**, 2149–53.

Demmig-Adams, B., Gilmore, A.M. and Adams, W.W. (1996) *In vivo* functions of carotenoids in higher plants. *FASEB Journal* **10**, 403–12.

DiMascio, P., Kaiser, S. and Sies, H. (1989) Lycopene as the most efficient biological carotenoid singlet oxygen quencher. *Archives of Biochemistry and Physics* **274**, 532–8.

Duester, G. (2000) Families of retinoid dehydrogenases regulating vitamin A function: production of visual pigment and retinoic acid. *European Journal of Biochemistry* **267**, 4315–24.

Duester, G. (2001) Genetic dissection of retinoid dehydrogenases. *Chemico-Biological Interactions* **130–132**, 469–80.

Eichler, O., Sies, H. and Stahl, W. (2002) Divergent optimum levels of lycopene, beta-carotene and lutein protecting against UVB irradiation in human fibroblastst. *Photochemistry and Photobiology* **75**, 503–6.

Eisenreich, W., Rohdich, F. and Bacher, A. (2001) Deoxyxylulose phosphate pathway to terpenoids. *Trends in Plant Science* **6**, 78–84.

Estévez, J.M., Cantero, A., Reindl, A., Reichler, S. and León, P. (2001) 1-Deoxy-D-xylulose-5-phosphate synthase, a limiting enzyme for plastidic isoprenoid biosynthesis in plants. *Journal of Biological Chemistry* **276**, 22901–9.

Fiore, A., Dall'osto, L., Fraser, P.D., Bassi, R. and Giuliano, G. (2006) Elucidation of the beta-carotene hydroxylation pathway in Arabidopsis thaliana. *FEBS Letters* **580**, 4718–22.

Fraser, P.D. and Bramley, P.M. (2004) The biosynthesis and nutritional uses of carotenoids. *Progress in Lipid Research* **43**, 228–65.

Gartner, C., Stahl, W. and Sies, H. (1997) Lycopene is more bioavailable from tomato paste than from fresh tomatoes. *American Journal of Clinical Nutrition* **66**, 116–22.

Giovannucci, E. (1999) Tomatoes, tomato-based products, lycopene, and cancer: review of the epidemiologic literature. *Journal of the National Cancer Institute* **91**, 317–31.

Giovannucci, E., Rimm, E.B., Liu, Y., Stampfer, M.J. and Willet, W.C. (2002) A prospective study of tomato products, lycopene, and prostate cancer risk. *Journal of the National Cancer Institute* **94**, 391–8.

Giuliano, G., Aquilani, R. and Dharmapuri, S. (2000) Metabolic engineering of plant carotenoids. *Trends in Plant Science* **5**, 406–9.

Gollnick, H.P.M., Hopfenmuller, W., Hemmes, C., Chun, S.C., Sundermeier, K. and Biesalski, H.K. (1996) Systemic beta carotene plus topical UV-sunscreen are an optimal protection against harmful effects of natural UV-sunlight: results of the Berlin-Eilath study. *European Journal of Dermatology* **6**, 200–5.

Goodrow, E.F., Wilson, T.A., Houde, S.C., Vishwanathan, R., Scollin, P.A., Handelman, G. and Nicolosi, R.J. (2006) Consumption of one egg per day increases serum lutein and zeaxanthin concentrations in older adults without altering serum lipid and lipoprotein cholesterol concentrations. *Journal of Nutrition* **136**, 2519–24.

Gruszecki, W.I. and Strzalka, K. (2005) Carotenoids as modulators of lipid membrane physical properties. *Biochimica et Biophysica Acta* **1740**, 108–15.

Handelman, G.J. (2001) The evolving role of carotenoids in human biochemistry. *Nutrition* **17**, 818–22.

Harrison, E.H. (2005) Mechanisms of digestion and absorption of dietary vitamin A. *Annual Review of Nutrition* **25**, 87–103.

Hennekens, C.H., Buring, J.E., Manson, J.E., Stampfer, M., Rosner, B., Cook, N.R., Belanger, C., LaMotte, F., Gaziano, J.M., Ridker, P.M., Willett, W. and Peto, R. (1996) Lack of effect of long-term supplementation with beta carotene on the incidence of malignant neoplasms and cardiovascular disease. *New England Journal of Medicine* **334**, 1145–9.

van het Hof, K.H., Brouwer, I.A., West, C.E., Haddeman, E., Steegers-Theunissen, R.P., van Dusseldorp, M., Weststrate, J.A., Eskes, T.K. and Hautvast, J.G. (1999) Bioavailability of lutein from vegetables is 5 times higher than that of beta-carotene. *American Journal of Clinical Nutrition* **70**, 261–8.

van het Hof, K.H., West, C.E., Weststrate, J.A. and Hautvast, J.G. (2000) Dietary factors that affect the bioavailability of carotenoids. *Journal of Nutrition* **130**, 503–6.

Hirschberg, J. (2001) Carotenoid biosynthesis in flowering plants. *Current Opinion in Plant Biology* **4**, 210–18.

Hoffmann, J., Linseisen, J., Riedl, J. and Wolfram, G. (1999) Dietary fiber reduces the antioxidative effect of a carotenoid and alphatocopherol mixture on LDL oxidation ex vivo in humans. *European Journal of Nutrition* **38**, 278–85.

Holden, J.M., Eldridge, A.L., Beecher, G.R., Buzzard, I.M., Bhagwat, S., Davis, C.S., Douglass, L.W., Gebhardt, S., Haytowitz, D. and Schake, S. (1999) Carotenoid content of U.S. foods: an update of the database. *Journal of Food Composition and Analysis* **12**, 169–96.

Huang, D.Y., Furukawa, A. and Ichikawa, Y. (1999) Molecular cloning of retinal oxidase/aldehyde oxidase cDNAs from rabbit and mouse livers and functional expression of recombinant mouse retinal oxidase cDNA in *Escherichia coli*. *Archives of Biochemistry and Physics* **364**, 264–72.

Huang, D.Y. and Ichikawa, Y. (1994) Two different enzymes are primarily responsible for retinoic acid synthesis in rabbit liver cytosol. *Biochemical and Biophysical Research Communications* **205**, 1278–83.

Hughes, D.A. (2001) Dietary carotenoids and human immune function. *Nutrition* **17**, 823–7.

Isaacson, T., Ronen, G., Zamir, D. and Hirschberg, J. (2002) Cloning of tangerine from tomato reveals a carotenoid isomerase essential for the production of beta-carotene and xanthophylls in plants. *Plant Cell* **14**, 333–42.

Jacques, P.F. (1999) The potential preventive effects of vitamins for cataract and age-related macular degeneration. *International Journal for Vitamin and Nutrition Research* **69**, 198–205.

Johnson, E.J. (2002) The role of carotenoids in human health. *Nutrition in Clinical Care* **5**, 56–65.

Johnson, E.J., Hammond, B.R., Yeum, K.J., Qin, J., Wang, X.D., Castaneda, C., Snodderly, D.M. and Russell, R.M. (2000) Relation among serum and tissue concentrations of lutein and zeaxanthin and macular pigment density. *American Journal of Clinical Nutrition* **71**, 1555–62.

Khachik, F., Spangler, C.J., Smith, J.C., Canfield, L.M., Steck, A. and Pfander, H. (1997) Identification, quantification, and relative concentrations of carotenoids and their metabolites in human milk and serum. *Analytical Chemistry* **69**, 1873–81.

Kiefer, C., Hessel, S., Lampert, J.M., Vogt, K., Lederer, M.O., Breithaupt, D.E., and von Lintig, J. (2001) Identification and characterization of a mammalian enzyme catalyzing the asymmetric oxidative cleavage of provitamin A. *Journal of Biological Chemistry* **276**, 14110–16.

Kim, J. and DellaPenna, D. (2006) Defining the primary route for lutein synthesis in plants: the role of Arabidopsis carotenoid beta-ring hydroxylase CYP97A3. *Proceedings of the National Academy of Sciences USA* **103**, 3474–9.

Kim, L., Rao, A.V. and Rao, L.G. (2002) Effect of lycopene on prostate LNCaP cancer cells in culture. *Journal of Medicinal Food* **5**, 181–7.

Kopsell, D.A. and Kopsell, D.E. (2006) Accumulation and bioavailability of dietary carotenoids in vegetable crops. *Trends in Plant Science* **11**, 499–507.

Kotake-Nara, E., Kushiro, M., Zhang, H., Sugawara, T., Miyashita, K. and Nagao, A. (2001) Carotenoids affect proliferation of human prostate cancer cells. *Journal of Nutrition* **131**, 3303–6.

Krinsky, N. I., Landrum, J. T. and Bone, R. A. (2003) Biologic mechanisms of the protective role of lutein and zeaxanthin in the eye. *Annual Review of Nutrition* 23, 171–201.

Lichtenthaler, H.K. (1999) The 1-deoxy-D-xylulose-5-phosphate pathway of isoprenoid biosynthesis in plants. *Annual Review of Plant Physiology and Plant Molecular Biology* **50**, 47–65.

Liden, M., Tryggvason, K. and Eriksson, U. (2003) Structure and function of retinol dehydrogenases of the short chain dehydrogenase/reductase family. *Molecular Aspects of Medicine* **24**, 403–9.

Lindqvist, A. and Andersson, S. (2002) Biochemical properties of purified recombinant human beta-carotene 15,15'-monooxygenase. *Journal of Biological Chemistry* **277**, 23942–8.

von Lintig, J., Hessel, S., Isken, A., Kiefer, C., Lampert, J.M., Voolstra, O. and Vogt, K. (2005) Towards a better understanding of carotenoid metabolism in animals. *Biochimica et Biophysica Acta* **1740**, 122–31.

Lyle, B.J., Mares-Perlman, J.A., Klein, B.E., Klein, R. and Greger, J.L. (1999) Antioxidant intake and risk of incident age-related nuclear cataracts in the Beaver Dam Eye Study. *American Journal of Epidemiology* **149**, 801–9.

Mahmoud, S.S. and Croteau, R.B. (2001) Metabolic engineering of essential oil yield and composition in mint by altering expression of deoxyxylulose phosphate reductoisomerase and menthofuran synthase. *Proceedings of the National Academy of Sciences USA* **98**, 8915–20.

Mannisto, S., Smith-Warner, S.A., Spiegelman, D., Albanes, D., Anderson, K., van den Brandt, P.A., Cerhan, J.R., Colditz, G., Feskanich, D., Freudenheim, J.L., Giovannucci, E., Goldbohm, R.A., Graham, S., Miller, A.B., Rohan, T.E., Virtamo, J., Willett, W. and Hunter, D.J. (2004) Dietary carotenoids and risk of lung cancer in a pooled analysis of seven cohort studies. *Cancer Epidemiology, Biomarkers and Prevention* **13**, 40–8.

Mares-Perlman, J.A., Millen, A.E., Ficek, T.L. and Hankinson, S.E. (2002) The body of evidence to support a protective role for lutein and zeaxanthin in delaying chronic disease. Overview. *Journal of Nutrition* **132**, 518S–524S.

Melendez-Martinez, A.J., Vicario, I.M. and Heredia, F.J. (2004) Nutritional importance of carotenoid pigments. *Archivos Latinoamericanos de Nutricion* **54**, 149–54 [in Spanish].

Miller, E.C., Giovannucci, E., Erdman, J.W., Jr, Bahnson, R., Schwartz, S.J. and Clinton, S.K. (2002) Tomato products, lycopene, and prostate cancer risk. *Urologic Clinics of North America* **29**, 83–93.

Muller, P., Li, X.P. and Niyogi, K.K. (2001) Non-photochemical quenching. A response to excess light energy. *Plant Physiology* **125**, 1558–66.

Nagao, A. (2004) Oxidative conversion of carotenoids to retinoids and other products. *Journal of Nutrition* **134**, 237S–240S.

Napoli, J.L. (1999) Interactions of retinoid binding proteins and enzymes in retinoid metabolism. *Biochimica et Biophysica Acta* **1440**, 139–62.

Nishino, H., Murakosh, M., Ii, T., Takemura, M., Kuchide, M., Kanazawa, M., Mou, X.Y., Wada, S., Masuda, M., Ohsaka, Y., Yogosawa, S., Satomi, Y. and Jinno, K. (2002) Carotenoids in cancer chemoprevention. *Cancer Metastasis Review* **21**, 257–64.

Omenn, G.S., Goodman, G.E., Thornquist, M.D., Balmes, J., Cullen, M.R., Glass, A., Keogh, J.P., Meyskens, F.L., Valanis, B., Williams, J.H., Jr, Barnhart, S., Cherniak, M.G., Brodkin, C.A. and Hammar, S. (1996a) Risk factors for lung cancer and for intervention effects in CARET, the Beta-Carotene and Retinol Efficacy Trial. *Journal of the National Cancer Institute* **88**, 1550–9.

Omenn, G.S., Goodman, G. E., Thornquist, M.D., Balmes, J., Cullen, M.R., Glass, A., Keogh, J.P., Meyskens, F.L., Valanis, B., Williams, J.H., Barnhart, S. and Hammar, S. (1996b) Effects of a combination of beta carotene and vitamin A on lung cancer and cardiovascular disease. *New England Journal of Medicine* **334**, 1150–5.

O'Neill, M.E., Carroll, Y., Corridan, B., Olmedilla, B., Granado, F., Blanco, I., van den Berg, H., Hininger, I., Rousell, A.-M., Chopra, M., Southon, S. and Thurnham, D.I. (2001) A European carotenoid database to assess carotenoid intakes and its use in a five-country comparative study. *British Journal of Nutrition* **85**, 499–507.

Orafanos, C.E., Zouboulis, C.C., Almond-Roesler, B. and Geilen, C.C. (1997) Current use and future potential role of retinoids in dermatology. *Drugs* **53**, 358–88.

Paine, J.A., Shipton, C.A., Chaggar, S., Howells, R.M., Kennedy, M.J., Vernon, G., Wright, S.Y., Hinchliffe, E., Adams, J.L., Silverstone, A.L. and Drake, R. (2005) Improving the nutritional value of Golden Rice through increased pro-vitamin A content. *Nature Biotechnology* **23**, 482–7.

Paiva, S.A. and Russell, R.M. (1999) Beta-carotene and other carotenoids as antioxidants. *Journal of the American College of Nutrition* **18**, 426–33.

Park, H., Kreunen, S.S., Cuttriss, A. J., DellaPenna, D. and Pogson, B.J. (2002) Identification of the carotenoid isomerase provides insight into carotenoid biosynthesis, prolamellar body formation, and photomorphogenesis. *Plant Cell* **14**, 321–32.

Parker, R.S., Swanson, J.E., You, C.S., Edwards, A.J. and Huang, T. (1999) Bioavailability of carotenoids in human subjects. *Proceedings of the Nutrition Society* **58**, 155–62.

Pattison, D.J., Harrison, R.A. and Symmons, D.P.M. (2004) The role of diet in susceptibility to rheumatoid arthritis: a systematic review. *Journal of Rheumatology* **31**, 1310–19.

Penniston, K.L. and Tanumihardjo, S.A. (2006) The acute and chronic toxic effects of vitamin A. *American Journal of Clinical Nutrition* **83**, 191–201.

Pryor, W.A., Stahl, W. and Rock, C.L. (2000) Beta carotene: from biochemistry to clinical trials. *Nutrition Review* **58**, 39–53.

Re, R., Fraser, P.D., Long, M., Bramley, P. M. and Rice-Evans, C. (2001) Isomerization of lycopene in the gastric milieu. *Biochemical and Biophysical Research Communications* **281**, 576–81.

Rice-Evans, C.A., Sampson, J., Bramley, P.M. and Holloway, D.E. (1997) Why do we expect carotenoids to be antioxidants *in vivo*? *Free Radical Research* **26**, 381–98.

Rigotti, A., Trigatti, B.L., Penman, M., Rayburn, H., Herz, J. and Krieger, M. (1997) A targeted mutation in the murine gene encoding the high density lipoprotein (HDL) receptor scavenger receptor class B type I reveals its key role in HDL metabolism. *Proceedings of the National Academy of Sciences USA* **94**, 12610–15.

Rissanen, T., Voutilainen, S., Nyyssonen, K. and Salonen, J.T. (2002) Lycopene, atherosclerosis, and coronary heart disease. *Experimental Biology and Medicine (Maywood)* **227**, 900–7.

Rock, C.L., Lovalvo, J.L., Emenhiser, C., Ruffin, M.T., Flatt, S.W. and Schwartz, S.J. (1998) Bioavailability of beta-carotene is lower in raw than in processed carrots and spinach in women. *Journal of Nutrition* **128**, 913–16.

Rock, C.L. and Swendseid, M.E. (1992) Plasma beta-carotene response in humans after meals supplemented with dietary pectin. *American Journal of Clinical Nutrition* **55**, 96–9.

Rodriguez-Amaya, D.B. (2003) Foods carotenoids: analysis, composition and alterations during storage and proessing of foods. *Forum of Nutrition* **56**, 35–7.

Rodríguez-Concepción, M. and Boronat, A. (2002) Elucidation of the methylerythritol phosphate pathway for isoprenoid biosynthesis in bacteria and plastids. A metabolic milestone achieved through genomics. *Plant Physiology* **130**, 1079–89.

Sandmann, G. (2001) Genetic manipulation of carotenoid biosynthesis: strategies, problems and achievements. *Trends in Plant Science* **6**, 14–17.

Seddon, J.M., Ajani, U.A., Sperduto, R.D., Hiller, R., Blair, N., Burton, T.C., Farber, M.D., Gragoudas, E.S., Haller, J. and Miller, D.T., et al. (1994) Dietary carotenoids, vitamins A, C, and E, and advanced age-related macular degeneration. Eye Disease Case-Control Study Group. *Journal of the American Medical Association* **272**, 1413–20.

Shiau, A., Mobarhan, S., Stacewicz-Sapuntzakis, M., Benya, R., Liao, Y., Ford, C., Bowen, P., Friedman, H. and Frommel, T.O. (1994) Assessment of the intestinal retention of beta-carotene in humans. *Journal of the American College of Nutrition* **13**, 369–75.

Snellen, E.L., Verbeek, A.L., Van Den Hoogen, G.W., Cruysberg, J.R. and Hoyng, C.B. (2002) Neovascular age-related macular degeneration and its relationship to antioxidant intake. *Acta Ophthalmologica Scandinavica* **80**, 368–71.

Snodderly, D.M. (1995) Evidence for protection against age-related macular degeneration by carotenoids and antioxidant vitamins. *American Journal of Clinical Nutrition* **62**, 1448S–1461S.

Solomons, N.W. (2001) Vitamin A and carotenoids. In: *Present Knowledge in Nutrition* (ed. B.A. Bowman and R.M. Russell), pp. 127–45. Washington, DC: ILSI Press.

Stahl, W., Heinrich, U., Jungmann, H., Sies, H. and Tronnier, H. (2000) Carotenoids and carotenoids plus vitamin E protect against ultraviolet light-induced erythema in humans. *American Journal of Clinical Nutrition* **71**, 795–8.

Stahl, W. and Sies, H. (1992) Uptake of lycopene and its geometrical isomers is greater from heat-processed than from unprocessed tomato juice in humans. *Journal of Nutrition* **122**, 2161–6.

Stahl, W. and Sies, H. (2005) Bioactivity and protective effects of natural carotenoids. *Biochimica et Biophysica Acta* **1740**, 101–7.

Tapiero, H., Townsend, D.M. and Tew, K.D. (2004) The role of carotenoids in the prevention of human pathologies. *Biomedicine and Pharmacotherapy* **58**, 100–10.

Tian, L., Musetti, V., Kim, J., Magallanes-Lundback, M. and DellaPenna, D. (2004) The *Arabidopsis* LUT1 locus encodes a member of the cytochrome p450 family that is required for carotenoid epsilon-ring hydroxylation activity. *Proceedings of the National Academy of Sciences USA* **101**, 402–7.

West, K.P.J. (2003) Vitamin A deficiency disorders in children and women. *Food and Nutrition Bulletin* **24**, S78–90.

Wright, M.E., Mayne, S.T., Swanson, C.A., Sinha, R. and Alavanja, M.C. (2003) Dietary carotenoids, vegetables, and lung cancer risk in women: the Missouri women's health study (United States). *Cancer Causes and Control* **14**, 85–96.

Yan, W., Jang, G.F., Haeseleer, F., Esumi, N., Chang, J., Kerrigan, M., Campochiaro, M., Campochiaro, P., Palczewski, K. and Zack, D.J. (2001) Cloning and characterization of a human beta,beta-carotene-15,15'-dioxygenase that is highly expressed in the retinal pigment epithelium. *Genomics* **72**, 193–202.

Ye, X., Al-Babili, S., Kloti, A., Zhang, J., Lucca, P., Beyer, P. and Potrykus, I. (2000) Engineering the provitamin A (beta-carotene) biosynthetic pathway into (carotenoid-free) rice endosperm. *Science* **287**, 303–5.

Yeum, K.J. and Russell, R.M. (2002) Carotenoid bioavailability and bioconversion. *Annual Review of Nutrition* **22**, 483–504.

Ylonen, K., Alfthan, G., Groop, L., Saloranta, C., Aro, A. and Virtanen, S.M. (2003) Dietary intakes and plasma concentrations of carotenoids and tocopherols in relation to glucose metabolism in subjects at high risk of type 2 diabetes: the Botnia Dietary Study. *American Journal of Clinical Nutrition* **77**, 1434–41.

You, C.S., Parker, R.S., Goodman, K.J., Swanson, J.E. and Corso, T.N. (1996) Evidence of cis-trans isomerization of 9-cis-beta-carotene during absorption in humans. *American Journal of Clinical Nutritionition* **64**, 177–83.

Yuan, J.M., Stram, D.O., Arakawa, K., Lee, H.P. and Yu, M.C. (2003) Dietary cryptoxanthin and reduced risk of lung cancer: the Singapore Chinese Health Study. *Cancer Epidemiology, Biomarkers and Prevention* **12**, 890–8.

Chapter 4

Polyphenols

David Vauzour, Katerina Vafeiadou
and Jeremy P. E. Spencer

Introduction

In recent years there has been intense interest in the potential health effects of dietary polyphenols. Polyphenols are found ubiquitously in plants and are therefore abundant in the human diet. Increased polyphenol consumption has been associated with a reduced risk of development of a range of chronic diseases, such as cancer and cardiovascular and neurodegenerative disorders. Initially the antioxidant property of polyphenols was believed to underlie their beneficial effects *in vivo*. However, they are subject to extensive metabolism in the small intestine, the liver and in the colon following oral ingestion, and the resulting circulating metabolites have reduced antioxidant potential. Despite this, other potential mechanisms of action have emerged for polyphenols, which include their interaction with cell signalling pathways and modulation of mitochondrial function. In this chapter we aim to: (1) provide an overview of the different classes of polyphenols, (2) describe their biosynthesis within plants, (3) provide an understanding of the metabolism and biotransformation of polyphenols within the body following ingestion and (4) highlight their potential mechanisms of action in the body, notably their antioxidant and non-antioxidant activities.

Polyphenol structure

Polyphenols represent a wide variety of compounds that possess multiple hydroxyl groups on aromatic rings. Thousands of molecules possessing polyphenol structure have been identified in plants. These compounds are classified into different groups based on the number of phenol rings and the way in which these rings interact.

Phenolic acids and stilbenes

Phenolic acids are abundant in the diet and may be classified into two different classes: hydroxybenzoic acids (HBA) and hydroxycinnamic acids (HCA) based on C1-C3 and

Phytonutrients, First Edition. Edited by Andrew Salter, Helen Wiseman and Gregory Tucker.
© 2012 Blackwell Publishing Ltd. Published 2012 by Blackwell Publishing Ltd.

(A)

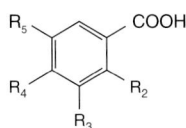

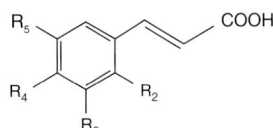

(1) Benzoic acids	R₂	R₃	R₄	R₅	(2) Cinnamic acids
p-Hydroxybenzoic acid	H	H	OH	H	p-Coumaric acid
Protocatechuic acid	H	OH	OH	H	Cafeic acid
Vanillic acid	H	OCH₃	OH	H	Ferulic acid
Gallic acid	H	OH	OH	OH	
Syringic acid	H	OCH₃	OH	OCH₃	Sinapic acid
Salicylic acid	OH	H	H	H	
Gentisic acid	OH	H	H	OH	

(B)

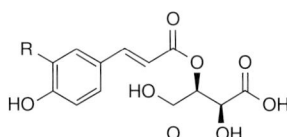

Hydroxycinnamic tartric esters	R
trans-caftaric acid	OH
trans-coutaric acid	H
trans-fertaric acid	OCH₃

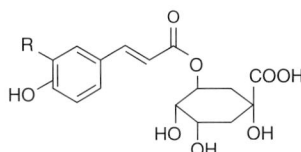

Hydroxycinnamic quinic esters	R
Chlorogenic qcid	OH
p-coumaroylquinic acid	H
Feruoylquinic acid	OCH₃

Figure 4.1 Chemical structures of the main phenolic acids (A) and their derivatives (B) encountered in plants.

C3-C6 skeletons respectively. Variations in the structure lie in the hydroxylation and methoxylation pattern of the aromatic cycle (Figure 4.1A). The most common phenolic acids are not present in plants in a free state but occur as simple esters of glucose, tartaric acid and quinic acid (Herrmann 1989). HBA are derivatives of the hydroxybenzoic acids such as p-hydroxybenzoic, protocatechuic and gallic acids and are mostly present in the form of glucosides and some esters with glucose. However, gallic acid is mainly esterified to quinic acid or catechins and is usually present in polymeric forms as soluble tannins (Herrmann 1989). The most common HCA is caffeic acid and occurs in foods mainly as chlorogenic acid (an ester of caffeic acid with quinic acid) or caftaric acid (an ester of caffeic acid with tartaric acid) (Figure 4.1B) (Macheix and Fleuriet 1998).

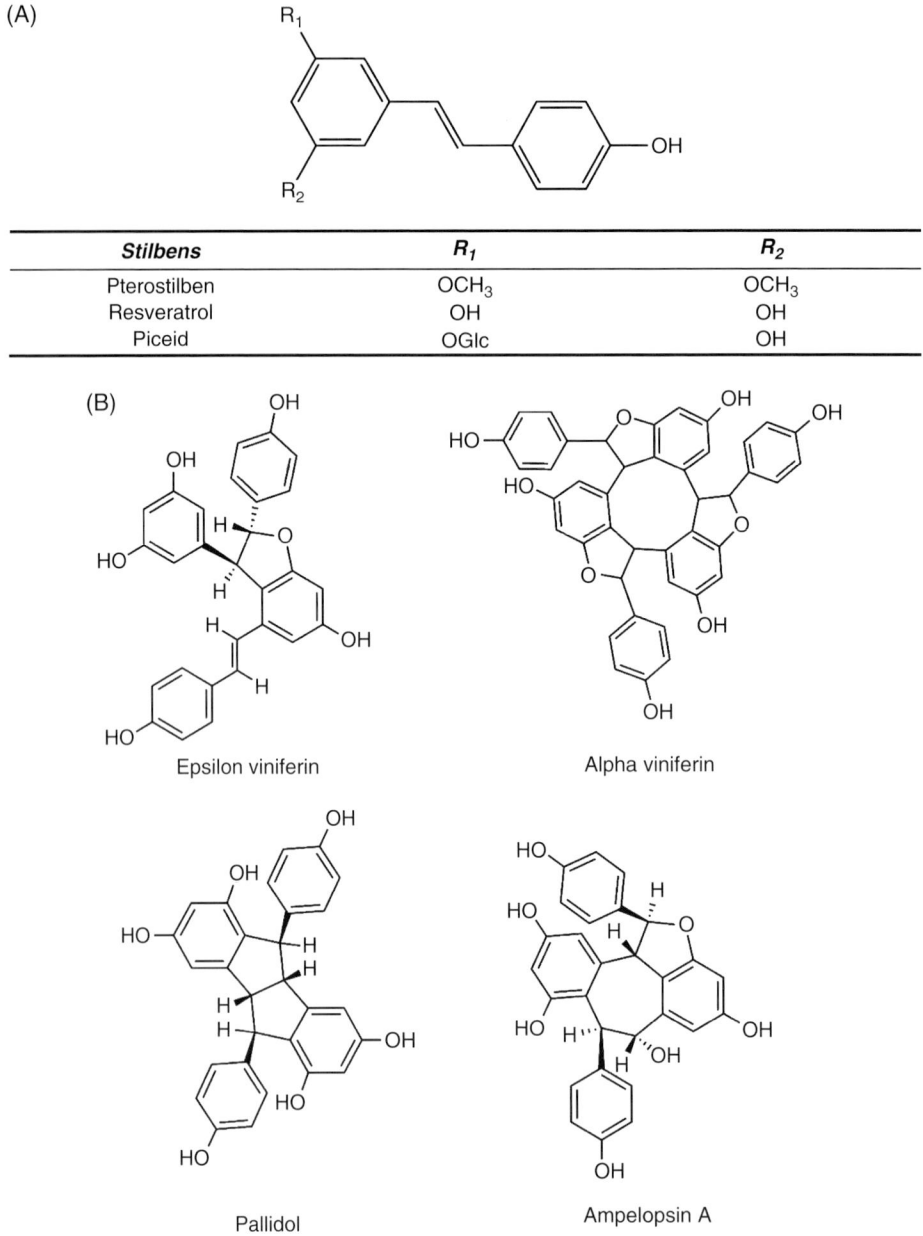

(A)

Stilbens	R_1	R_2
Pterostilben	OCH_3	OCH_3
Resveratrol	OH	OH
Piceid	OGlc	OH

(B)

Epsilon viniferin

Alpha viniferin

Pallidol

Ampelopsin A

Figure 4.2 Chemical structure of stilbenes (A) and some resveratrol polymers (B).

Stilbenes possess a 1,2-diarylethenes structure based on the C6-C2-C6 backbone and are usually synthesised in plants in response to infection or injury (Langcake 1981). The stilbene resveratrol can be found in the *cis* or *trans* configurations, either glucosylated (piceid) (Figure 4.2A) or in lower concentrations as the parent molecule of a family of polymers such as viniferins, pallidol or ampelopsin A (Langcake and Pryce 1977) (Figure 4.2B).

Flavonoids

Flavonoids are polyphenolic compounds that share a common structure consisting of two aromatic rings (A and B), which are bound together by three carbon atoms, forming an oxygenated heterocycle (ring C) (Figure 4.3A). Based on the variation in the type of heterocycle, flavonoids may be divided into seven subclasses: flavonols, flavones, flavanones, flavanonols, flavanols, anthocyanidins, and isoflavones. Individual differences within each group arise from the variation in number and arrangement of the hydroxyl groups and their alkylation and/or glycosylation.

Flavonols and flavones share a similar structure based on the 2-phenylchromen-4-one skeleton. Hydroxylation on position 3 of this structure gives rise to the 3-hydroxyflavones also called flavonols. The diversity of these compounds stems from the different positions of the phenolic -OH groups (Figure 4.3B). Flavanols, also referred as flavan-3-ols, have a structure based on the 2-phenyl-3,4-dihydro-2H-chromen-3-ol skeleton. Variations in structures lie in the hydroxylation pattern of the B ring and the creation of ester bonds with gallic acid in position 3 (Figure 4.3C). The lack of a double bond at the 2–3 position and the presence of a 3-hydroxyl group on the C ring create two centres of asymmetry. This latter gives rise to four different structures with the (−)-epicatechin (2R,3R-3,5,7,3′,4′-pentahydroxyflavan) and the (+)-catechin (2R,3S-3,5,7,3′,4′-pentahydroxy-flavan) being the most common optical isomers found in nature. Moreover, flavanols are also encountered as oligomers or polymers, and referred to as condensed tannins or proanthocyanidins (because they release anthocyanidins when heated under acidic condi-tions) (Bate-Smith 1954, 1953). These compounds differ in the nature based on their constitutive units (e.g. catechins and epicatechin), their sequence and the positions of interflavanic linkages (C4-C6 or C4-C8 in the B-type series, with additional C2-O-C7 or C2-O-C5 bonds in A-type structures (Cheynier 2005). Anthocyanidins are the aglycone forms of the anthocyanins and have a structure based on the flavylium (2-phenylchrome-nylium) ion skeleton. These compounds are encountered as glycoside forms and are water-soluble flavonoid pigments that appear red to blue according to pH. Individual structures arise from the variation in number and arrangement of the hydroxyl and meth-oxy groups (Figure 4.3D). Flavanones and flavanonols share a similar structure based on the 2,3-dihydro-2-phenylchromen-4-one skeleton. Hydroxylation in position 3 of the C-ring allows the differentiation of flavanonols from flavanones. (Figure 4.3E). Finally, isoflavones are a subclass of the isoflavonoids that have a structure based on the 3-phe-nylchromen-4-one skeleton. Isoflavonoids have a greater structural variability and higher presence as aglycones in plants than other classes of flavonoids (Head 1998). More than 600 isoflavones have been identified to date and are classified according to the oxidation level of the central pyran ring (Figure 4.3F).

(A)

(B)

(C)

Flavonols

	R_1	R_2	R_3
Kaempferol	OH	H	H
Quercetin	OH	OH	H
Myricetin	OH	OH	OH
Isorhamnetin	OH	OCH$_3$	H

Flavones

Luteolin	H	OH	H
Apigenin	H	H	H

Flavanols

	R_1	R_4
Catechin	OH	H
Epicatechin	OH	H
EGC	OH	OH
ECG	gallate	H
EGCG	gallate	OH

(D)

Anthocyanidins

	R_1	R_2
Pelargonidin	H	H
Cyanidin	OH	H
Delphinidin	OH	OH
Paeonidin	OCH$_3$	H
Petunidin	OCH$_3$	OH
Malvidin	OCH$_3$	OCH$_3$

(E)

Flavanones

	R_1	R_2	R_3
Naringenin	H	H	OH
Hesperetin	H	OCH$_3$	H

Flavanonols

Taxifolin	OH	OH	OH
Astilbin	O-rhamnosyl	OH	OH
Engeletin	O-rhamnosyl	H	OH

(F)

Isoflavones

	R_1	R_2
Genistein	OH	OH
Daidzein	OH	H

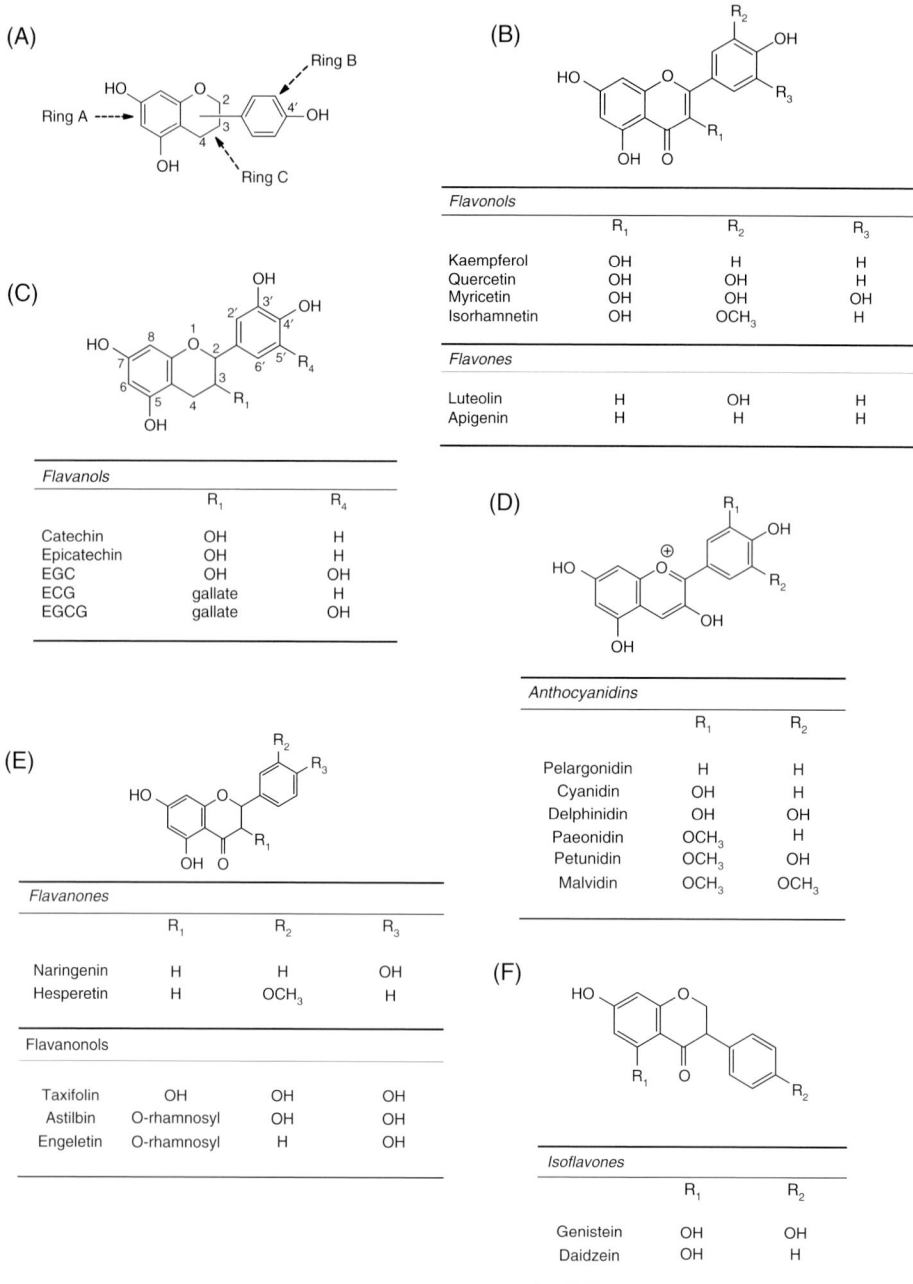

Figure 4.3   The structures of the main classes of flavonoids. The major differences between the individual groups reside in the hydroxylation pattern of the ring-structure, the degree of saturation of the C-ring and the substitution of in the 3-position: (A) general structure of flavonoids, (B) structure of flavonols and flavones, (C) structure of flavanols, also referred as flavan-3-ols, (D) structure of anthocyanidins, (E) structure of flavanones and flavanonols and (F) structure of isoflavones.

Biosynthetic routes within the plant

Shikimic precursor and benzoic acid biosynthesis

The shikimate pathway is a common route for the aromatic amino acids and many aromatic secondary metabolites. During this seven-step pathway, many branch points are encountered, serving as starting points for biosynthesis of secondary products. The formation of shikimic acid begins with a coupling of phosphoenolpyruvate (PEP) and D-erythrose-4-phosphate (E-4-P) following an aldol-type condensation to give the D-arabino-heptulosonic acid 7-phosphate (DAHP). The enzymatic synthesis of DAHP is catalysed by the DAHP synthase *(a)*, an enzyme that can be activated by numerous environmental stimuli such as light, mechanical wounding, or elicitation by microorganisms (Dyer et al. 1989; Henstrand et al. 1992; McCue and Conn 1989). Intervention of the 3-dehydroquinate synthase *(b)* on DAHP allows formation of the 3-dehydroquinic acid (DHQ), the carbocyclic precursor of the flavonoid B-ring, by an oxidation, a ß-elimination of inorganic phosphate and an intramolecular aldol condensation (Widlanski et al. 1989). A reduction of DHQ leads to quinic acid, a natural compound found as a free form or as esters (Dewick 2002). Shikimic acid itself is formed from DHQ via 3-dehydroshikimic acid by dehydration and reduction steps catalysed by DHQ dehydratase *(c)* and the NADP-dependent shikimate dehydrogenase *(d)* respectively. In plants, these two steps of the shikimate pathway are catalysed by the bifunctional DHQ dehydratase-shikimate dehydrogenase (Singh and Christendat 2006). The simple phenolic acids protocatechuic acid (3,4-dihydroxybenzoic acid) and gallic acid (3,4,5-trihydroxybenzoic acid) can be formed by branchpoint reactions from 3-dehydroshikimic acid, which involve dehydration and enolisation, or, for gallic acid, dehydrogenation and enolisation (Dewick 1992; Dewick 2002) (Figure 4.4A).

Cinnamic acid biosynthesis

Chorismic acid, the end product of the shikimate pathway, plays an important role and constitutes the start point of cinnamic acid biosynthesis. It is obtained by the following phosphoryllation of shikimic acid by the shikimate kinase enzyme *(a)*, to yield shikimate 3-phosphate. Condensation of a new molecule of phosphoenolpyruvate (PEP), as an enol ether side chain, with the shikimate 3-phosphate gives 3-enolpyruvylshikimic acid 3-phosphate (EPSP). This reaction is catalysed by the enzyme EPSP synthase *(b)*. The last step of chorismic acid biosynthesis resides in the 1,4-elimination of phosphoric acid catalysed by chorismate synthase *(c)* and requires reduced flavin (Hawkes et al. 1990). Pathways to the aromatic amino acids L-phenylalanine and L-tyrosine via prephenic acid may vary according to the organism and only two routes are involved (Figure 4.4B):

The first route involves a sigmatropic rearrangement of chorismic acid to yield prephenic acid in a reaction catalysed by chorismate mutase *(d)*. Access to L-Phe or L-Tyr requires transamination of phenyl-pyruvic acid and/or hydroxyl-phenyl-pyruvic acid (routes *(f)* and *(g)*), along with the aminotransferase enzymes (routes *(h)* and *(i)*) (Figure 4.4B). The second route involves first a transamitation of prephenic acid thus transformed into arogenic acid. This reaction is catalysed by the prephenate aminotransferase *(e)*.

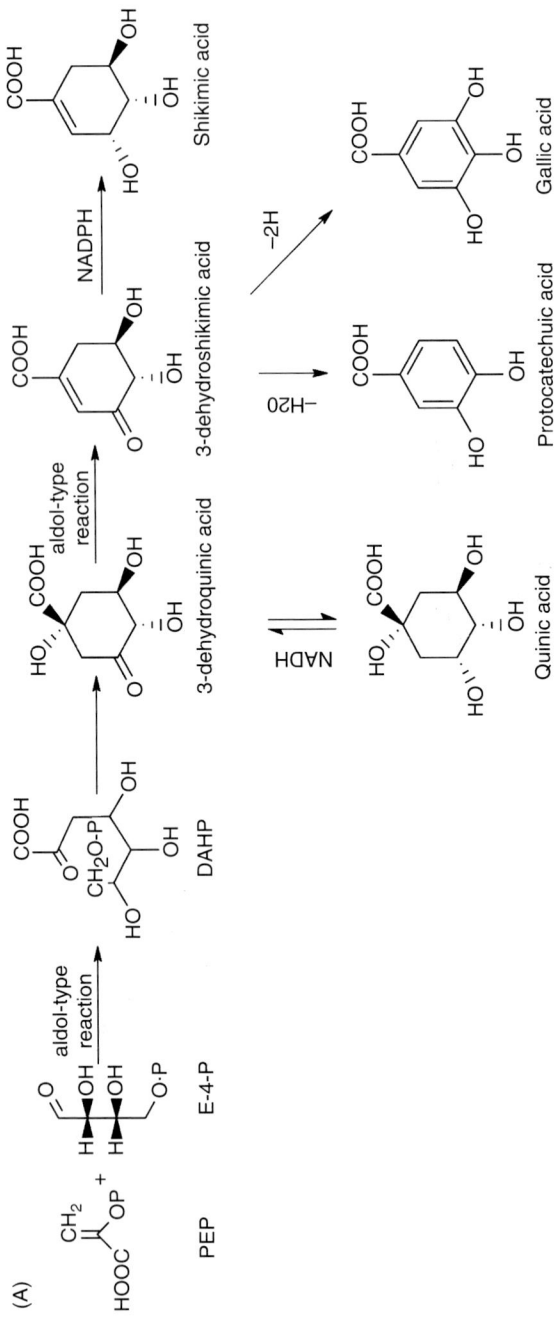

Figure 4.4 Polyphenols biosynthetic pathways. (A) Shikimic precursor and benzoic acid biosynthesis.

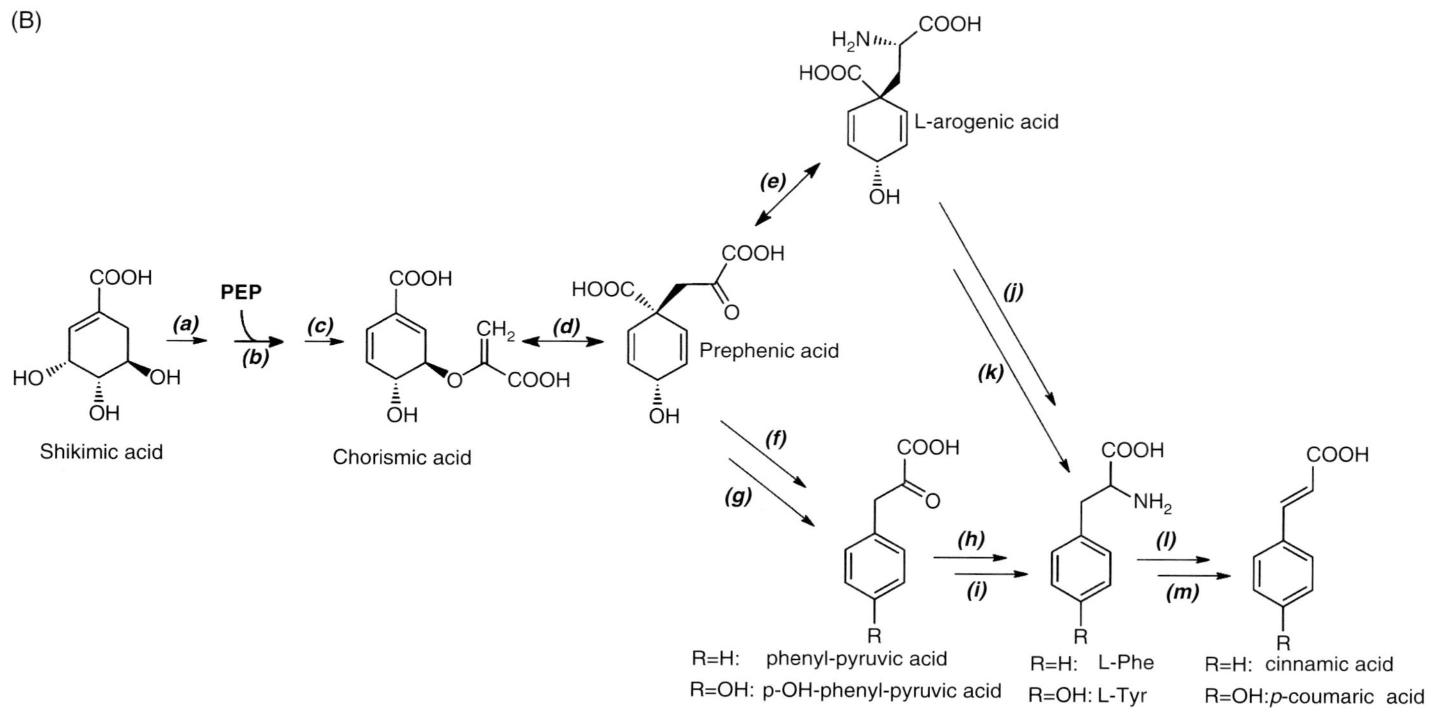

(B)

Figure 4.4 *(cont'd)* (B) Cinnamic acids biosynthesis; **(a)** shikimate kinase, **(b)** 3-enolpyruvylshikimic acid 3-phosphate synthase, **(c)** chorismate synthase, **(d)** chorismate mutase, **(e)** prephenate aminotransferase, **(f)** and **(g)** prephenate dehydratase and dehydrogenase, **(h** and **i)** phenylalanine and tyrosine aminotransferase, **(j** and **k)** arogenate dehydratase and dehydrogenase, **(l** and **m)** phenylalanin and tyrosine ammonia lyase.

(C)

C6 - C3

Cinnamic acid   *p*-hydroxy-cinnamic acid

oxidation →

"Benzoic acids"
C6 + C1

Salicylic acid

(D)

4-hydroxycinnamic acid

CoASH
activation →
SCoA

4-hydroxycinnamoyl-CoA

3 × Malonyl-CoA

Aldol reaction →

Decarboxylation
hydrolysis →
CO₂

Resveratrol

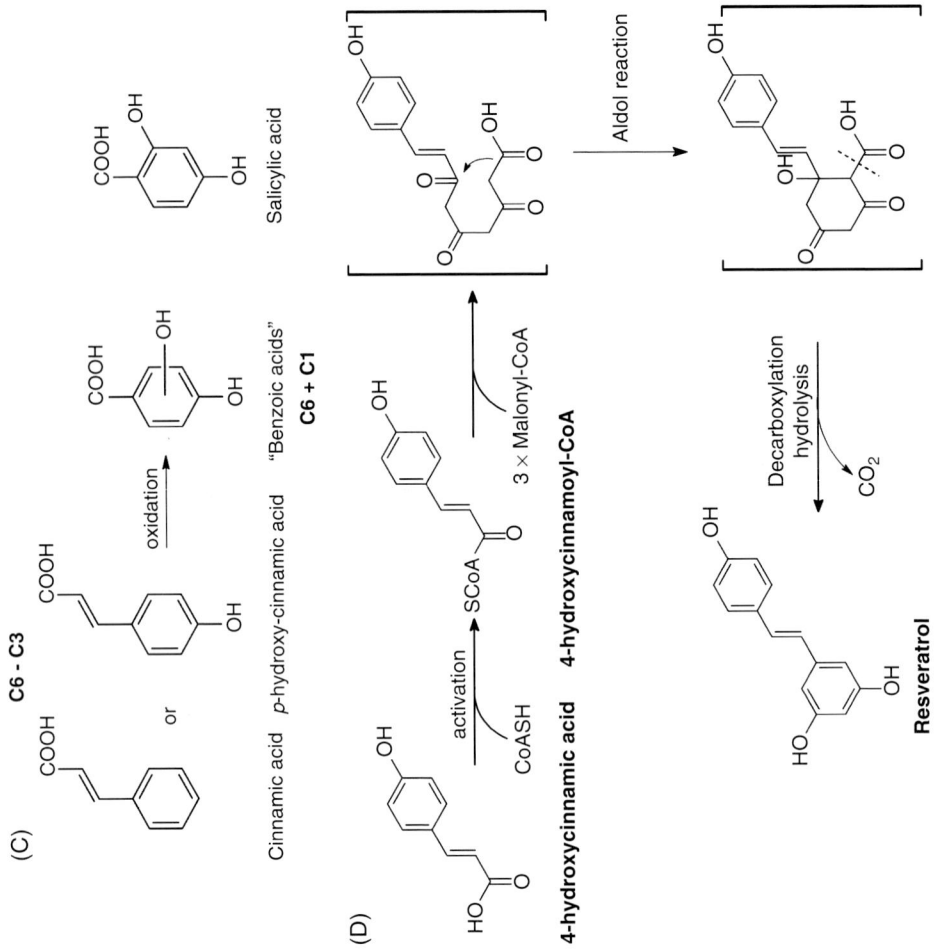

Figure 4.4 *(cont'd)* (C) Benzoic acids biosynthesis through cinnamic acid oxidation. (D) Stilbenes biosynthesis.

Arogenic acid is then transformed into L-Phe following dehydratation-decarboxylation (catalysed by the arogenate dehydratase *(j)*) or L-Tyr by dehydrogenation-decarboxylation (catalysed by the arogenate dehydrogenase *(k)*) (Figure 4.4B). L-Phe and L-Tyr, as C6-C3 building blocks, represent the precursors for a broad range of molecules. At this stage, other enzymes step in: ammonia lyase enzymes. These latter catalyse the *trans* elimination of ammonia on L-Phe and L-Tyr. For L-Phe, this would give cinnamic acid (catalysed by the phenylalanin ammonia lyase (PAL) *(l)*) whilst L-Tyr could yield *p*-coumaric acid (catalysed by the tyrosine ammonia lyase (TAL) *(m)*) (See Figure 4.4B). Other cinnamic acids are obtained by further hydroxylation and methylation reactions giving rise to cinnamic acids such as caffeic, ferulic and sinapic acids

The formation of benzoic acids from intermediates in the shikimate pathway was described in the previous section. An alternative route exists, however, in which cinnamic acid derivatives are oxidised, losing two carbons from the side chain following a β-oxidation-like reaction. Even if the C6-C1 derivative is built up at this stage, reactions of hydroxylations and/or methylations can occur prior to chain shortening giving new compounds such as salicylic acid for example (Figure 4.4C).

Stilbene biosynthesis

Stilbenes are generated from an activated cinnamoyl-CoA starter unit. The enzyme stilbene synthase couple a cinnamoyl-CoA unit with three malonyl-CoA units. An aldol reaction, generating the aromatic ring, followed by a decarboxylation and hydrolysis give the stilbene resveratrol. Transformation from cinnamoyl-CoA/malonyl-CoA to a stilbene is catalysed by this single enzyme (Figure 4.4D).

Flavonoid biosynthesis

Flavonoids are secondary metabolites synthesised by plants. All flavonoids derive from a chalcone precursor, the product of the condensation of 4-coumaroyl CoA (a product of the centralphenyl-propanoid pathway) and three molecules of malonyl-CoA (formed from acetate via a cytoplasmatic form of acetyl CoA carboxylase) by the action of the enzyme chalcone synthase (CHS) (Dixon and Steele 1999; Winkel-Shirley 2001). Chalcone is isomerised to a flavanone by the enzyme chalcone flavanone isomerase (CHI). From these central intermediates, the pathway diverges into several side branches, each resulting in a different class of flavonoids. Flavones are synthesised by the flavone synthase (FSI/FS2) whilst isoflavones are formed by the isoflavone synthase (IFS). Flavanone 3-hydroxylase (F3H) catalyses the 3β-hydroxylation of (2S)-flavanones to dihydroflavonols. The latter are transformed into flavan-3,4-diols (leucoanthocyanidins) by the dihydroflavonol reductase (DFR) which is then converted to anthocyanidins by anthocyanidin synthase (ANS). The enzyme leucoanthocyanidin reductase (LAR) removes the hydroxyl in position 4 to produce the corresponding flavan-3-ol (e.g catechin from leucocyanidin) and the anthocyanidin reductase (ANR) converts anthocyanidin to the corresponding 2,3-flavan-3-ol (e.g. epicatechin from cyanidin). The formation of glucosides is catalysed by UDP glucose-flavonoid 3-*O*-glucosyl transferase (UFGT) which stabilises the anthocyanidins and flavonols by 3-*O*-glucosylation (Bohm 1998). The basic flavonoid biosynthesis pathway is

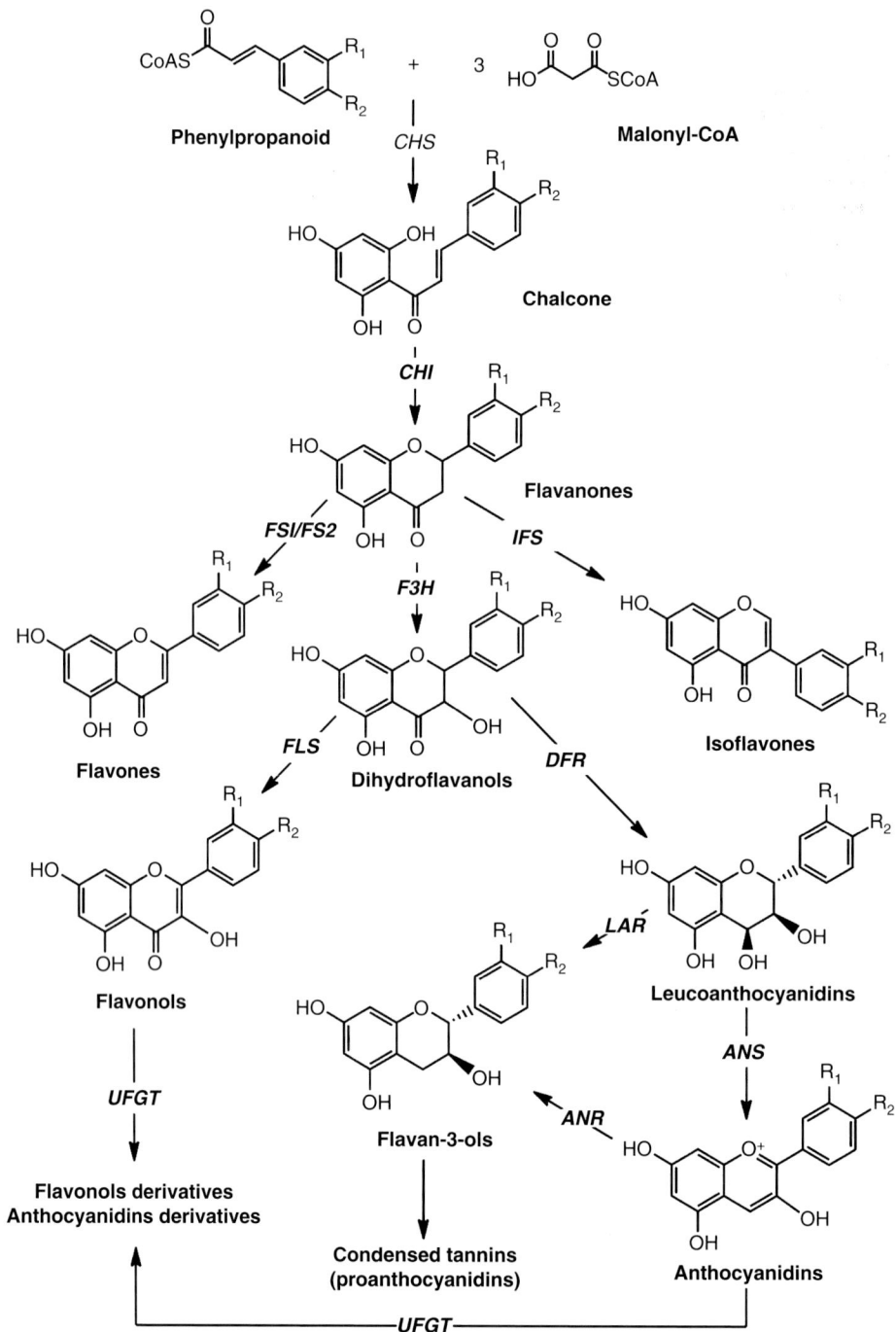

Figure 4.5 The biosynthesis of flavonoids in plants. All flavonoids are derived from chalcone precursors that are derived from phenylpropanoid and three malonyl- CoA and biosynthesised by chalcone synthase (CHS). Various enzymes act to bring about the formation of the various flavonoid classes: chalcone isomerase (CHI), flavone synthase (FSI/FS2), isoflavone synthase (IFS), flavanone 3-hydroxylase (F3H), dihydroflavonol reductase (DFR), anthocyanidin synthase (ANS), leucoanthocyanidin reductase (LAR), anthocyanidin reductase (ANR), UDP glucose-flavonoid 3-O-glucosyl transferase (UFGT), flavonol synthase (FLS).

conserved, although further modifications are possible in particular plant species. The flavonoid biosynthetic pathway responds to environmental and developmental factors by
altering the quantities and proportions of the compounds generated (Bais et al. 2003).

Each branch of the flavonoid pathway is independently regulated, thus ensuring that the
appropriate compounds are produced when and where they are required. This has significantly broadened the possibility of manipulating specific groups of phytochemicals by
metabolic engineering. Increases in the rate of gene transcription generally precede flavonoid production, suggesting that control of gene transcription might be a key element for
biosynthetic gene regulation (Davies and Schwinn 2006). For example, the expression of
DFR, ANS and FLS was significantly enhanced when the maize LC and C1 regulators of
anthocyanins were expressed from a fruit-specific promoter in tomato flesh (Bovy et al.
2002). These studies suggest that such regulation represents a potential new target for the
enhancement of flavonoid production within plants (Braun et al. 2001; Broun 2004). After
synthesis in the cytosol, flavonoids accumulate in vacuoles and cell walls (Winkel-Shirley
2001). A multidrug and toxin extrusion transporter (MATE) and a glutathione transporter
have been identified as mechanisms of transport into the vacuole, whereas transport into
the cell wall is via endoplasmic reticulum-derived vesicles. It is thought that different species use different mechanisms to distribute flavonoids within cells, or that more than one
mechanism is used in some species (Figure 4.5).

Major sources within the diet

Phenolic acids and stilbenes

Hydroxycinnamic acids are found in a variety of foods, the most common being caffeic
and ferulic acids and their derivatives (Table 4.1). They are mostly present in ester forms
bound to quinic, shikimic or tartaric acids. Caffeic acid is generally the most abundant
phenolic acid and is mainly found as the quinic ester, chlorogenic acid, in blueberries,
kiwis, plums and apples (Macheix et al. 1991). However, a very high intake of chlorogenic acid is common among coffee drinkers because of the very high concentrations
(50–150 mg) of chlorogenic acids in one cup (200 ml) of instant coffee (Clifford 1999).

Trans-resveratrol (Table 4.1) is the most commonly studied stilbene as a result of its
well-described anticarcinogenic properties. It has been shown to inhibit the metabolic
activation of carcinogens, to possess both antioxidant and anti-inflammatory properties,
to decrease cell proliferation and to induce apoptosis (Bianchini and Vainio 2003). Major
dietary sources of resveratrol include grapes, wine and peanuts. Resveratrol is found in
low concentrations (0.3–7 mg aglycones/L and 15 mg glycosides/L) in red wine and thus
is unlikely to produce protective effects at normal nutritional intakes.

Flavonoids

Flavonols

Flavonols are the most ubiquitous flavonoids in food, as they are present in almost all
fruit and vegetables. Quercetin, the main flavonol in our diet, is particularly abundant in
onions (0.3 mg/g fresh weight) (Hertog et al. 1992), and tea (10–25 mg/L) (Hertog et al.

Table 4.1   Polyphenol containing foods

	Source	Polyphenol content (mg/kg) or (mg/L) fresh weight
Phenolic acids	Blueberry, kiwi, plum, cherry, apple, coffee	100–2000
	Blackberry, raspberry, strawberry, blackcurrant, potato	20–300
Stilbenes	Grapes, grape juices, wine, peanuts	0–30
Flavonols	Onion, kale	300–1200
	Leek, cherry tomato, broccoli, blueberry blackcurrant, Apricot	50–300
	Apple, green bean, black grape, tomato, black tea, green tea	0–50
Flavones	Parsley	200–2000
	Celery	20–200
	Capsicum pepper	1–20
Flavanones	Orange, orange juice	200–1000
	Grapefruit, grapefruit juice	100–700
	Lemon juice	50–300
Flavanols	Chocolate, green tea	500–1000
	Beans, black tea	300–500
	Apricot, cherry, grape, peach, blackberry, apple, red wine, cider	10–300
Anthocyanins	Aubergine, blackberry, blackcurrant, blueberry, black grape, cherry	1000–5000
	Rhubarb	1000–2000
	Strawberry, red wine, plumb, red cabbage	10–1000
Isoflavones	Soya flour	1000–2000
	Soya beans, miso, tofu, tempeh, soya milk	10–1000

1993b) but also in reasonable concentrations in red wine, apples and berries. Other flavonols in the diet include kaempferol (broccoli), myricetin (berries) and isorhamnetin (onion). These compounds are present in plants in glycosylated forms, where the associated sugar moiety is predominantly glucose or rhamnose, although, other sugars may also be attached (Table 4.1). The daily intake of quercetin was estimated to range between 3 and 38 mg in the seven countries study (Hertog et al. 1995), whereas in the United States, the estimated intake of flavonols, of which quercetin constituted 73%, was 20–22 mg/day (Sampson et al. 2002).

Flavanones

Flavanones are the main type of flavonoids present in citrus fruit and juices. The highest concentrations are found in the solid parts of the fruit particularly the albedo and the membranes but concentrations up to 200–600 mg/L of flavanones have also been found in the juice (Tomas-Barberan and Clifford 2000). Flavanones are generally glycosylated, but the main aglycones are hesperetin and naringenin in oranges. The main flavonoid of grapefruit is naringenin. Other sources include tomatoes and aromatic plants such as mint (Table 4.1). Average intakes in Finland were estimated to be 8.3 mg/day for naringenin and 28.3 mg/day for hesperetin (Kumpulainen et al. 1999).

Flavanols

Flavanols are a unique class of flavonoids because they exist in both the monomeric form (catechins) and the polymer form (proanthocyanidins). In contrast to other classes of flavonoids, flavonols are not glycosylated in food, and they usually occur as aglycones or gallate esters on the 3-position of the flavonoid ring. Catechin and epicatechin are the main flavanols, and are found in various fruit such as apples and apricots and are also present at high concentrations in red wine and cocoa. Gallocatechin, epigallocatechin and epigallocatechin gallate are found in seeds of certain leguminous plants, in grapes and at a high concentration in tea (Table 4.1). The daily intake of catechin in monomeric form as well as dimers and trimers has been estimated to be 18–50 mg/day with the main sources being tea, chocolate, apples, pears and grapes (Arts et al. 2000a, b).

Flavones

Flavones are much less common than other flavonoids in the human diet. The main sources of dietary intake are herbs such as parsley and celery. They exist mainly as glycosides of luteolin and apigenin. A group of polymethoxylated flavones such as tangeretin, which are considered the most hydrophobic forms of flavonoids, exist in essential oils derived from citrus fruits (Table 4.1).

Anthocyanins

Anthocyanins are a class of water-soluble flavonoids, which are abundant in some vegetables and fruit, particularly berries to which they impart a pink, red, blue or purple colour, and exist mainly as glycosides. High intake of anthocyanidin relates to the high concentrations found in vegetables and fruit; for example, a serving of 200 g aubergine or black grapes can provide up to 1500 mg of anthocyanins, and a 300 ml glass of red wine can contain 100 mg of anthocyanins (Manach et al. 2004). The mean dietary intake in Finland has been estimated to be 82 mg/day, with the main sources being berries, red wine and juices (Manach et al. 2005) (Table 4.1).

Isoflavones

Isoflavones are naturally occurring plant components having a 1,2-diarylpropane structure. These compounds belong to the phytoestrogens class having a similar chemical structure to mammalian oestrogens. They are present in several legumes but soya beans have been identified as the principal dietary source for humans. The isoflavone content of soybeans varies depending on the variety of soybean, the year harvested, geographic location and plant part. Non-soy legumes such as lentils and other types of beans do not contain appreciable amounts of isoflavones (Franke 1997). Isoflavones are present in plants either as the aglycone (mainly genistein or daidzein) or as different glycosides, including their β–glucosides, namely genistin and daidzin or their methoxylated derivatives, namely biochanin A and formononetin (Ruiz-Larrea et al. 1997) (Table 4.1).

Metabolic fate of dietary polyphenols

Although polyphenols and in particular flavonoids have been identified as powerful anti-oxidants *in vitro,* their ability to act as effective antioxidants *in vivo* will be dependent on the extent of their biotransformation (Vitaglione et al. 2005) and conjugation during absorption from the gastrointestinal (GI) tract, in the liver and finally in the cells. Native polyphenols in the diet are subjected to extensive metabolism following oral ingestion. In the upper gastrointestinal tract, dietary polyphenols act as substrates for various enzymes and are subject to extensive metabolism by glucosidase enzymes, phase I enzymes (hydrolysing and oxidising), such as cytochrome P450, and phase II enzymes (conjugating and detoxifying) found both in the small intestine and the liver. Further transformations have been reported in the colon, where the enzymes of the gut microflora act to breakdown flavonoids to simple phenolic acids, which may also be absorbed and further metabolised in the liver (Figure 4.6).

Gastrointestinal tract metabolism

Modifications of polyphenol structure may occur at many points in the GI tract. In the upper GI tract saliva has been found to cause degalloylation of flavanol gallate esters, such as epigallocatechin gallate (Yang et al. 1999) but to have little effect on the stability of green tea catechins (Tsuchiya et al. 1997). The quercetin rutinoside, rutin, is hydrolysed by cell-free extracts of human salivary cultures (Laires et al. 1989) and by streptococci isolated from the mouths of normal individuals (Parisis and Pritchard 1983), but quercetin-3-rhamnoside (quercitrin) is not susceptible to hydrolysis suggesting that only rutin-glycosidase-elaborating organisms occur in saliva (Macdonald et al. 1983). An interaction of flavanols and procyanidins with salivary proteins has been shown and indicates that (+)-catechin has a higher affinity for proline-rich proteins than (–)-epicatechin and C(4)-C(8) linked procyanidin dimers bind more strongly than their C(4)-C(6) counterparts (De Freitas and Mateus 2001). This polyphenol–protein binding in the form adsorption with high molecular weight salivary proteins, bacterial cells and mucous materials may be one explanation for the observed decrease in quercetin mutagenicity after incubation with saliva (Nishioka et al. 1981).

There are many factors that influence the extent and rate of absorption of ingested compounds by the small intestine (Lin et al. 1999). These include, physiochemical factors such as molecular size, lipophilicity, solubility, pKa, and biological factors including gastric and intestinal transit time, lumen pH, membrane permeability and first pass metabolism (Higuchi et al. 1981; Ho et al. 1983). Procyanidin oligomers ranging from a dimer to decamer (isolated from *Theobroma cacao*), have been observed to be unstable under conditions of low pH similar to that present in the gastric juice of the stomach

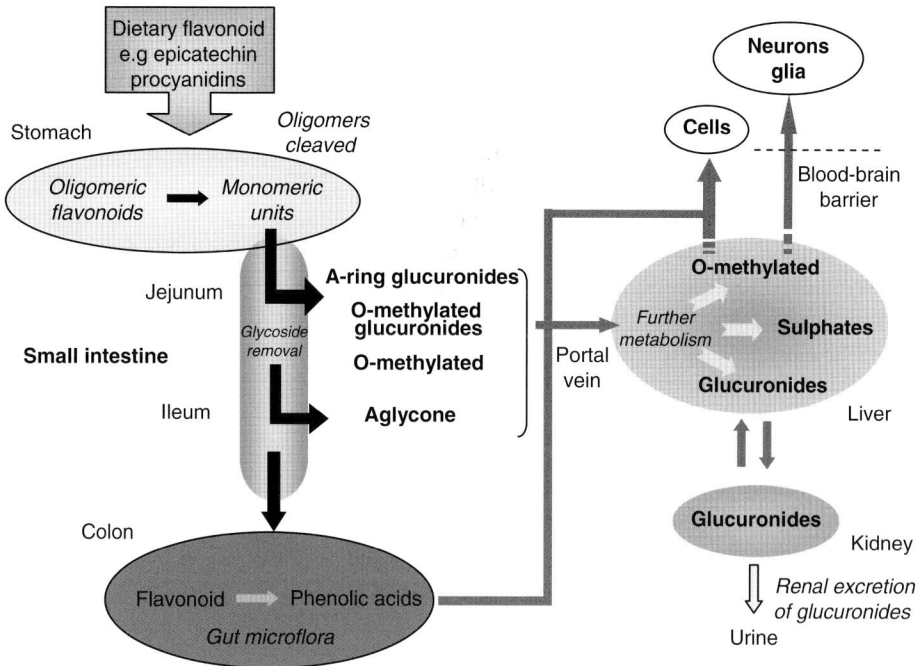

Figure 4.6   Summary of the formation of gastrointestinal tract and hepatic metabolites and conjugates of polyphenols in humans. Cleavage of oligomeric flavonoids such as procyanidins may occur in the stomach in environment of low pH. All classes of flavonoids undergo extensive metabolism in the jejunum and ileum of the small intestine and resulting metabolites enter the portal vein and undergo further metabolism in the liver. Colonic microflora degrades flavonoids into smaller phenolic acids that may also be absorbed. The fate of flavonoids is renal excretion, although, some may enter cells and tissues. See plate section for colour version of this figure.

(Spencer et al. 2001d). During incubation of the procyanidins with simulated gastric juice, oligomers rapidly decompose to epicatechin monomeric and dimeric units but also to other oligomeric units primarily, although other oligomeric units, such as trimer and tetramer were also formed (Spencer et al. 2000). Thus, absorption of flavanols and procyanidins, for example after consumption of chocolate or cocoa, are likely to be influenced by pre-absorption events in the gastric lumen within the residence time. However, consideration needs to be given to the food matrix, which may influence the pH environment of the procyanidins and their subsequent decomposition. Monomeric flavonoid glycosides have been observed to be stable in the acidic environment of the stomach and are not observed to be undergoing non-enzymatic deglycosylation (Gee et al. 1998). Because glycosides derivatives of polyphenols are relatively polar molecules, their passive diffusion across the membranes of the small intestinal brush border is unlikely. However, many studies have suggested that flavonoid glycosides are subject to the action of β-glucosidases prior to their absorption in the jejunum and ileum (Ioku et al. 1998; Hollman et al. 1999a; Spencer et al. 1999; Gee et al. 2000; Morand et al. 2000; Day and Williamson 2001; Walle et al. 2000b) and it is generally believed that the removal of the glycosidic moiety is necessary before absorption of the flavonoid can take place. The majority of polyphenol glycosides, and in some instances the aglycones, present in plant-derived foods are extensively conjugated and metabolised during absorption in the small intestine and then again in the liver. In particular there is strong evidence for the extensive phase I de-glycosylation and phase II metabolism (by UDP-glucuronosyltransferases, sulphotransferases and catechol-*O*-methyltransferases (COMT)) to yield glucuronides, sulphates and *O*-methylated derivatives. Indeed, in the jejunum and ileum of the small intestine there is efficient glucuronidation of nearly all polyphenols to differing extents by the action of UDP-glucuronosyltransferase enzymes. For catechol containing B-ring flavonoids there is also extensive *O*-methylation by the action of COMT. Unabsorbed polyphenols will reach the large intestine where they will be further metabolised by the enzymes of the gut microflora to simple phenolic acids.

Colonic metabolism

Studies have suggested that the extent of absorption of dietary polyphenols in the small intestine is relatively small (10–20%) (Kuhnle et al. 2000a, b). The implications of this low absorption in the small intestine means that the majority of ingested polyphenols, including those absorbed and conjugated in the enterocytes and/or the liver before transport back out into the lumen either directly or via the bile (Crespy et al. 1999), will reach the large intestine where they encounter colonic microflora. The colon contains approximately 10^{12} micro-organisms/cm^3, which has an enormous catalytic and hydrolytic potential, and this enzymatic degradation of flavonoids by the colonic microflora results in a huge array of new metabolites. For example, bacterial enzymes may catalyse many reactions including hydrolysis, dehydroxylation, demethylation, ring cleavage and decarboxylation as well as rapid de-conjugation (Scheline 1999). Unlike human enzymes, the bacteria of the large intestine catalyse the breakdown of the flavonoid backbone itself to simpler molecules such as phenolic acids. Specific metabolites have been observed in urine after consumption of a variety of phenolics. For example, the glycine conjugate of benzoic acid, hippuric acid, is primarily derived from plant phenolics and aromatic amino acids through the action of intestinal bacteria and, consequently, the level of hippuric acid would be expected to increase in the urine of individuals consuming diets rich in flavanols or polyphenols in general. It must be noted however, that hippuric acid could possibly derive from other sources such as quinic acid or, in quantitative terms, more importantly from the aromatic amino acids tryptophan, tyrosine and phenylalanine, as well as from the use of benzoic acid as a food preservative.

The 5,7,3′,4′-hydroxylation pattern of flavan-3-ols is believed to enhance ring opening after hydrolysis (Spencer et al. 2001c) and metabolism of flavanols by enzymes of the microflora of the large intestine results in many metabolites: 3,4-dihydrophenylacetic acid, 3-hydroxyphenylacetic acid, homovanillic acid and their conjugates derived from the B-ring (Scheline 1999) and phenolic acids from the C-ring. Flavanols, because of their structures (no C-4 carbonyl group), can also degrade to the specific metabolites phenylvalerolactones. Phenylpropionic acids (which may undergo further metabolism to benzoic acids) may also be the products of flavanol metabolism in animal studies, which demonstrates fission of the A-ring (Scheline 1999). The metabolism of flavan-3-ol

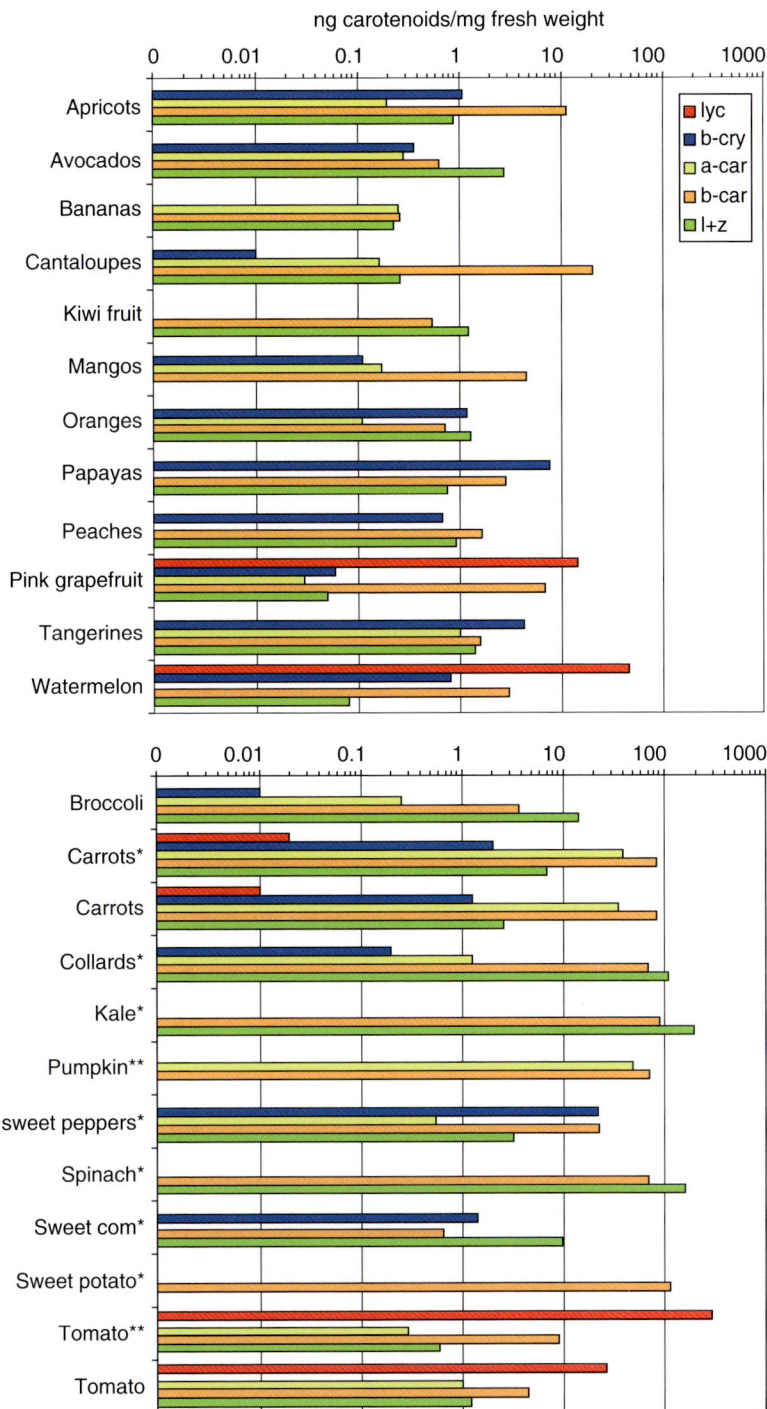

Figure 3.2 Carotenoid levels in fruits and vegetables. Data were collected from the United States Department of Agriculture (USDA) and Nutrition Coordination Center (NCC) Carotenoid Database (Holden et al., 1999) and correspond to raw foods unless indicated with an asterisc (cooked) or two asteriscs (canned). Note that the carotenoid content scale is logarithmic. lyc, lycopene; b-cry, β-cryptoxanthin; a-car, α-carotene; b-car, β-carotene; l+z, lutein and zeaxanthin.

Phytonutrients, First Edition. Edited by Andrew Salter, Helen Wiseman and Gregory Tucker.
© 2012 Blackwell Publishing Ltd. Published 2012 by Blackwell Publishing Ltd.

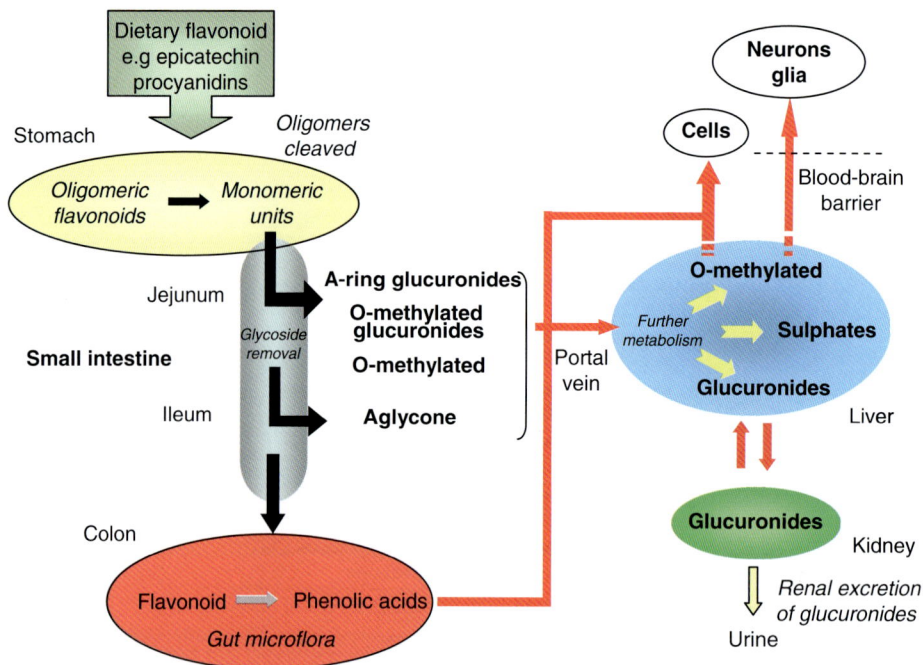

Figure 4.6 Summary of the formation of gastrointestinal tract and hepatic metabolites and conjugates of polyphenols in humans. Cleavage of oligomeric flavonoids such as procyanidins may occur in the stomach in environment of low pH. All classes of flavonoids undergo extensive metabolism in the jejunum and ileum of the small intestine and resulting metabolites enter the portal vein and undergo further metabolism in the liver. Colonic microflora degrades flavonoids into smaller phenolic acids that may also be absorbed. The fate of flavonoids is renal excretion, although some may enter cells and tissues.

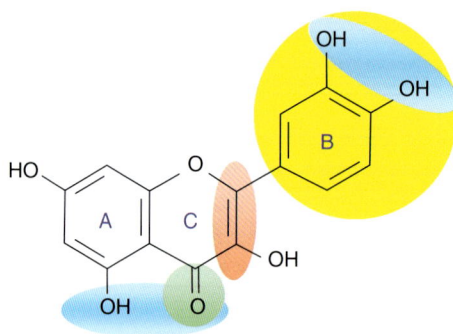

Figure 4.7 Structure of the flavonol quercetin showing features important in defining the classical antioxidant potential of flavonoids. The most important of these is the catechol or dihydroxylated B-ring (shaded yellow). Other important features include the presence of unsaturation in the C-ring (shaded red) and the presence of a 4-oxo function in the C-ring (shaded green). The catechol group and other functions may also ascribe an ability to chelate transition metal ions such as copper and iron (shaded blue).

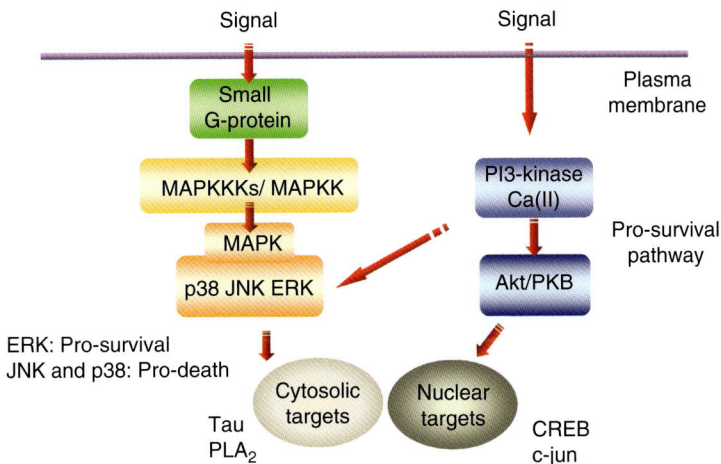

Figure 4.8 Diagrammatic representation of the MAP kinase and Akt/PKB signalling pathways. Extracellular signal-related kinase (ERK), c-jun amino-terminal kinase (JNK) and p38 are involved in growth, differentiation, development, apoptosis and inflammation. ERK and JNK are generally considered as having opposing actions in cells with signalling through ERK usually regarded as pro-signalling and JNK pro-apoptotic. The serine/threonine kinase, Akt/PKB, is one of the main downstream effectors of phosphatidylinositol 3-kinase (PI3-kinase) and a pivotal kinase in cell survival.

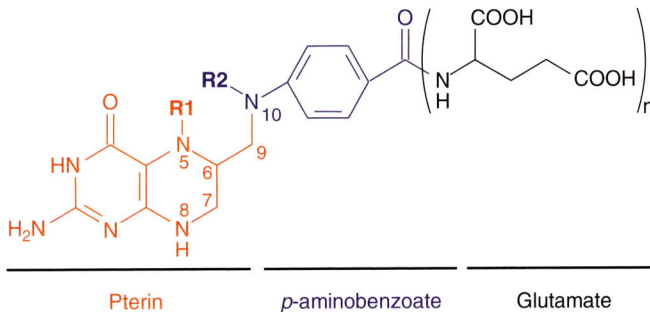

Folates	R1	R2
5-formyl-THF	CHO	H
10-formyl-THF	H	CHO
5,10-methenyl-THF	$=CH^{+-}$	
5,10-methylene-THF	$-CH_2-$	
5-methyl-THF	CH_3	H
5-formimino-THF	CH=NH	H

Figure 6.1 Chemical structure of tetrahydrofolate and its C1-substituted derivatives. Cellular folates are substituted at the N-5 and/or N-10 positions by C1-units of different oxidation states and usually contain 5 to 8 glutamate residues.

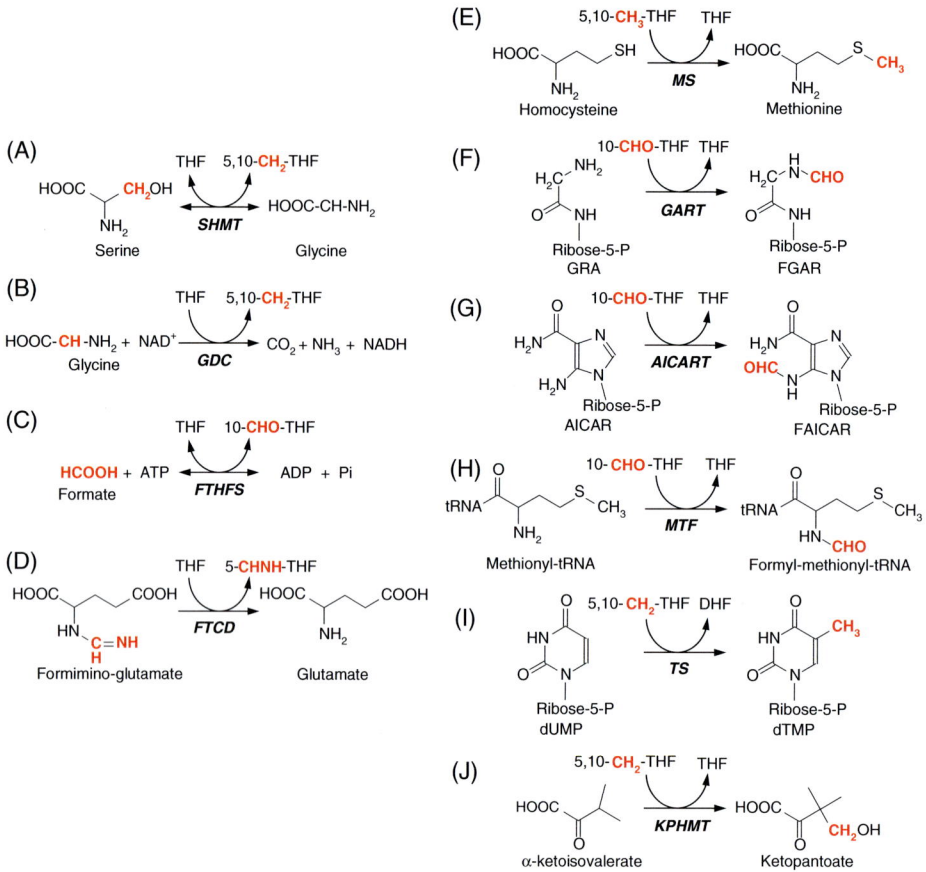

Figure 6.2 Key reactions of C1 metabolism. Reactions involved in the generation of C1-substituted folates are described on the left column and the anabolic reactions utilizing folates on the right. A, serine-glycine interconversion catalyzed by serine hydroxymethyl transferase (SHMT); B, catabolism of glycine catalyzed by the glycine decarboxylase complex (GDC); C, synthesis of 10-formyl-THF by 10-formyl-THF synthetase (FTHFS); D, synthesis of 5-formimino-THF by the formiminotransferase domain of the bifunctional enzyme glutamate formiminotransferase / formimino-THF cyclodeaminase (FTCD); E, methylation of homocysteine to methionine catalyzed by methionine synthase (MS); F and G, purine ring synthesis involves two formylation reactions catalyzed by glycinamide ribonucleotide transformylase (GART) and aminoimidazole carboximide ribonucleide transformylase (AICART); H, formylation of methionyl-tRNA catalyzed by methionyl-tRNA transformylase (MTF); I, methylation of dUMP to dTMP catalyzed by thymidylate synthase (TS), note that this reaction produces dihydrofolate (DHF); J, synthesis of ketopantoate, precursor of pantothenate, from α-ketoisovalerate catalyzed by ketopantoate hydroxymethyl transferase (KPHMT).

oligomers may also take place in the colon. Colonic-derived metabolites of flavanols have been detected in human plasma and urine after a single ingestion of green tea (Li et al. 2000), which suggests that there may be significant metabolism by gut microflora in the colon. Flavonols such as quercetin-3-rhamnoglucoside and quercetin-3-rhamnoside may also undergo metabolism by the colonic flora with *Bacteroides distasonis, B. uniformis* and *B. ovatus* capable of cleaving the sugar using α-rhamnosidase and β-glucosidase to liberate quercetin aglycone (Bokkenheuser et al. 1987) and other phenolic metabolites (Baba et al. 1983). Other bacteria, such as *Enterococcus casseliflavus,* have been observed to degrade quercetin-3-glucoside (Schneider et al. 1999), luteolin-7-glucoside, rutin, quercetin, kaempferol, luteolin, eriodictyol, naringenin, taxifolin and phloretin (Schneider and Blaut 2000) to phenolic acids and *E. ramulus* is capable of degrading the aromatic ring system of quercetin producing the transient intermediate, phloroglucinol (Schneider et al. 1999). Other flavonoid glycosides, hesperidin, naringin and poncirin are also metabolised to phenolic acids, via aglycones, by human intestinal microflora that produce α-rhamnosidase, exo-β-glucosidase, endo-β-glucosidase and/or β-glucuronidase enzymes (Kim et al. 1998). In addition, baicalin, puerarin and daidzin were transformed to their aglycones by the bacteria producing β-glucuronidase, C-glycosidase and β-glycosidase, respectively.

Role in human health

High intake of fruits and vegetables which are rich in polyphenolic compounds has been associated in many epidemiological studies with decreased risk in a range of diseases including cardiovascular disease (Kuriyama et al. 2006), specific forms of cancer (Kuriyama et al. 2006; Sun et al. 2006) and neurodegenerative diseases (Checkoway et al. 2002). In support of these observations, polyphenols, and in particular flavonoids, have been shown to exert beneficial effects in many human, animal and *in vitro* studies (Schroeter et al. 2001; Magee and Rowland 2004; Ambra et al. 2006; Beltz et al. 2006; Samy et al. 2006). With respect to cardiovascular disease, flavonoids may alter lipid metabolism (Zern et al. 2005), inhibit low-density lipoprotein (LDL) oxidation (Jeong et al. 2005), inhibit atherosclerotic lesion formation (Fuhrman et al. 2005) and platelet aggregation (Hubbard et al. 2006), decrease inflammation and vascular cell adhesion molecule expression (Ludwig et al. 2004) and improve endothelial function (Nagaya et al. 2004; Hallund et al. 2006). The anticarcinogenic effects of polyphenols may include inhibition of cell proliferation (Wang et al. 2000) and induction of apoptosis (Mantena et al. 2006), modulation of phase I and II detoxification enzyme activity (Valerio, Jr. et al. 2001; Bacon et al. 2003), inhibition of angiogenesis and prevention of tumour invasion (Cao and Cao 1999; Piao et al. 2006). With respect to neurodegeneration, polyphenols may benefit memory performance and cognitive function and prevent cognitive losses associated with ageing and even reverse certain age-related declines (Joseph et al. 1998, 1999). Neuroprotective mechanisms of flavonoids and other polyphenols include modulation of neuronal and mitochondrial function (Schroeter et al. 2001; Smith et al. 2002) as well as inhibition of inflammatory processes involved in neurodegeneration (Kim et al. 2001; Chen et al. 2005).

Although polyphenols are known to exert beneficial effects in multiple diseases, the exact molecular and cellular mechanisms of these effects are currently unclear. For years it has been postulated that the beneficial effects of polyphenols are a result of their antioxidant capacity. This ability of flavonoids to act as hydrogen donating antioxidants was used to explain their protective effects against oxidative stress and disease incidence (Hertog et al. 1993a; Rice-Evans et al. 1995; Higdon and Frei 2003). However, recent evidence suggests that their antioxidant capacity *per se* cannot be the only explanation for their bioactivity and that mechanisms other than the classical antioxidant properties, such as modulation of signalling pathways, may as well contribute to their postulated beneficial effects (Williams et al. 2004). The antioxidant and non-antioxidant activities of polyphenols will be described in detail in the following sections.

Flavonoids as classical antioxidants

Flavonoids are antioxidants *in vitro* due to the hydrogen donating properties of their phenolic hydroxyl groups, which are attached to the ring structures. The hydrogen donating properties of flavonoids depend mainly on the number and arrangement of hydroxyl groups in the molecule. Structurally important features which define this antioxidant activity are the hydroxylation pattern, in particular the 3′,4′-dihydroxyl catechol group in the B-ring, the planarity of the molecule and the presence of 2,3-unsaturation in conjugation with a 4-oxo-function in the C-ring (Figure 4.7). Therefore, flavonoids, such as quercetin, that have an O-dihydroxy catechol group in the B-ring are more powerful antioxidants and scavengers of free radicals than other flavonoids, such as naringenin, that lack the specific dihydroxylation pattern. As a result, the main focus on flavonoid research has been directed towards their antioxidant capacity. The flavonoid ability to act as classical electron (or hydrogen) donating antioxidants (Hertog et al. 1993a; Hertog and Hollman 1996; Rice-Evans et al. 1996; Hollman et al. 1999b) to scavenge a variety of

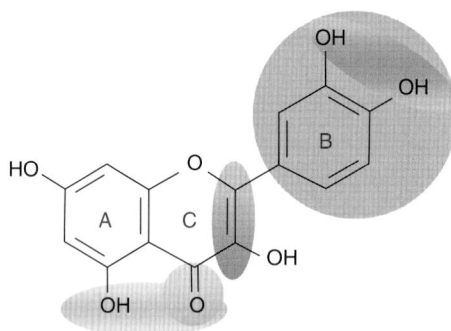

Figure 4.7 Structure of the flavonol quercetin showing features important in defining the classical antioxidant potential of flavonoids. The most important of these is the catechol or dihydroxylated B-ring (shaded yellow). Other important features include the presence of unsaturation in the C-ring (shaded red) and the presence of a 4-oxo function in the C-ring (shaded green). The catechol group and other functions may also ascribe an ability to chelate transition metal ions such as copper and iron (shaded blue). See plate section for colour version of this figure.

reactive species, such as hydroxyl radicals, superoxide and peroxyl radicals (Rice-Evans 2001; Garcia-Alonso et al. 2005; Kruk et al. 2005) has been extensively reported in several *in vitro* investigations.

In addition, the *in vitro* antioxidant efficacy of flavonoids has been described for the protection against oxidative damage to a variety of cellular biomolecules. For example, flavonoids may inhibit LDL oxidation (Green et al. 1993; Hubac et al. 1994; Yannai et al. 1998; Yamamoto et al. 1999) as well as protein and DNA oxidation (Duthie et al. 1997; Duthie and Dobson 1999) *in vitro*. Since LDL oxidation is a crucial initial step in atherosclerosis progression (Heinecke 2006), investigations have also focused on the potential of flavonoids to inhibit LDL peroxidation *ex vivo*. Although some of these studies have demonstrated a protective effect of flavonoids against LDL oxidation (Ishikawa et al. 1997; Hirano et al. 2000; Wan et al. 2001), others have failed to do so (de Rijke et al. 1996; Vissers et al. 2001), suggesting that more studies are warranted in order to elucidate the potential protective effects of flavonoids against LDL oxidation *ex vivo*. Flavonoids may also scavenge reactive nitrogen species in the form of peroxynitrite (Justesen 2000, 2001; Rice-Evans 2001) and limit dopamine oxidation mediated by peroxynitrite in a structure-dependent way involving oxidation or nitration of the flavonoid ring system (Weisshaar and Jenkins 1998). Furthermore, their antioxidant properties may also include their ability to chelate transition metal ions (Morel et al. 1994; Bailey et al. 1998). For instance, the iron-chelating properties of tea catechins have been suggested to play a key role in the neuroprotective effects of flavonoids in *in vitro* cell culture models (Levites et al. 2002a, b). Several other *in vitro* investigations have demonstrated that flavonoids may also protect against oxidative damage by their potential to quench singlet oxygen (Tournaire et al. 1993; Devasagayam et al. 1995; Halliwell et al. 2005; Mukai et al. 2005).

Although evidence from *in vitro* studies suggests that flavonoids may exert antioxidant effects, data on the effects of flavonoids on oxidative damage *in vivo* are conflicting and should be interpreted with caution. Flavonoids have been postulated to increase the plasma total antioxidant capacity in several *in vivo* investigations (Rietveld and Wiseman 2003). Many studies on humans have investigated the effects of flavonoid-enriched diets on F_2-isoprostanes, a biomarker of lipid peroxidation *in vivo* (Wiseman et al. 2000; Sanchez-Moreno et al. 2003; Montuschi et al. 2004). Some of these have reported a decrease in F_2-isoprostane concentration after orange juice and soy intake (O'Reilly et al. 2001; van den Berg et al. 2001), whereas others failed to show any significant effect on F_2-isoprostanes *in vivo* (Widlansky et al. 2005). Similarly, evidence on the effects of flavonoids on markers of DNA damage *in vivo* is contradictory. Black tea consumption failed to exert any reduction in urinary 8-hydroxy-2'-deoxyguanosine, a marker of oxidative DNA damage (Thompson et al. 1999), whereas in a study by Thomspon et al. (2005) fruit and vegetable consumption resulted in a decrease in lymphocyte 8-hydroxy-2'-deoxyguanosine levels, suggesting a beneficial effect of flavonoids on markers of oxidative damage *in vivo* (Freese et al. 1999; bu-Amsha et al. 2001; Hodgson et al. 2002). Likewise, there is a range of studies that have produced conflicting results on the effects of flavonoids on markers of oxidative stress in humans (Halliwell et al. 2004), further demonstrating a lack of systemic antioxidant effects of flavonoids *in vivo*. Furthermore, it should be noted that F_2-isoprostanes and 8-hydroxy-2'-deoxyguanosine are not considered to be ideal biomarkers of oxidative stress and, as argued by Halliwell et al. (2004), the establishment of generally accepted biomarkers of oxidative damage is an absolute necessity before conclusions on the bioactivity of polyphenols as antioxidants *in vivo* can be made (Rice-Evans et al. 1996).

Although flavonoids may react with reactive oxygen species and display potent anti-oxidant effects in *in vitro* models, it is clear that their efficiency as antioxidants *in vivo* will mainly depend on the form that is bioavailable to the cells and tissues. Therefore, understanding of the absorption and metabolism of flavonoids, and polyphenols in general, as well as identification of the structures of their *in vivo* metabolites, is absolutely necessary to resolve the bioefficiency of flavonoids as dietary antioxidants.

Non-antioxidant activities of flavonoids

Since oxidative stress may play a pivotal role in the development of most diseases, it has been sensible to hypothesise that the beneficial effects of flavonoids against age-related disease are mostly attributed to their antioxidant properties (Spencer et al. 2001a, 2003). However, as mentioned earlier, some studies have speculated that the hydrogen donating activity of flavonoids is not the sole explanation for their cellular effects (Morand et al. 1998). This argument is based on several lines of reasoning. First, as discussed earlier in this chapter, flavonoids undergo extensive metabolism *in vivo* resulting in a structural alteration which is accompanied by a significant loss in their antioxidant activity. There has been some evidence that after ingestion of dietary flavonoids, the resulting metabolites may exert antioxidant activity in biological fluids (Turner et al. 2004; Pollard et al. 2006). However, it is well established that sulphated and glucuronidated forms of flavonoids have a significantly lower capacity for donating hydrogen ions and scavenging free radicals compared to the parent compounds (Turner et al. 2004). Furthermore, flavonoids probably undergo intracellular metabolism such as conjugation with thiols (especially glutathione) and oxidative metabolism, which may also alter their redox capacity (Manach and Donovan 2004). Secondly, the concentration of flavonoids and their metabolites that may accumulate *in vivo* in plasma and in organs, such as the brain, are not more than 1 μmol/L (Halliwell et al. 2000), which is much lower than the concentration recorded for well-known small molecule antioxidants such as ascorbic acid and α-tocopherol (Schroeter et al. 2000). Consequently, it is probable that flavonoids, at the concentration found *in vivo,* cannot compete with other antioxidants such as ascorbate and α-tocopherol that are present in the circulation. In support of this, *in vitro* investigations in neuron cells have shown that flavonoids may protect neurons against oxidative stress more effectively than ascorbate, even when the latter was used at 10-fold higher concentrations, further supporting non-antioxidant activity (Conseil et al. 1998). Thirdly, evidence exists that flavonoids possess more biological activities that are suggestive for additional cellular mechanisms of action. For example, flavonoids have the ability to bind to the ATP-binding sites of proteins (Di Pietro et al. 1975), such as mitochondrial ATPase (Barzilai and Rahamimoff 1983), calcium membrane ATPase (Gamet-Payrastre et al. 1999), protein kinase C (Boege et al. 1996) and topoisomerase (Medina et al. 1997). In addition, flavonoids bind to the benzodiazepine binding sites of GABA-A and adenosine receptors (Spencer et al. 2001a) and may also directly interact with mitochondria (Laughton et al. 1991; Lin et al. 2000; Van Hoorn et al. 2002) and affect the activity of enzymes such as cyclooxygenase, lipoxygenase and xanthine oxidase (Williams et al. 2004).

Interactions with cell signalling pathways

Recent evidence from *in vitro* studies indicates that a number of biological effects of flavonoids may be mediated by interactions with signalling proteins central to intracellular signal transduction pathways (Kong et al. 2000). Specifically, flavonoids have been reported to exert cellular effects through selective actions at different components of a number of protein kinase and lipid kinase signalling cascades, such as PI3-kinase, Akt/PKB tyrosine kinase, PKC and members of the MAP kinase family (Schroeter et al. 2001, 2002). The interaction of flavonoids with the MAP kinase pathway is of great significance since MAP signalling cascades are important enzymes involved in gene expression, cell proliferation and cell death (Chang and Karin 2001). The MAP kinase signalling pathway comprises the extracellular signal-related kinase (ERK), c-jun amino-terminal kinase (JNK) and p38 kinases. In general activation of the ERK pathway is regulated by growth factors and is associated with cell survival, whereas that of JNK and p38 is activated by inflammatory stimuli and stress and is involved in cell death (Torii et al. 2004; Sumbayev and Yasinska 2005). In particular, oxidative stress may influence the MAPK signalling pathways by activation of pro-apoptotic signalling proteins such as JNK, which may initiate the apoptotic mechanism within the cells (Kwon et al. 2003) (Figure 4.8). Interestingly, flavonoids have close structural homology with pharmacological inhibitors of cell signalling cascades, such as PD98059, a MAPK inhibitor and LY294002, a phosphatidylinositol-3 kinase (PI3) inhibitor which was modelled on the structure of quercetin (Vlahos et al. 1994). LY294002 and quercetin fit into the ATP binding pocket of the enzyme and it seems that the number and substitution of hydroxyl groups on the B ring

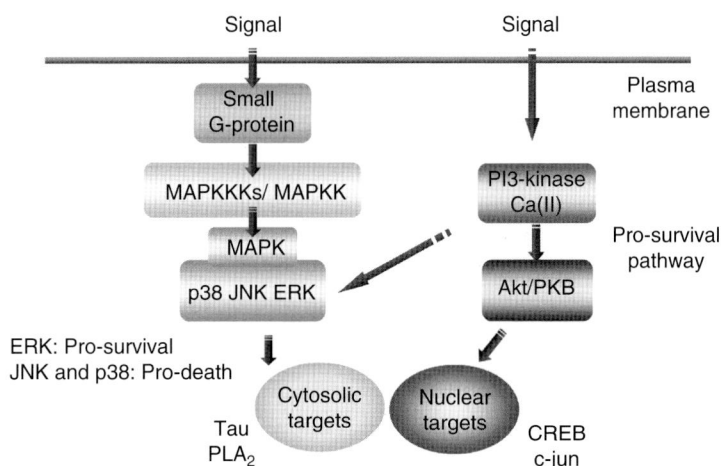

Figure 4.8   Diagrammatic representation of the MAP kinase and Akt/PKB signalling pathways. Extracellular signal-related kinase (ERK), c-jun amino-terminal kinase (JNK) and p38 are involved in growth, differentiation, development, apoptosis and inflammation. ERK and JNK are generally considered as having opposing actions in cells with signalling through ERK usually regarded as pro-signalling and JNK pro-apoptotic. The serine/threonine kinase, Akt/PKB, is one of the main downstream effectors of phosphatidylinositol 3-kinase (PI3-kinase) and a pivotal kinase in cell survival. See plate section for colour version of this figure.

and the degree of unsaturation of the C2-C3 bond are important determinants of this particular bioactivity. Similarly to the PI3 inhibitor LY294002, quercetin and other flavonoids have been shown to inhibit PI3-kinase activity (Agullo et al. 1997; Gamet-Payrastre et al. 1999), with inhibition directed at the ATP-binding site of the kinase (Vlahos et al. 1994). There are a number of potential sites within signalling pathways where flavonoids or their metabolites may interact. For instance, flavonoids may inhibit oxidative stress-induced apoptosis by preventing the activation of JNK, for example by influencing one of the many upstream MAPKKK activating proteins that transduce signals to JNK. Flavonoids may also act by maintaining calcium homeostasis, which is important in MAPK activation (Zippel et al. 2000; Montero et al. 2004). Alternatively, they may interact directly with mitochondria, for example by modulating the mPT, which controls cytochrome c release during apoptosis (Green and Reed 1998), or by modulating other mitochondrial associated pro-apoptotic factors such as DIABLO/smac (Srinivasula et al. 2001).

Importantly, the intracellular concentrations of flavonoids required to affect cell signalling pathways are considerably lower than those required to impact cellular antioxidant capacity, and flavonoid metabolites may still retain their ability to interact with cell signalling proteins, even if their antioxidant activity is diminished (Spencer et al. 2003). For example, both epicatechin and its *in vivo* metabolite 3′-O-methyl-epicatechin have been shown to elicit strong protective effects against oxidised LDL-induced neuronal cell death by inhibiting JNK, c-jun and caspase-3 activation (Schroeter et al. 2001; Spencer et al. 2001b). Interestingly, both components had no effect on the oxidised LDL-mediated increase in intracellular oxidative stress, suggesting that protection in this model is not mediated directly by antioxidant effects. Neuroprotective effects of flavonoids which include modulation of signalling pathways have been also shown for epigallocatechin gallate (EGCG) that induced stimulation of the cell survival PKC and modulated cell survival/cell cycle genes such as *Bax, Bad, Bcl-2, Bcl-w* and *Bcl-x(L)* (Levites et al. 2002a). EGCG has also been shown to protect neurons against oxidative stress-induced injury by activating the (PI3K)/Akt-dependent anti-apoptotic pathway and by inhibiting glycogen synthase kinase-3 (GSK-3) activity, which is known to be involved in cell death (Koh et al. 2004). It is also possible that polyphenols may inhibit neuroinflammatory processes via modulation of signalling cascades. This has been proposed for resveratrol, which suppressed phosphorylation of p38 in lipopolysaccharide (LPS)-activated microglia, suggesting that polyphenols may also modulate signalling cascades, such as MAPK, that participate in the pro-inflammatory responses in microglial cells (Bhat et al. 1998; Bi et al. 2005).

Flavonoids may also affect growth-related signal transduction pathways involved in the progression of cancer. For example, EGCG has been shown to induce apoptotic cell death in human leukaemia U937 cells by modulating JNK, p38, ASK1 and MAP kinase kinase (MKK), signalling cascades (Saeki et al. 2002), whereas EGCG-induced G2 cell cycle arrest in breast cancer cells was induced by phosphorylation of JNK and p38 signalling pathways, further suggesting a regulation of MAPK as a protective mechanism of action of flavonoids in cancer (Deguchi et al. 2002). Other flavonoids, such as isoflavones, may also exert anticarcinogenic effects through modulation of signalling cascades. For instance, genistein has been shown to induce apoptosis and cell cycle arrest in leukaemic cells by mechanisms including modulation of MAPK pathways (Shen et al. 2007).

Furthermore, polyphenols may also exert beneficial effects in cardiovascular disease through modulation of endothelial signalling (Kyaw et al. 2004). For example, quercetin may inhibit cell proliferation and migration in smooth muscle cells by downregulating JNK and ERK pathways (Yoshizumi et al. 2002; Moon et al. 2003) and may also induce haem oxygenase 1 (HO-1) expression, which is known to inhibit atherosclerosis progression, through p38 activation in aortic smooth muscle cells (Lin et al. 2004). Red wine polyphenols may also inhibit migration of smooth muscle cells by inhibiting PI3K and p38 phosphorylation, further supporting the theory that polyphenols may exert anti-atherogenic effects through inhibition of distinct signalling pathways (Iijima et al. 2002).

Other potential mechanisms of action

In terms of other possible modes of action, flavonoids may aid detoxification of potential carcinogens by modulation of the drug metabolising enzymes such as cytochrome (CYP) P450 enzyme, whose CYP1A form has been associated with the metabolism of many chemical carcinogens found in the environment and diet (Gonzalez and Gelboin 1994) and UDP-glucuronosyltransferases (UGTs), which catalyses the glucuronidation of both endogenous toxins and xenobiotics (Radominska-Pandya et al. 1999). For instance, green tea extract has been shown to increase the expression of CYP1A in human gastrointestinal epithelial cell lines (Netsch et al. 2006), whereas quercetin may induce CYP1A expression in MCF-7 cancer cells (Ciolino et al. 1999). In addition, the flavonoid chrysin may cause an induction of intestinal UGT in human intestinal Caco-2 cells (Galijatovic et al. 2001) and in human hepatoma Hep G2 cells (Walle et al. 2000a), suggesting an important role of flavonoids in detoxification systems.

Conclusion

The results of numerous studies in cell culture suggest that flavonoids may affect chronic disease by selectively inhibiting kinases (Hou et al. 2004). Specifically, there is now convincing evidence to suggest that flavonoids and more importantly their *in vivo* metabolites, such as the methylated forms may interact with cell signalling pathways involved in growth, differentiation and apoptosis and that these interactions may mediate their cellular effects. This hypothesis is further supported by the fact that the antioxidant properties of flavonoids seem unlikely to be the only explanation for their reported beneficial effects because extensive metabolism in the gastrointestinal tract significantly reduces their antioxidant capacity and results in plasma concentrations much lower than that of the established antioxidants such as ascorbate and α-tocopherol. Nevertheless, it should be noted that the interactions of flavonoids with cell signalling cascades mainly depend on the cell type and the disease studied, and the actions of flavonoids at different sites may have beneficial or detrimental effects. Therefore, an understanding of the exact molecular and cellular mechanisms of flavonoid action and, more importantly, the *in vivo* metabolite forms at different sites is crucial in evaluating the potential beneficial effects of polyphenols against chronic and age-related diseases.

Summary

Phenolics are ubiquitously found in plants and constitute a major part of a daily human diet. Lots of data has emerged on the potential health effects of several classes of phenolic compounds, and in particular flavonoids, in a number of chronic and age-related diseases. Over recent years we have gained an understanding of how polyphenols are metabolised within the body and now it is essential to understand the mode of action of the bioavailable forms of phenolic compounds. Phenolics exert strong bioactivity and it is now evident that they may exert their beneficial effects through a range of mechanisms more complex than previously thought. Whether these mechanisms include antioxidants effects and/or modulation of cell signalling pathways need to be further investigated to establish the role of phenolics in chronic disease prevention. In particular, emphasis should be given to the potential mechanisms of action of circulating phenolic compounds that can reach the target tissues and are able to penetrate the cells and thus exert a biological effect at a cellular level. Nevertheless, more well-designed human studies that measure appropriate biomarkers are warranted to assess the role of phenolic compounds in health and disease. The outcomes of these studies may ultimately be used to make dietary recommendations about the efficiency of phenolics in preventing chronic disease development or progression.

Acknowledgements

The authors are funded by the Biotechnology and Biological Sciences Research Council (BB/F008953/1; BB/C518222/1; BB/G005702/1) and the Medical Research Council (G0400278/NI02).

References

Agullo, G., Gamet-Payrastre, L., Manenti, S., Viala, C., Remesy, C., Chap, H. and Payrastre, B. (1997) Relationship between flavonoid structure and inhibition of phosphatidylinositol 3-kinase: a comparison with tyrosine kinase and protein kinase C inhibition. *Biochemical Pharmacology* **53**, 1649–57.

Ambra, R., Rimbach, G., de Pascual, T.S., Fuchs, D., Wenzel, U., Daniel, H., and Virgili, F. (2006) Genistein affects the expression of genes involved in blood pressure regulation and angiogenesis in primary human endothelial cells. *Nutrition Metabolism and Cardiovascular Disease* **16**, 35–43.

Arts, I.C.W., van de Putte, B. and Hollman, P.C.H. (2000a) Catechin contents of foods commonly consumed in The Netherlands. 1. Fruits, vegetables, staple foods, and processed foods 166. *Journal of Agricultural and Food Chemistry* **48**, 1746–51.

Arts, I.C.W., van de Putte, B. and Hollman, P.C.H. (2000b) Catechin contents of foods commonly consumed in The Netherlands. 2. Tea, wine, fruit juices, and chocolate milk 167. *Journal of Agricultural and Food Chemistry* **48**, 1752–7.

Baba, S., Furuta, T., Fujioka, M. and Goromaru, T. (1983) Studies on drug metabolism by use of isotopes XXVII: urinary metabolites of rutin in rats and the role of intestinal microflora in the metabolism of rutin. *Journal of Pharmocological Science* **72**, 1155–8.

Bacon, J.R., Williamson, G., Garner, R.C., Lappin, G., Langouet, S. and Bao, Y. (2003) Sulforaphane and quercetin modulate PhIP-DNA adduct formation in human HepG2 cells and hepatocytes. *Carcinogenesis* **24**, 1903–11.

Bailey, D.G., Malcolm, J., Arnold, O. and Spence, J.D. (1998) Grapefruit juice-drug interactions [Full text delivery]. *British Journal of Clinical Pharmacology* **46**, 101–10.

Bais, H.P., Walker, T.S., Kennan, A.J., Stermitz, F.R. and Vivanco, J.M. (2003) Structure-dependent phytotoxicity of catechins and other flavonoids: flavonoid conversions by cell-free protein extracts of *Centaurea maculosa* (spotted knapweed) roots 2169. *Journal of Agricultural and Food Chemistry* **51**, 897–901.

Barzilai, A. and Rahamimoff, H. (1983) Inhibition of Ca^{2+}-transport ATPase from synaptosomal vesicles by flavonoids. *Biochimica et Biophysica Acta* **730**, 245–54.

Bate-Smith, E. (1953) Colour reactions of flowers attributed to flavanols and carotenoid oxides. *Journal of Experimental Botany* **4**, 1–9.

Bate-Smith, E. (1954) Leuco-anthocyanins. I. Detection and identification of anthocyanidins formed from leuco-anthocyanins in plant tissues. *Biochemical Journal* **58**, 122–5.

Beltz, L.A., Bayer, D.K., Moss, A.L. and Simet, I.M. (2006) Mechanisms of cancer prevention by green and black tea polyphenols. *Anticancer Agents in Medical Chemistry* **6**, 389–406.

van den Berg, R., van Vliet, T., Broekmans, W.M., Cnubben, N.H., Vaes, W.H., Roza, L., Haenen, G.R., Bast, A. and van den Berg, H. (2001) A vegetable/fruit concentrate with high antioxidant capacity has no effect on biomarkers of antioxidant status in male smokers. *Journal of Nutrition* **131**, 1714–22.

Bhat, N.R., Zhang, P., Lee, J.C. and Hogan, E.L. (1998) Extracellular signal-regulated kinase and p38 subgroups of mitogen-activated protein kinases regulate inducible nitric oxide synthase and tumor necrosis factor-alpha gene expression in endotoxin-stimulated primary glial cultures. *Journal of Neuroscience* **18**, 1633–41.

Bi, X.L., Yang, J.Y., Dong, Y.X., Wang, J.M., Cui, Y.H., Ikeshima, T., Zhao, Y.Q. and Wu, C.F. (2005) Resveratrol inhibits nitric oxide and TNF-alpha production by lipopolysaccharide-activated microglia. *International Immunopharmacology* **5**, 185–93.

Bianchini, F. and Vainio, H. (2003) Wine and resveratrol: mechanisms of cancer prevention? *European Journal of Cancer Prevention* **12**, 417–25.

Boege, F., Straub, T., Kehr, A., Boesenberg, C., Christiansen, K., Andersen, A., Jakob, F. and Kohrle, J. (1996) Selected novel flavones inhibit the DNA binding or the DNA religation step of eukaryotic topoisomerase I. *Journal of Biological Chemistry* **271**, 2262–70.

Bohm, B. (1998) *Introduction to Flavonoids*. Singapore: Harwood Academic.

Bokkenheuser, V.D., Shackleton, C.H. and Winter, J. (1987) Hydrolysis of dietary flavonoid glycosides by strains of intestinal Bacteroides from humans. *Biochemical Journal* **248**, 953–6.

Bovy, A., de Voss, R., Kemper, M., Schijlen, E., Almenar, P.M., Muir, S., Collins, G., Robinson, S., Verhoeyen, M., Hughes, S., Santos-Buelga, C. and van Tunen, A. (2002) High-flavonol tomatoes resulting from the heterologous expression of the maize transcription factor genes LC and C1. *Plant Cell* **14**, 2509–26.

Braun, E.L., Dias, A.P., Matulnik, T.J. and Grotewold, E. (2001) *Transcription Factors and Metabolic Engineering: Novel Applications For Ancient Tools*. Oxford: Pergamon-Elsevier Science.

Broun, P. (2004) Transcription factors as tools for metabolic engineering in plants. *Current Opinion in Plant Biology* **7**, 202–9.

bu-Amsha, C.R., Burke, V., Mori, T.A., Beilin, L.J., Puddey, I.B. and Croft, K.D. (2001) Red wine polyphenols, in the absence of alcohol, reduce lipid peroxidative stress in smoking subjects. *Free Radical Biology and Medicine* **30**, 636–42.

Cao, Y. and Cao, R. (1999) Angiogenesis inhibited by drinking tea. *Nature* **398**, 381.

Chang, L. and Karin, M. (2001) Mammalian MAP kinase signalling cascades. *Nature* **410**, 37–40.

Checkoway, H., Powers, K., Smith-Weller, T., Franklin, G.M., Longstreth, W.T., Jr and Swanson, P.D. (2002) Parkinson's disease risks associated with cigarette smoking, alcohol consumption, and caffeine intake. *American Journal of Epidemiology* **155**, 732–8.

Chen, J.C., Ho, F.M., Pei-Dawn, L.C., Chen, C.P., Jeng, K.C., Hsu, H.B., Lee, S.T., Wen, T.W. and Lin, W.W. (2005) Inhibition of iNOS gene expression by quercetin is mediated by the inhibition of IkappaB kinase, nuclear factor-kappa B and STAT1, and depends on heme oxygenase-1 induction in mouse BV-2 microglia. *European Journal of Pharmacology* **521**, 9–20.

Cheynier, V. (2005) Polyphenols in foods are more complex than often thought. *American Journal of Clinical Nutrition* **81**, 223S–229S.

Ciolino, H.P., Daschner, P.J. and Yeh, G.C. (1999) Dietary flavonols quercetin and kaempferol are ligands of the aryl hydrocarbon receptor that affect CYP1A1 transcription differentially. *Biochemical Journal* **340** (Part 3), 715–22.

Clifford, M.N. (1999) Chlorogenic acids and other cinnamates – nature, occurrence and dietary burden. *Journal of the Science of Food and Agriculture* **79**, 362–72.

Conseil, G., Baubichon-Cortay, H., Dayan, G., Jault, J.M., Barron, D. and Di Pietro, A. (1998) Flavonoids: a class of modulators with bifunctional interactions at vicinal ATP- and steroid-binding sites on mouse P-glycoprotein. *Proceedings of the National Academy of Sciences USA* **95**, 9831–6.

Crespy, V., Morand, C., Manach, C., Besson, C., Demigne, C. and Remesy, C. (1999) Part of quercetin absorbed in the small intestine is conjugated and further secreted in the intestinal lumen. *American Journal of Physiology* **277**, G120–G126.

Davies, K.M. and Schwinn, K.E. (2006) Molecular biology and biotechnology of flavonoid biosynthesis. In: *Flavonoids: Chemistry, Biochemistry, and Applications* (eds O.M. Andersen and K.R. Markham), pp. 143–218. Boca Raton, FL: CRC Press.

Day, A.J. and Williamson, G. (2001) Biomarkers for exposure to dietary flavonoids: a review of the current evidence for identification of quercetin glycosides in plasma. *British Journal of Nutrition* **86** (Suppl 1), 105–10.

De Freitas, V. and Mateus, N. (2001) Structural features of procyanidin interactions with salivary proteins. *Journal of Agriculture and Food Chemistry* **49**, 940–5.

Deguchi, H., Fujii, T., Nakagawa, S., Koga, T. and Shirouzu, K. (2002) Analysis of cell growth inhibitory effects of catechin through MAPK in human breast cancer cell line T47D. *International Journal of Oncology* **21**, 1301–5.

Devasagayam, T.P., Subramanian, M., Singh, B.B., Ramanathan, R. and Das, N.P. (1995) Protection of plasmid pBR322 DNA by flavonoids against single-stranded breaks induced by singlet molecular oxygen. *Journal of Photochemistry and Photobiology B: Biology* **30**, 97–103.

Dewick, P.M. (1992) The biosynthesis of shikimate metabolites. *Natural Product Reports* **9**, 153–81.

Dewick, P.M. (2002) The shikimate pathway: aromatic amino acids and phenylpropanoids. In: *Medicinal Natural Products: A Biosynthetic Approach,* 2nd edn, pp. 121–66. Chichester: John Wiley & Sons Ltd.

Di Pietro, A., Godinot, C., Bouillant, M L. and Gautheron, D C. (1975) Pig heart mitochondrial ATPase: properties of purified and membrane-bound enzyme. Effects of flavonoids. *Biochimie* **57**, 959–67.

Dixon, R.A. and Steele, C.L. (1999) Flavonoids and isoflavonoids – a gold mine for metabolic engineering. *Trends in Plant Science* **4**, 394–400.

Duthie, S.J., Collins, A.R., Duthie, G.G. and Dodson, V.L. (1997) Quercetin and myricetin protect against hydrogen peroxide-induced DNA damage (strand breaks and oxidised pyrimidines) in human lymphocytes. *Mutation Research – Genetic Toxicology and Environmental Mutagenesis* **393**, 223–31.

Duthie, S.J. and Dobson, V.L. (1999) Dietary flavonoids protect human colonocyte DNA from oxidative attack *in vitro*. *European Journal of Nutrition* **38**, 28–34.

Dyer, W.E., Henstrand, J.M., Handa, A.K. and Herrmann, K.M. (1989) Wounding induces the first enzyme of the shikimate pathway in Solanaceae. *Proceedings of the National Academy of Sciences USA* **86**, 7370–73.

Franke, A. (1997) Isoflavone content of breast milk and soy formulas: benefits and risks. *Clinical Chemistry* **43**, 850–1.

Freese, R., Basu, S., Hietanen, E., Nair, J., Nakachi, K., Bartsch, H. and Mutanen, M. (1999) Green tea extract decreases plasma malondialdehyde concentration but does not affect other indicators of oxidative stress, nitric oxide production, or hemostatic factors during a high-linoleic acid diet in healthy females. *European Journal of Nutrition* **38**, 149–57.

Fuhrman, B., Volkova, N., Coleman, R. and Aviram, M. (2005) Grape powder polyphenols attenuate atherosclerosis development in apolipoprotein E deficient (E0) mice and reduce macrophage atherogenicity. *Journal of Nutrition* **135**, 722–8.

Galijatovic, A., Otake, Y., Walle, U.K. and Walle, T. (2001) Induction of UDP-glucuronosyltransferase UGT1A1 by the flavonoid chrysin in Caco-2 cells – potential role in carcinogen bioinactivation. *Pharmaceutical Research* **18**, 374–9.

Gamet-Payrastre, L., Manenti, S., Gratacap, M.P., Tulliez, J., Chap, H. and Payrastre, B. (1999) Flavonoids and the inhibition of PKC and PI 3-kinase. *General Pharmacology* **32**, 279–86.

Garcia-Alonso, M., Rimbach, G., Sasai, M., Nakahara, M., Matsugo, S., Uchida, Y., Rivas-Gonzalo, J.C. and De Pascual-Teresa, S. (2005) Electron spin resonance spectroscopy studies on the free radical scavenging activity of wine anthocyanins and pyranoanthocyanins. *Molecular Nutrition and Food Research* **49**, 1112–19.

Gee, J.M., Dupont, M.S., Day, A.J., Plumb, G.W., Williamson, G. and Johnson, I.T. (2000) Intestinal transport of quercetin glycosides in rats involves both deglycosylation and interaction with the hexose transport pathway. *Journal of Nutrition* **130**, 2765–71.

Gee, J.M., Dupont, M.S., Rhodes, M.J.C. and Johnson, I.T. (1998) Quercetin glucosides interact with the intestinal glucose transport pathway. *Free Radical Biology and Medicine* **25**, 19–25.

Gonzalez, F.J. and Gelboin, H.V. (1994) Role of human cytochromes P450 in the metabolic activation of chemical carcinogens and toxins. *Drug Metabolism Reviews* **26**, 165–83.

Green, D.R. and Reed, J.C. (1998) Mitochondria and apoptosis. *Science* **281**, 1309–12.

Green, E.S., Cooper, C.E., Davies, M.J. and Rice-Evans, C. (1993) Antioxidant drugs and the inhibition of low-density lipoprotein oxidation. *Biochemical Society Transactions* **21**, 362–6.

Halliwell, B., Long, L.H., Yee, T.P., Lim, S. and Kelly, R. (2004) Establishing biomarkers of oxidative stress: the measurement of hydrogen peroxide in human urine. *Current Medicinal Chemistry* **11**, 1085–92.

Halliwell, B., Rafter, J. and Jenner, A. (2005) Health promotion by flavonoids, tocopherols, tocotrienols, and other phenols: direct or indirect effects? Antioxidant or not? *American Journal of Clinical Nutrition* **81**, 268S–276S.

Halliwell, B., Zhao, K. and Whiteman, M. (2000) The gastrointestinal tract: a major site of antioxidant action? *Free Radical Research* **33**, 819–30.

Hallund, J., Bugel, S., Tholstrup, T., Ferrari, M., Talbot, D., Hall, W.L., Reimann, M., Williams, C.M. and Wiinberg, N. (2006) Soya isoflavone-enriched cereal bars affect markers of endothelial function in postmenopausal women. *British Journal of Nutrition* **95**, 1120–26.

Hawkes, T.R., Lewis, T., Coggins, J.R., Mousdale, D.M., Lowe, D.J. and Thorneley, R.N. (1990) Chorismate synthase. Pre-steady-state kinetics of phosphate release from 5-enolpyruvylshikimate 3-phosphate. *Biochemical Journal* **265**, 899–902.

Head, K.A. (1998) Isoflavones and other soy constituents in human health and disease. *Alternative Medicine Review* **3**, 433–50.

Heinecke, J.W. (2006) Lipoprotein oxidation in cardiovascular disease: chief culprit or innocent bystander? *Journal of Experimental Medicine* **203**, 813–16.

Henstrand, J.M., McCue, K.F., Brink, K., Handa, A.K., Herrmann, K.M. and Conn, E.E. (1992) Light and fungal elicitor induce 3-deoxy-d-arabino-heptulosonate 7-phosphate synthase mRNA in suspension cultured cells of parsley (*Petroselinum crispum* L.). *Plant Physiology* **98**, 761–3.

Herrmann, K. (1989) Occurrence and content of hydroxycinnamic acid and hydroxybenzoic acid compounds in foods. *Critical Reviews in Food Science and Nutrition* **28**, 315–47.

Hertog, M.G., Feskens, E.J., Hollman, P.C., Katan, M.B. and Kromhout, D. (1993a) Dietary anti-oxidant flavonoids and risk of coronary heart disease: the Zutphen Elderly Study. *Lancet* **342**, 1007–11.

Hertog, M.G. and Hollman, P.C. (1996) Potential health effects of the dietary flavonol quercetin. *European Journal of Clinical Nutrition* **50**, 63–71.

Hertog, M.G.L., Hollman, P.C.H. and Katan, M.B. (1992) Content of potentially anticarcinogenic flavonoids of 28 vegetables and 9 fruits commonly consumed in the Netherlands. *Journal of Agricultural and Food Chemistry* **40**, 2379–83.

Hertog, M.G.L., Hollman, P.C.H. and Vandeputte, B. (1993b) Content of potentially anticarcino-genic flavonoids of tea infusions, wines, and fruit juices. *Journal of Agricultural and Food Chemistry* **41**, 1242–6.

Hertog, M.G.L., Kromhout, D., Aravanis, C., Blackburn, H., Buzina, R., Fidanza, F., Giampaoli, S., Jansen, A., Menotti, A., Nedeljkovic, S., Pekkarinen, M., Simic, B.S., Toshima, H., Feskens, E.J.M., Hollman, P.C.H. and Katan, M.B. (1995) Flavonoid intake and long-term risk of coronary-heart-disease and cancer in the 7 Countries Study. *Archives of Internal Medicine* **155**, 381–6.

Higdon, J.V. and Frei, B. (2003) Tea catechins and polyphenols: health effects, metabolism, and antioxidant functions. *Critical Reviews in Food Science and Nutrition* **43**, 89–143.

Higuchi, W.I., Ho, N.F., Park, J.Y. and Komiya, I. (1981) Rate-limiting steps and factors in drug absorption. In: *Drug Absorption* (eds L.F. Prescott and W.S. Nimno), pp. 35–60. New York: ADIS Press.

Hirano, R., Osakabe, N., Iwamoto, A., Matsumoto, A., Natsume, M., Takizawa, T., Igarashi, O., Itakura, H. and Kondo, K. (2000) Antioxidant effects of polyphenols in chocolate on low-density lipoprotein both *in vitro* and *ex vivo*. *Journal of Nutritional Science and Vitaminology (Tokyo)* **46**, 199–204.

Ho, N.F., Park, J.Y., Ni, P.F. and Higuchi, W.I. (1983) Advancing quantitative and mechanistic approaches in interfacing gastrointestinal drug absorption studies in animals and humans. In: *Animal Models for Oral Drug Delivery. In Situ and In vivo Approaches* (eds W. Crouthamel and A.C. Sarapu), pp. 27–106 Washington DC: American Pharmaceutics Association.

Hodgson, J.M., Croft, K.D., Mori, T.A., Burke, V., Beilin, L.J. and Puddey, I.B. (2002) Regular inges-tion of tea does not inhibit *in vivo* lipid peroxidation in humans. *Journal of Nutrition* **132**, 55–8.

Hollman, P.C., Bijsman, M.N., van Gameren, Y., Cnossen, E.P., de Vries, J.H. and Katan, M.B. (1999a) The sugar moiety is a major determinant of the absorption of dietary flavonoid glyco-sides in man. *Free Radical Research* **31**, 569–73.

Hollman, P.C., Feskens, E.J. and Katan, M.B. (1999b) Tea flavonols in cardiovascular disease and cancer epidemiology. *Proceedings of the Society for Experimental Bioogy andl Medicine* **220**, 198–202.

Hou, Z., Lambert, J.D., Chin, K. V. and Yang, C.S. (2004) Effects of tea polyphenols on signal transduction pathways related to cancer chemoprevention. *Mutation Research* **555**, 3–19.

Hubac, C., Ferran, J., Tremolieres, A. and Kondorosi, A. (1994) Luteolin uptake by rhizobium-meliloti—evidence for several steps including an active extrusion process. *Microbiology-UK* **140**, 2769–74.

Hubbard, G.P., Wolffram, S., de Vos R., Bovy, A., Gibbins, J.M. and Lovegrove, J.A. (2006) Ingestion of onion soup high in quercetin inhibits platelet aggregation and essential components of the collagen-stimulated platelet activation pathway in man: a pilot study. *British Journal of Nutrition* **96**, 482–8.

Iijima, K., Yoshizumi, M., Hashimoto, M., Akishita, M., Kozaki, K., Ako, J., Watanabe, T., Ohike, Y., Son, B., Yu, J., Nakahara, K. and Ouchi, Y. (2002) Red wine polyphenols inhibit vascular smooth muscle cell migration through two distinct signaling pathways. *Circulation* **105**, 2404–10.

Ioku, K., Pongpiriyadacha, Y., Konishi, Y., Takei, Y., Nakatani, N. and Terao, J. (1998) beta-Glucosidase activity in the rat small intestine toward quercetin monoglucosides. *Bioscience, Biotechnology and Biochemistry* **62**, 1428–31.

Ishikawa, T., Suzukawa, M., Ito, T., Yoshida, H., Ayaori, M., Nishiwaki, M., Yonemura, A., Hara, Y. and Nakamura, H. (1997) Effect of tea flavonoid supplementation on the susceptibility of low-density lipoprotein to oxidative modification. *American Journal of Clinical Nutrition* **66**, 261–6.

Jeong, Y.J., Choi, Y.J., Kwon, H.M., Kang, S.W., Park, H.S., Lee, M. and Kang, Y.H. (2005) Differential inhibition of oxidized LDL-induced apoptosis in human endothelial cells treated with different flavonoids. *British Journal of Nutrition* **93**, 581–91.

Joseph, J.A., Shukitt-Hale, B., Denisova, N. A., Bielinski, D., Martin, A., McEwen, J.J. and Bickford, P.C. (1999) Reversals of age-related declines in neuronal signal transduction, cognitive, and motor behavioral deficits with blueberry, spinach, or strawberry dietary supplementation. *Journal of Neuroscience* **19**, 8114–21.

Joseph, J. A., Shukitt-Hale, B., Denisova, N.A., Prior, R.L., Cao, G., Martin, A., Taglialatela, G. and Bickford, P. C. (1998) Long-term dietary strawberry, spinach, or vitamin E supplementation retards the onset of age-related neuronal signal-transduction and cognitive behavioral deficits. *Journal of Neuroscience* **18**, 8047–55.

Justesen, U. (2000) Negative atmospheric pressure chemical ionisation low-energy collision activation mass spectrometry for the characterisation of flavonoids in extracts of fresh herbs. *Journal of Chromatography A* **902**, 369–79.

Justesen, U. (2001) Collision-induced fragmentation of deprotonated methoxylated flavonoids, obtained by electrospray ionization mass spectrometry. *Journal of Mass Spectrometry* **36**, 169–78.

Kim, D.H., Jung, E.A., Sohng, I.S., Han, J.A., Kim, T.H. and Han, M.J. (1998) Intestinal bacterial metabolism of flavonoids and its relation to some biological activities. *Archives Pharmacal Research* **21**, 17–23.

Kim, H., Kim, Y.S., Kim, S. Y. and Suk, K. (2001) The plant flavonoid wogonin suppresses death of activated C6 rat glial cells by inhibiting nitric oxide production. *Neuroscience Letters* **309**, 67–71.

Koh, S.H., Kim, S.H., Kwon, H., Kim, J.G., Kim, J.H., Yang, K.H., Kim, J., Kim, S.U., Yu, H.J., Do, B.R., Kim, K.S. and Jung, H.K. (2004) Phosphatidylinositol-3 kinase/Akt and GSK-3 mediated cytoprotective effect of epigallocatechin gallate on oxidative stress-injured neuronal-differentiated N18D3 cells. *Neurotoxicology* **25**, 793–802.

Kong, A.N., Yu, R., Chen, C., Mandlekar, S. and Primiano, T. (2000) Signal transduction events elicited by natural products: role of MAPK and caspase pathways in homeostatic response and induction of apoptosis. *Archives of Pharmacal Research* **23**, 1–16.

Kruk, I., boul-Enein, H.Y., Michalska, T., Lichszteld, K. and Kladna, A. (2005) Scavenging of reactive oxygen species by the plant phenols genistein and oleuropein. *Luminescence* **20**, 81–9.

Kuhnle, G., Spencer, J.P.E., Chowrimootoo, G., Schroeter, H., Debnam, E.S., Srai, S.K.S., Rice-Evans, C. and Hahn, U. (2000a) Resveratrol is absorbed in the small intestine as resveratrol glucuronide. *Biochemical and Biophysical Research Communications* **272**, 212–17.

Kuhnle, G., Spencer, J.P.E., Schroeter, H., Shenoy, B., Debnam, E.S., Srai, S.K., Rice-Evans, C. and Hahn, U. (2000b) Epicatechin and catechin are O-methylated and glucuronidated in the small intestine. *Biochemical and Biophysical Research Communications* **277**, 507–12.

Kumpulainen, J.T., Lehtonen, M. and Mattila, P. (1999) Trolox equivalent antioxidant capacity of average flavonoid intake in Finland. In: *Natural Antioxidants and Anticarcinogens in Nutrition, Health and Disease* (eds J.T. Kumpulainen and J.T. Salonen), pp. 141–50. Cambridge: Royal Society of Chemistry.

Kuriyama, S., Shimazu, T., Ohmori, K., Kikuchi, N., Nakaya, N., Nishino, Y., Tsubono, Y. and Tsuji, I. (2006) Green tea consumption and mortality due to cardiovascular disease, cancer, and all causes in Japan: the Ohsaki study. *Journal of the American Medical Association* **296**, 1255–65.

Kwon, Y.W., Masutani, H., Nakamura, H., Ishii, Y. and Yodoi, J. (2003) Redox regulation of cell growth and cell death. *Biological Chemistry* **384**, 991–6.

Kyaw, M., Yoshizumi, M., Tsuchiya, K., Izawa, Y., Kanematsu, Y. and Tamaki, T. (2004) Atheroprotective effects of antioxidants through inhibition of mitogen-activated protein kinases. *Acta Pharmacologica Sinica* **25**, 977–85.

Laires, A., Pacheco, P. and Rueff, J. (1989) Mutagenicity of rutin and the glycosidic activity of cultured cell-free microbial preparations of human faeces and saliva. *Food and Chemical Toxicology* **27**, 437–43.

Langcake, P. (1981) Disease resistance of *Vitis* spp. and the production of the stress metabolites resveratrol, e-viniferin, a-viniferin and pterostilbene. *Physiological Plant Pathology* **18**, 213–26.

Langcake, P. and Pryce, R. J. (1977) The production of resveratrol and the viniferins by grapevines in response to ultraviolet irradiation. *Phytochemistry* 16.

Laughton, M.J., Evans, P. J., Moroney, M.A., Hoult, J.R. and Halliwell, B. (1991) Inhibition of mammalian 5-lipoxygenase and cyclo-oxygenase by flavonoids and phenolic dietary additives. Relationship to antioxidant activity and to iron ion-reducing ability. *Biochemical Pharmacology* **42**, 1673–81.

Levites, Y., Amit, T., Youdim, M.B. and Mandel, S. (2002a) Involvement of protein kinase C activation and cell survival/ cell cycle genes in green tea polyphenol (−)-epigallocatechin 3-gallate neuroprotective action. *Journal of Biological Chemistry* **277**, 30574–80.

Levites, Y., Youdim, M.B., Maor, G. and Mandel, S. (2002b) Attenuation of 6-hydroxydopamine (6-OHDA)-induced nuclear factor-kappaB (NF-kappaB) activation and cell death by tea extracts in neuronal cultures. *Biochemical Pharmacology* **63**, 21–29.

Li, C., Lee, M. J., Sheng, S. Q., Meng, X. F., Prabhu, S., Winnik, B., Huang, B. M., Chung, J. Y., Yan, S. Q., Ho, C. T. and Yang, C. S. (2000) Structural identification of two metabolites of catechins and their kinetics in human urine and blood after tea ingestion. *Chemical Research In Toxicology* **13**, 177–184.

Lin, H.C., Cheng, T.H., Chen, Y.C. and Juan, S.H. (2004) Mechanism of heme oxygenase-1 gene induction by quercetin in rat aortic smooth muscle cells. *Pharmacology* **71**, 107–112.

Lin, J.H., Chiba, M. and Baillie, T.A. (1999) Is the role of the small intestine in first-pass metabolism overemphasized? *Pharmacological Reviews* **51**, 135–58.

Lin, J.K., Chen, P.C., Ho, C.T. and Lin-Shiau, S.Y. (2000) Inhibition of xanthine oxidase and suppression of intracellular reactive oxygen species in HL-60 cells by theaflavin-3,3′-digallate, (−)-epigallocatechin-3-gallate, and propyl gallate. *Journal of Agricultural and Food Chemistry* **48**, 2736–43.

Ludwig, A., Lorenz, M., Grimbo, N., Steinle, F., Meiners, S., Bartsch, C., Stangl, K., Baumann, G. and Stangl, V. (2004) The tea flavonoid epigallocatechin-3-gallate reduces cytokine-induced VCAM-1 expression and monocyte adhesion to endothelial cells. *Biochemical and Biophysical ResearchCommunications* **316**, 659–65.

McCue, K.F. and Conn, E.E. (1989) Induction of 3-deoxy-D-arabino-heptulosonate-7-phosphate synthase activity by fungal elicitor in cultures of *Petroselinum crispum. Proceedings of the National Academy of Sciences USA* **86**, 7374–7.

Macdonald, I.A., Mader, J.A. and Bussard, R.G. (1983) The role of rutin and quercitrin in stimulating flavonol glycosidase activity by cultured cell-free microbial preparations of human feces and saliva. *Mutation Research* **122**, 95–102.

Macheix, J.J., Sapis, J.C. and Fleuriet, A. (1991) Phenolic compounds and polyphenoloxidase in relation to browning in grapes and wines. *Critical Reviews in Food Science and Nutrition* **30**, 441–86.

Macheix, J. and Fleuriet, A. (1998) Phenolic acids in fruits. In: *Flavonoids in Health and Disease* (eds C.A. Rice-Evans and L. Packer), pp. 35–59. New York: Marcel Dekker.

Magee, P.J. and Rowland, I.R. (2004) Phyto-oestrogens, their mechanism of action: current evidence for a role in breast and prostate cancer. *British Journal of Nutrition* **91**, 513–31.

Manach, C. and Donovan, J.L. (2004) Pharmacokinetics and metabolism of dietary flavonoids in humans. *Free Radical Research* **38**, 771–85.

Manach, C., Scalbert, A., Morand, C., Remesy, C. and Jimenez, L. (2004) Polyphenols: food sources and bioavailability. *American Journal of Clinical Nutrition* **79**, 727–47.

Manach, C., Williamson, G., Morand, C., Scalbert, A. and Remesy, C. (2005) Bioavailability and bioefficacy of polyphenols in humans. I. Review of 97 bioavailability studies. *American Journal of Clinical Nutrition* **81**, 230S–242S.

Mantena, S.K., Baliga, M.S. and Katiyar, S.K. (2006) Grape seed proanthocyanidins induce apoptosis and inhibit metastasis of highly metastatic breast carcinoma cells. *Carcinogenesis* **27**, 1682–91.

Medina, J.H., Viola, H., Wolfman, C., Marder, M., Wasowski, C., Calvo, D. and Paladini, A.C. (1997) Overview – flavonoids: a new family of benzodiazepine receptor ligands. *Neurochemical Research* **22**, 419–25.

Montero, M., Lobaton, C.D., Hernandez-Sanmiguel, E., Santodomingo, J., Vay, L., Moreno, A. and Alvarez, J. (2004) Direct activation of the mitochondrial calcium uniporter by natural plant flavonoids. *Biochemical Journal* **384**, 19–24.

Montuschi, P., Barnes, P.J. and Roberts, L.J. (2004) Isoprostanes: markers and mediators of oxidative stress. *FASEB Journal* **18**, 1791–800.

Moon, S.K., Cho, G.O., Jung, S.Y., Gal, S.W., Kwon, T.K., Lee, Y.C., Madamanchi, N.R. and Kim, C.H. (2003) Quercetin exerts multiple inhibitory effects on vascular smooth muscle cells: role of ERK1/2, cell-cycle regulation, and matrix metalloproteinase-9. *Biochemical and Biophysical Research Communications* **301**, 1069–78.

Morand, C., Crespy, V., Manach, C., Besson, C., Demigne, C. and Remesy, C. (1998) Plasma metabolites of quercetin and their antioxidant properties. *American Journal of Physiology* **275**, R212–19.

Morand, C., Manach, C., Crespy, V. and Remesy, C. (2000) Respective bioavailability of quercetin aglycone and its glycosides in a rat model. *Biofactors* **12**, 169–74.

Morel, I., Lescoat, G., Cillard, P. and Cillard, J. (1994) Role of flavonoids and iron chelation in antioxidant action. *Methods in Enzymology* **234**, 437–43.

Mukai, K., Nagai, S. and Ohara, K. (2005) Kinetic study of the quenching reaction of singlet oxygen by tea catechins in ethanol solution. *Free Radical Biology and Medicine* **39**, 752–61.

Nagaya, N., Yamamoto, H., Uematsu, M., Itoh, T., Nakagawa, K., Miyazawa, T., Kangawa, K. and Miyatake, K. (2004) Green tea reverses endothelial dysfunction in healthy smokers. *Heart* **90**, 1485–6.

Netsch, M.I., Gutmann, H., Schmidlin, C.B., Aydogan, C. and Drewe, J. (2006) Induction of CYP1A by green tea extract in human intestinal cell lines. *Planta Medica* **72**, 514–20.

Nishioka, H., Nishi, K. and Kyokane, K. (1981) Human saliva inactivates mutagenicity of carcinogens. *Mutat Research* **85**, 323–33.

O'Reilly, J.D., Mallet, A.I., McAnlis, G.T., Young, I.S., Halliwell, B., Sanders, T.A. and Wiseman, H. (2001) Consumption of flavonoids in onions and black tea: lack of effect on F2-isoprostanes and autoantibodies to oxidized LDL in healthy humans. *American Journal of Clinical Nutrition* **73**, 1040–44.

Parisis, D.M. and Pritchard, E.T. (1983) Activation of rutin by human oral bacterial isolates to the carcinogen-mutagen quercetin. *Archives of Oral Biology* **28**, 583–90.

Piao, M., Mori, D., Satoh, T., Sugita, Y. and Tokunaga, O. (2006) Inhibition of endothelial cell proliferation, *in vitro* angiogenesis, and the down-regulation of cell adhesion-related genes by genistein. Combined with a cDNA microarray analysis. *Endothelium* **13**, 249–66.

Pollard, S.E., Kuhnle, G.G., Vauzour, D., VafeiAdou, K., Tzounis, X., Whiteman, M., Rice-Evans, C. and Spencer, J.P. (2006) The reaction of flavonoid metabolites with peroxynitrite. *Biochemical and Biophysical Research Communications* **350**, 960–68.

Radominska-Pandya, A., Czernik, P.J., Little, J.M., Battaglia, E. and Mackenzie, P.I. (1999) Structural and functional studies of UDP-glucuronosyltransferases. *Drug Metabolism Reviews* **31**, 817–99.

Rice-Evans, C. (2001) Flavonoid antioxidants. *Current Medicinal Chemistry* **8**, 797–807.

Rice-Evans, C.A., Miller, N.J., Bolwell, P.G., Bramley, P.M. and Pridham, J.B. (1995) The relative antioxidant activities of plant-derived polyphenolic flavonoids. *Free Radical Research* **22**, 375–83.

Rice-Evans, C.A., Miller, N.J. and Paganga, G. (1996) Structure–antioxidant activity relationships of flavonoids and phenolic acids. *Free Radical Biology and Medicine* **20**, 933–56.

Rietveld, A. and Wiseman, S. (2003) Antioxidant effects of tea: evidence from human clinical trials. *Journal of Nutrition* **133**, 3285S–3292S.

de Rijke, Y.B., Demacker, P.N., Assen, N.A., Sloots, L.M., Katan, M.B. and Stalenhoef, A.F. (1996) Red wine consumption does not affect oxidizability of low-density lipoproteins in volunteers. *American Journal of Clinical Nutrition* **63**, 329–34.

Ruiz-Larrea, M.B., Mohan, A.R., Paganga, G., Miller, N.J., Bolwell, G.P. and Rice-Evans, C.A. (1997) Antioxidant activity of phytoestrogenic isoflavones. *Free Radical Research* **26**, 63–70.

Saeki, K., Kobayashi, N., Inazawa, Y., Zhang, H., Nishitoh, H., Ichijo, H., Saeki, K., Isemura, M. and Yuo, A. (2002) Oxidation-triggered c-Jun N-terminal kinase (JNK) and p38 mitogen-activated protein (MAP) kinase pathways for apoptosis in human leukaemic cells stimulated by epigallocatechin-3-gallate (EGCG): a distinct pathway from those of chemically induced and receptor-mediated apoptosis. *Biochemical Journal* **368**, 705–20.

Sampson, L., Rimm, E., Hollman, P.C.H., de Vries, J.H.M. and Katan, M.B. (2002) Flavonol and flavone intakes in US health professionals. *Journal of the American Dietetic Association* **102**, 1414–20.

Samy, R.P., Gopalakrishnakone, P. and Ignacimuthu, S. (2006) Anti-tumor promoting potential of luteolin against 7,12-dimethylbenz(a)anthracene-induced mammary tumors in rats. *Chemico-biological Interactions* **164**, 1–14.

Sanchez-Moreno, C., Cano, M.P., de Ancos, B., Plaza, L., Olmedilla, B., Granado, F. and Martin, A. (2003) Effect of orange juice intake on vitamin C concentrations and biomarkers of antioxidant status in humans. *American Journal of Clinical Nutrition* **78**, 454–60.

Scheline, R.R. (1999) Metabolism of oxygen heterocyclic compounds. In: *CRC Handbook of Mammalian Metabolism of Plant Compounds*, pp. 243–295. Boca Raton, FL: CRC Press.

Schneider, H. and Blaut, M. (2000) Anaerobic degradation of flavonoids by *Eubacterium ramulus*. *Archives of Microbiology* **173**, 71–5.

Schneider, H., Schwiertz, A., Collins, M.D. and Blaut, M. (1999) Anaerobic transformation of quercetin-3-glucoside by bacteria from the human intestinal tract. *Archives of Microbiology* **171**, 81–91.

Schroeter, H., Boyd, C., Spencer, J.P., Williams, R.J., Cadenas, E. and Rice-Evans, C. (2002) MAPK signaling in neurodegeneration: influences of flavonoids and of nitric oxide. *Neurobiology of Aging* **23**, 861–80.

Schroeter, H., Spencer, J.P., Rice-Evans, C. and Williams, R.J. (2001) Flavonoids protect neurons from oxidized low-density-lipoprotein-induced apoptosis involving c-Jun N-terminal kinase (JNK), c-Jun and caspase-3. *Biochemical Journal* **358**, 547–57.

Schroeter, H., Williams, R.J., Matin, R., Iversen, L. and Rice-Evans, C.A. (2000) Phenolic antioxidants attenuate neuronal cell death following uptake of oxidized low-density lipoprotein. *Free Radical Biology and Medicine* **29**, 1222–33.

Shen, J., Tai, Y.C., Zhou, J., Stephen Wong, C.H., Cheang, P.T., Fred Wong, W.S., Xie, Z., Khan, M., Han, J.H. and Chen, C.S. (2007) Synergistic antileukemia effect of genistein and chemotherapy in mouse xenograft model and potential mechanism through MAPK signaling. *Experimental Hematology* **35**, 75–83.

Singh, S.A. and Christendat, D. (2006) Structure of *Arabidopsis* dehydroquinate dehydratase-shikimate dehydrogenase and implications for metabolic channeling in the shikimate pathway. *Biochemistry* **45**, 7787–96.

Smith, J.V., Burdick, A.J., Golik, P., Khan, I., Wallace, D. and Luo, Y. (2002) Anti-apoptotic properties of *Ginkgo biloba* extract EGb 761 in differentiated PC12 cells. *Cellular and Molecular Biology (Noisy-le-Grand, France)* **48**, 699–707.

Spencer, J.P., Schroeter, H., Crossthwaithe, A.J., Kuhnle, G., Williams, R.J. and Rice-Evans, C. (2001a) Contrasting influences of glucuronidation and O-methylation of epicatechin on hydrogen peroxide-induced cell death in neurons and fibroblasts. *Free Radical Biology and Medicine* **31**, 1139–46.

Spencer, J.P., Schroeter, H., Kuhnle, G., Srai, S.K., Tyrrell, R.M., Hahn, U. and Rice-Evans, C. (2001b) Epicatechin and its *in vivo* metabolite, 3'-O-methyl epicatechin, protect human fibroblasts from oxidative-stress-induced cell death involving caspase-3 activation. *Biochemical Journal* **354**, 493–500.

Spencer, J.P.E., Chaudry, F., Pannala, A.S., Srai, S.K., Debnam, E. and Rice-Evans, C. (2000) Decomposition of cocoa procyanidins in the gastric milieu. *Biochemical and Biophysical Research Communications* **272**, 236–41.

Spencer, J.P.E., Chowrimootoo, G., Choudhury, R., Debnam, E.S., Srai, S. K. and Rice-Evans, C. (1999) The small intestine can both absorb and glucuronidate luminal flavonoids. *FEBS Letters* **458**, 224–30.

Spencer, J.P.E., Rice-Evans, C. and Williams, R. J. (2003) Modulation of pro-survival Akt/protein kinase B and ERK1/2 signaling cascades by quercetin and its *in vivo* metabolites underlie their action on neuronal viability. *Journal of Biological Chemistry* 278, 34783–34793.

Spencer, J.P.E., Schroeter, H., Rechner, A. and Rice-Evans, C. (2001d) Bioavailability of flavan-3-ols and procyanidins: gastrointestinal tract influences and their relevance to bioactive forms *in vivo*. *Antioxidants and Redox Signaling* **3**, 1023–40.

Spencer, J.P.E., Schroeter, H., Shenoy, B., Srai, S. K., Debnam, E.S. and Rice-Evans, C. (2001c) Epicatechin is the primary bioavailable form of the procyanidin dimers B2 and B5 after transfer across the small intestine. *Biochemical and Biophysical Research Communications* **285**, 588–93.

Srinivasula, S.M., Hegde, R., Saleh, A., Datta, P., Shiozaki, E., Chai, J., Lee, R.A., Robbins, P.D., Fernandes-Alnemri, T., Shi, Y. and Alnemri, E.S. (2001) A conserved XIAP-interaction motif in caspase-9 and Smac/DIABLO regulates caspase activity and apoptosis. *Nature* **410**, 112–16.

Sumbayev, V.V. and Yasinska, I.M. (2005) Regulation of MAP kinase-dependent apoptotic pathway: implication of reactive oxygen and nitrogen species. *Archives of Biochemistry and Biophysics* **436**, 406–12.

Sun, C.L., Yuan, J.M., Koh, W.P. and Yu, M.C. (2006) Green tea, black tea and breast cancer risk: a meta-analysis of epidemiological studies. *Carcinogenesis* **27**, 1310–15.

Thompson, H.J., Heimendinger, J., Gillette, C., Sedlacek, S.M., Haegele, A., O'Neill, C. and Wolfe, P. (2005) *In vivo* investigation of changes in biomarkers of oxidative stress induced by plant food rich diets. Journal of Agricultural and Food Chemistry **53**, 6126–32.

Thompson, H. J., Heimendinger, J., Haegele, A., Sedlacek, S.M., Gillette, C., O'Neill, C., Wolfe, P. and Conry, C. (1999) Effect of increased vegetable and fruit consumption on markers of oxidative cellular damage. *Carcinogenesis* **20**, 2261–6.

Tomas-Barberan, F.A. and Clifford, M.N. (2000) Dietary hydroxybenzoic acid derivatives – nature, occurrence and dietary burden. *Journal of the Science of Food and Agriculture* **80**, 1024–32.

Torii, S., Nakayama, K., Yamamoto, T. and Nishida, E. (2004) Regulatory mechanisms and function of ERK MAP kinases. *Journal of Biochemistry (Tokyo)* **136**, 557–61.

Tournaire, C., Croux, S., Maurette, M.T., Beck, I., Hocquaux, M., Braun, A.M. and Oliveros, E. (1993) Antioxidant activity of flavonoids: efficiency of singlet oxygen (1 delta g) quenching. *Journal of Photochemistry and Photobiology B: Biology* **19**, 205–15.

Tsuchiya, H., Sato, M., Kato, H., Okubo, T., Juneja, L.R. and Kim, M. (1997) Simultaneous determination of catechins in human saliva by high- performance liquid chromatography. *Journal of Chromatography B* **703**, 253–8.

Turner, R., Baron, T., Wolffram, S., Minihane, A.M., Cassidy, A., Rimbach, G. and Weinberg, P.D. (2004) Effect of circulating forms of soy isoflavones on the oxidation of low density lipoprotein. *Free Radical Research* **38**, 209–16.

Valerio, L.G., Jr, Kepa, J.K., Pickwell, G.V. and Quattrochi, L.C. (2001) Induction of human NAD(P)H:quinone oxidoreductase (NQO1) gene expression by the flavonol quercetin. *Toxicology Letters* **119**, 49–57.

Van Hoorn, D.E., Nijveldt, R.J., Van Leeuwen, P.A., Hofman, Z., M'Rabet, L., De Bont, D.B. and Van, N.K. (2002) Accurate prediction of xanthine oxidase inhibition based on the structure of flavonoids. *European Journal of Pharmacology* **451**, 111–18.

Vissers, M.N., Zock, P.L., Leenen, R., Roodenburg, A.J., van Putte, K.P. and Katan, M.B. (2001) Effect of consumption of phenols from olives and extra virgin olive oil on LDL oxidizability in healthy humans. *Free Radical Research* **35**, 619–29.

Vitaglione, P., Sforza, S., Galaverna, G., Ghidini, C., Caporaso, N., Vescovi, P.P., Fogliano, V. and Marchelli, R. (2005) Bioavailability of trans-resveratrol from red wine in humans. *Molecular Nutrition and Food Research* **49**, 495–504.

Vlahos, C.J., Matter, W.F., Hui, K.Y. and Brown, R.F. (1994) A specific inhibitor of phosphatidylinositol 3-kinase, 2-(4-morpholinyl)-8-phenyl-4H-1-benzopyran-4-one (LY294002). *Journal of Biological Chemistry* **269**, 5241–8.

Walle, T., Otake, Y., Galijatovic, A., Ritter, J.K. and Walle, U.K. (2000a) Induction of UDP-glucuronosyltransferase UGT1A1 by the flavonoid chrysin in the human hepatoma cell line hep G2. *Drug Metababolism and Disposition* **28**, 1077–82.

Walle, T., Otake, Y., Walle, U.K. and Wilson, F.A. (2000b) Quercetin glucosides are completely hydrolyzed in ileostomy patients before absorption. *Journal of Nutrition* **130**, 2658–61.

Wan, Y., Vinson, J.A., Etherton, T.D., Proch, J., Lazarus, S.A. and Kris-Etherton, P.M. (2001) Effects of cocoa powder and dark chocolate on LDL oxidative susceptibility and prostaglandin concentrations in humans. *American Journal of Clinical Nutrition* **74**, 596–602.

Wang, W., Heideman, L., Chung, C.S., Pelling, J.C., Koehler, K.J. and Birt, D.F. (2000) Cell-cycle arrest at G2/M and growth inhibition by apigenin in human colon carcinoma cell lines. *MolecularCarcinogenosis* **28**, 102–10.

Weisshaar, B. and Jenkins, G.I. (1998) Phenylpropanoid biosynthesis and its regulation. *Current Opinion in Plant Biology* **1**, 251–7.

Widlanski, T., Bender, S.L. and Knowles, J.R. (1989) Dehydroquinate synthase: the use of substrate analogues to probe the late steps of the catalyzed reaction. *Biochemistry* **28**, 7572–82.

Widlansky, M.E., Duffy, S.J., Hamburg, N.M., Gokce, N., Warden, B.A., Wiseman, S., Keaney, J. F., Jr, Frei, B. and Vita, J.A. (2005) Effects of black tea consumption on plasma catechins and markers of oxidative stress and inflammation in patients with coronary artery disease. *Free Radical Biology and Medicine* **38**, 499–506.

Williams, R.J., Spencer, J.P. and Rice-Evans, C. (2004) Flavonoids: antioxidants or signalling molecules? *Free Radical Biology and Medicine* **36**, 838–49.

Winkel-Shirley, B. (2001) Flavonoid biosynthesis. A colorful model for genetics, biochemistry, cell biology, and biotechnology. *Plant Physiology* **126**, 485–93.

Wiseman, H., O'Reilly, J.D., Adlercreutz, H., Mallet, A.I., Bowey, E.A., Rowland, I.R. and Sanders, T.A. (2000) Isoflavone phytoestrogens consumed in soy decrease F(2)-isoprostane concentrations and increase resistance of low-density lipoprotein to oxidation in humans. *American Journal of Clinical Nutrition* **72**, 395–400.

Yamamoto, N., Moon, J.H., Tsushida, T., Nagao, A. and Terao, J. (1999) Inhibitory effect of quercetin metabolites and their related derivatives on copper ion-induced lipid peroxidation in human low-density lipoprotein [Full text delivery]. *Archives of Biochemistry and Biophysics* **372**, 347–54.

Yang, C.S., Lee, M.J. and Chen, L. (1999) Human salivary tea catechin levels and catechin esterase activities: implication in human cancer prevention studies. *Cancer Epidemiol, Biomarkers and Prevention* **8**, 83–9.

Yannai, S., Day, A.J., Williamson, G. and Rhodes, M.J.C. (1998) Characterization of flavonoids as monofunctional or bifunctional inducers of quinone reductase in murine hepatoma cell lines. *Food and Chemical Toxicology* **36**, 623–30.

Yoshizumi, M., Tsuchiya, K., Suzaki, Y., Kirima, K., Kyaw, M., Moon, J.H., Terao, J. and Tamaki, T. (2002) Quercetin glucuronide prevents VSMC hypertrophy by angiotensin II via the inhibition of JNK and AP-1 signaling pathway. *Biochemical and Biophysical Research Communications* **293**, 1458–65.

Zern, T.L., Wood, R.J., Greene, C., West, K.L., Liu, Y., Aggarwal, D., Shachter, N.S. and Fernandez, M.L. (2005) Grape polyphenols exert a cardioprotective effect in pre- and postmenopausal women by lowering plasma lipids and reducing oxidative stress. *Journal of Nutrition* **135**, 1911–17.

Zippel, R., Balestrini, M., Lomazzi, M. and Sturani, E. (2000) Calcium and calmodulin are essential for Ras-GRF1-mediated activation of the Ras pathway by lysophosphatidic acid. *ExperimentalCell Research* **258**, 403–8.

Chapter 5

Vitamins C and E

David Gray, John Brameld and Gregory Tucker

Introduction

Vitamins C and E represent the major dietary antioxidants and are both essential components of the human diet. Whilst they both demonstrate antioxidant activities, their other properties are very different. Vitamin C is a water soluble compound whilst vitamin E is fat soluble. This means that they operate in completely different micro-environments within the cell. This does not mean, however, that these two antioxidants do not cooperate. Vitamin E is found associated with cell membranes and protects the lipids from oxidation. In doing so it becomes a free radical itself which must in turn be reduced back to its active form. It is thought that one mechanism for this is by interaction with the water soluble vitamin C at the membrane surface. This in turn generates the free radical form of vitamin C, monodehydroascorbate (MDHA). At this point, however, the vitamin C is relatively unusual compared to many other dietary antioxidants, in that two molecules of MDHA can disproportionate to regenerate an active vitamin C and a molecule of dehydroascorbate (DHA). Thus vitamin C has the potential to act as a chain terminator in free radical reactions.

Vitamin C: structure and chemistry

The exact structure of vitamin C, or ascorbic acid, was determined by Haworth in 1932. Compared to many other vitamins, vitamin C is a relatively simple molecule being the aldone-1,4-lactone of L-galacturonic acid. The chemical structure of ascorbic acid is shown in Figure 5.1. Delocalisation of electrons over the C_2-C_3 region results in the molecule acting as an acid, the hydrogen of the C_3 hydroxyl group dissociating with a pKa of 4.13. Thus at physiological pH the ascorbic acid exists as a monovalent anion (L-ascorbate). Ascorbate can donate electrons to a wide range of substrates and as such is readily oxidised into the radical monodehydroascorbate (MDHA). Further oxidation results in the production of dehydroascorbate (DHA) as shown in Figure 5.1. The MDHA and DHA can both be reduced back to ascorbate by enzymatic means in both plants and animals.

Phytonutrients, First Edition. Edited by Andrew Salter, Helen Wiseman and Gregory Tucker.
© 2012 Blackwell Publishing Ltd. Published 2012 by Blackwell Publishing Ltd.

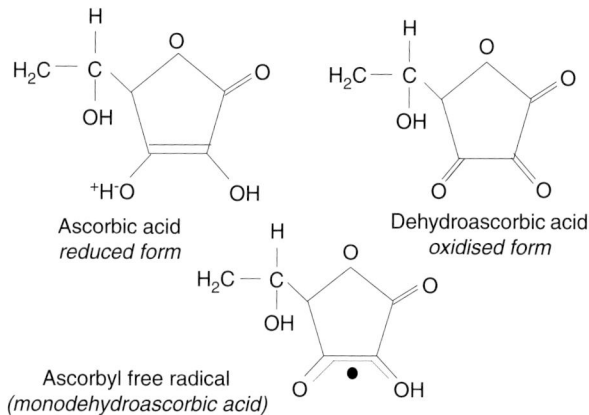

Figure 5.1   Structures of L-ascorbic acid, monodehydroascorbate (MDHA) and dehydroascorbate (DHA).

Alternatively, the DHA can undergo irreversible degradation to a range of products such as oxalate and L-threonate (Green and Fry 2005). Ascorbate is stable as a dry powder and is only readily oxidised once in solution. This coupled with the fact that ascorbate can be relatively easily synthesised chemically means that it is widely used as an additive in foods, often to act as an antioxidant to protect against browning.

Vitamin C is an important component in the diet for two main reasons. First, it is a key component in the general oxidant defence system of the body and secondly, because of its ability to participate in one electron reactions, it serves as a vital cofactor in many enzyme reactions.

Similarly to vitamin E, the main function of vitamin C is thought to be as an antioxidant, but in aqueous environments. However, unlike vitamin E, vitamin C also has specific roles as a cofactor in a number of biological reactions, all relating to its capacity as a reductant/antioxidant. Vitamin C is essential for the biosynthesis of collagen, L-carnitine and the catecholamines, adrenaline and noradrenaline. Like vitamin E, the effects of vitamin C deficiency are dependent to some extent on the other antioxidants present, although the other antioxidants are unable to act as cofactors in the synthesis of collagen, carnitine and catecholamines. Thus vitamin C deficiency results in scurvy, which was systematically studied by James Lind, a naval surgeon, in the 1750s. James Lind found that the disease could be prevented by daily consumption of fresh citrus fruits, such as limes – a potential source of the nickname 'Limeys' given to British sailors.

Dietary sources of vitamin C

Vitamin C is unusual as a micronutrient because it is often present in quite large amounts within plants (up to 100 mg/100 g). Levels are very variable between both tissues and species, and are also affected by the physiological status of the plant and environmental conditions (Logan et al. 1996; Lee and Kader 2000). Levels of vitamin C are normally high in green photosynthetic tissues such as leaves, as well as in fruit and other storage

Table 5.1 Dietary sources of vitamin C

Food	Range or average of Vitamin C content (mg/100g)
Fruit (raw)	
Blackcurrants	150–230
Strawberries	77
Kiwi fruit	59
Oranges	44–79
Grapefruit	36
Apples	6–14
Plums	4
Vegetables	
Green peppers (raw)	120
Brussels sprouts (boiled)	60
Cabbage (boiled)	20
Sweet potato (boiled)	17
Tomatoes (raw)	17
Carrots (raw)	4–6
Breakfast cereals	
Bran flakes	66
Cheerios	51
Corn flakes	0
Meat and meat products	
Liver (calf, fried)	19
Chicken (roasted)	0
Pork (grilled)	0
Lamb (stewed)	0

Source: data obtained from Food Standards Agency (2002).

organs (Loewus and Loewus 1987). Senescent processes in plants tend to be associated with a loss of vitamin C (Borraccino et al. 1994) and thus levels of ascorbate tend to decrease during the postharvest storage of crops such as spinach (Bergquist et al. 2006). These losses can normally be ameliorated by low-temperature storage during postharvest handling.

The main dietary sources of vitamin C are fruit and vegetables (see Table 5.1), and these commodities demonstrate a very wide range of levels from around 11 mg/100 g in potato tubers to around 220 mg/100 g in persimmon fruit (Lee and Kader 2000). In addition, it is also quite common practice to add vitamin C to many processed foods and beverages to increase shelf life. Dairy products, nuts, meat and fish are considered poor sources as they contain virtually no vitamin C, but liver contains as much vitamin C as a tomato fruit.

Vitamin C: biosynthesis and metabolism in plants

Vitamin C is synthesised by a wide range of living organisms. All plants are thought to be capable of synthesising this vitamin as can many animals. Interestingly, in the animal kingdom there are some specific exceptions to this ability to synthesise this vitamin,

Glucose-6-Phosphate
↓↑
Fructose-6-Phosphate
↓↑
D-Mannose-6-Phosphate
↓↑
D-Mannose-1-Phosphate
↓↑   GTP-Mannose Pyrophosphorylase
GDP-D-Mannose
↓↑   GTP-Mannose-3,5-epimerase
GDP-L-Galactose
↓   L-Galactose Guanyltransferase
L-Galactose-1-Phosphate
↓   L-Galactose-1-P Phosphatase
L-Galactose
↓   L-Galactose dehydrogenase
L-Galactono-1,4-lactone
↓   L-Galactono-1,4-lactone
                      dehydrogenase
L-Ascorbate (Vitamin C)

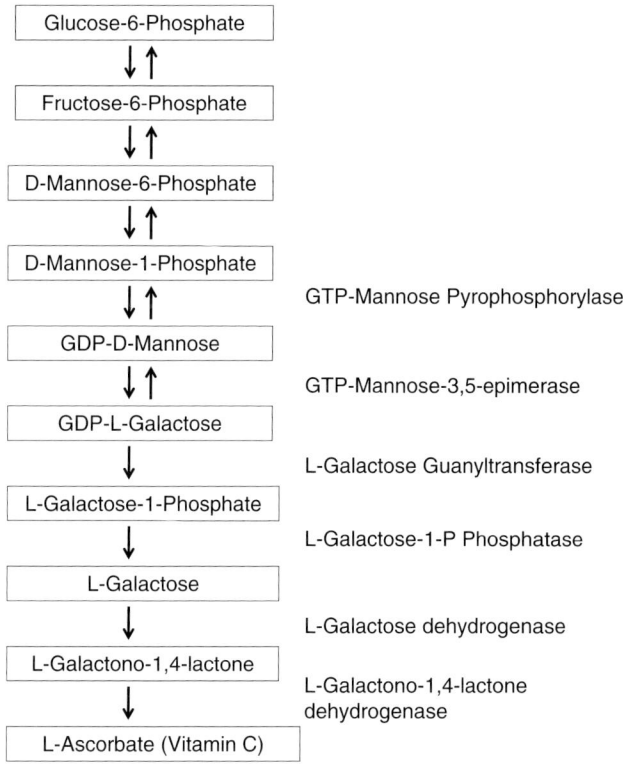

Figure 5.2   The L-galactose pathway for biosynthesis of vitamin C in plants.

including humans and other primates, bats, several birds and teleost fish. Thus it is an essential vitamin in the human diet. Fungi (yeasts) tend to synthesise a close homologue D-erythroascorbate. Despite this it is apparent that these organisms use very different biosynthetic routes.

The biosynthetic pathway for vitamin C was first described in mammals in the 1960s (Burns 1960). This pathway seems to be common to all animals capable of synthesising vitamin C and occurs in either the liver or kidney. Early investigations demonstrated, using radiotracer experiments, that glucose was the precursor for this nutrient in rats and that the carbon skeleton underwent 'inversion' during the process. The fact that mammals, such as humans and other primates, are unable to synthesise this vitamin lies in a mutation in the gene encoding the final enzyme in this biosynthetic pathway, namely L-gulono-1,4-lactone oxidase (Sato and Udenfriend 1978).

The biosynthetic pathway in plants was clearly identified as being different to that in animals since it was demonstrated that whilst glucose could still act as a precursor in plants, there was no accompanying inversion of the carbon skeleton. In 1998 Wheeler et al. published a biosynthetic pathway for ascorbate in plants. This has been termed the Smirnoff–Wheeler pathway and is summarised in Figure 5.2. Much of the pathway, i.e. from glucose-6-phosphate to GDP-galactose, is also involved in the generation of activated sugar residues for cell wall biosynthesis and protein glycosylation. The formation of L-galactose and subsequent reactions seem to be dedicated to ascorbate synthesis and indeed this has come to be known as the L-galactose pathway. Since the L-galactose pathway was first described, details concerning the genetics and biochemistry of all the steps involved have become available, and indeed all the genes involved in the dedicated part of the pathway have been cloned.

The identification of the genes involved in the L-galactose pathway has been aided by the availability of several mutants deficient in vitamin C accumulation. These were originally selected from mutants which had lost their antioxidant protection against reactive oxygen species (Conklin et al. 1999) and subsequently an EMS-mutagenised population of *Arabidopsis thaliana* plants was screened using a more selective method and six mutant lines were identified with reduced vitamin accumulation (Conklin et al. 2000). These were found to cover four loci (vtc1–4) which have been mapped: vtc1 and 3 to chromosome 2, vtc2 to chromosome 4, and vtc4 to chromosome 3.

Phosphomannose isomerase converts fructose-6-phosphate into mannose-6-phosphate. The activity of this enzyme is low in many plants and as such may be limiting. The next enzyme in the pathway is phosphomannose mutase which produces D-mannose-1-phosphate. The next reaction involves GDP-mannose pyrophosphorylase which catalyses the formation of GDP-mannose from D-mannose-1-phosphate. This was the first biosynthetic step to be associated with one of the vtc mutations. A gene for this enzyme (*vtc 1*) has been identified in *A. thaliana* (Conklin et al. 1999). GDP-mannose 3,5 epimerase is the next enzyme in the pathway. The conversion of GDP-D-mannose to GDP-L-galactose is an important step as it could be taken to represent the first dedicated step in the biosynthesis of ascorbate. Again this enzyme has been characterised from *A. thaliana* and shown to be a 84-kD dimer. The gene for this enzyme has also been identified in *A. thaliana* (Wolucka et al. 2001. The enzyme catalyzing the conversion of GDP-L-galactose to L-galactose-1-phosphate was the last to be characterised (Laing et al. 2007). This reaction is catalysed by the enzyme L-galactose quanyltransferase and has been shown to be equated with the vtc-2 mutant. The next step in the pathway is catalysed by the enzyme L-galactose-1-phosphate phosphatase. This enzyme converts L-galactose-1-phosphate into L-galactose and has been characterised from kiwi fruit (Laing et al. 2004) and a corresponding gene identified; this gene has been equated with the vtc-4 mutant in *A. thaliana*. L-galactose dehydrogenase, the next enzyme in the pathway, which converts L-galactose into L-galactono-1,4-lactone, has been cloned from *A. thaliana* using RT-PCR (Wolucka et al. 2001). The gene for the last enzyme in the pathway, L-galactono-1-4-lactone dehydrogenase, has been cloned from a variety of plant sources, such as sweet potato (Imai et al. 1998) and *A. thaliana*. This gene encodes a 66 kD mitochondrial enzyme which seems to use flavin as its prosthetic group.

Whilst the Smirnoff–Wheeler L-galactose pathway probably represents the major route for ascorbate synthesis in plants, the occurrence of other minor pathways cannot be excluded. These are thought to be able to convert glucose to ascorbate via myo-inositol or use galacturonate as precursors (Mapson and Isherwood 1956; Agius et al. 2003). These other pathways, and their relationship to the L-galactose pathway, are outlined in Figure 5.3.

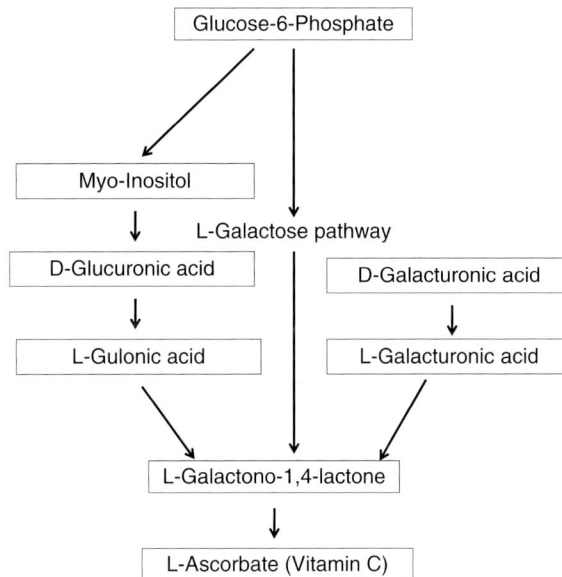

Figure 5.3   Vitamin C biosynthesis pathways in plants.

Factors, other than the rate of synthesis, that might influence the accumulation of ascorbate in a tissue include its rate of turnover, and this may be particularly true during the postharvest storage and handling of commodities such as fruit and vegetables. This turnover rate can vary considerably between tissues, thus in pea seedlings this has been estimated as 13% per hour (Pallanca and Smirnoff 2000) whilst in *Arabidopsis* it is 40% in 22 hours (Conklin et al. 1997). Whilst the biosynthetic pathway for vitamin C synthesis in plants has been well described, the pathway involved in its degradation is not well understood (Green and Fry 2005). The first step in the turnover of ascorbate is its conversion to DHA and, indeed, during the storage of spinach, the loss of ascorbate is accompanied by an increase in the level of DHA (Gil et al. 1999). This is not necessarily a problem in terms of nutritional value since once absorbed the DHA can be reduced back to ascorbic acid in the body. However, it does point out the importance of measuring both ascorbic acid and DHA in commodities to assess their nutritional value. The next steps in the degradation of the DHA are essentially irreversible and as such represent a loss of the nutrient from the diet. The DHA can be converted to 2,3-diketo-L-gulonate or enter more complex pathways and be converted to oxalate (Kostman et al. 2001) and/or tartrate (Loewus 1999). Indeed this may represent the biosynthetic pathway for these two compounds in plant tissues. Ascorbate can also accumulate in the apoplast, or extracellular spaces of the tissues, and may then be degraded by another pathway into L-threonate and L-tartrate (Green and Fry 2005). Although the precise details of these pathways are unclear, it does seem that this degradation can proceed either enzymatically or non-enzymatically. One enzyme that has been intensively studied is ascorbate oxidase (Pignocchi et al. 2003). This enzyme is located in the apoplast, converts ascorbate to DHA and is thought to play a major role in determining the redox balance of the apoplast.

Postharvest loss of ascorbate is particularly prevalent in green leafy vegetables and is generally less pronounced in fruits (Lee and Kader 2000). Kalt et al. (1999) monitored the levels of ascorbate in four varieties of berry stored for 8 days. They demonstrated that the ascorbate level remained constant during storage for strawberry and highbush blueberries whilst a decline was detected in raspberry and lowbush blueberry fruit. Gil et al. (2006) monitored levels of ascorbate in a range of minimally processed fruit over a 6-day period. They found losses of less than 5% for mango, strawberry and watermelon pieces, 10% in pineapple pieces and 25% in cantaloupe melon cubes. In contrast, spinach stored postharvest for 7 days exhibited a very significant loss of ascorbate, and although some of this was accumulating as DHA, the loss of total dietary 'vitamin C' was still very significant compared to that in fruit (Gil et al. 1999).

Vitamin C functions in plants

The function of ascorbate in plants can be considered in three major areas. First, ascorbate can function as a radical scavenger or as an antioxidant, in particular for scavenging reactive oxygen species (ROS) in chloroplasts, mitochondria and peroxisomes. Secondly, the MDHA generated in this scavenging role can interact directly with electron transport chains and act as an electron acceptor. Thirdly, ascorbate can act as a cofactor in several key enzymic reactions. These functions will only be considered in a very superficial manner in this review. For more details the reader is referred to the reviews by Horemans et al. (2000b) and Davey et al. (2000).

Ascorbate is a very useful antioxidant as, unlike many other potential physiological antioxidants, it can serve to terminate free radical reactions. Ascorbate is present in many plant cells at millimolar concentrations, although this can vary with species, tissues and even environmental factors. This means that ascorbate often represents a major antioxidant species in these tissues. The major radicals generated within cells are the ROS, which include superoxide, singlet oxygen, hydrogen peroxide and the hydroxyl radical. Chloroplasts, mitochondria and peroxisomes in plants all produce ROS as part of their normal metabolism. Indeed ROS production is thought to be essential in many aspects of plant metabolism such as responses to pathogen attack. However, these radicals are highly reactive and the hydroxyl radical in particular is capable of causing damage to DNA, proteins and lipids. The plant thus possesses a range of 'antioxidant defences' in which ascorbate plays a significant role.

Chloroplasts are potentially particularly susceptible to such radical damage because photosynthesis generates large amounts of oxygen in the immediate vicinity of a very powerful oxidation/reduction system. The ROS generated by the reaction of oxygen with the photosynthetic electron chain is rapidly converted to hydrogen peroxide by the action of the enzyme superoxide dismutase. Accumulation of this hydrogen peroxide would inhibit photosynthesis. The chloroplasts thus contain a number of ascorbate peroxidases. These enzymes carry out the following reaction:

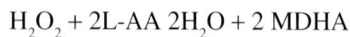

$$H_2O_2 + 2L\text{-}AA \quad 2H_2O + 2\ MDHA$$

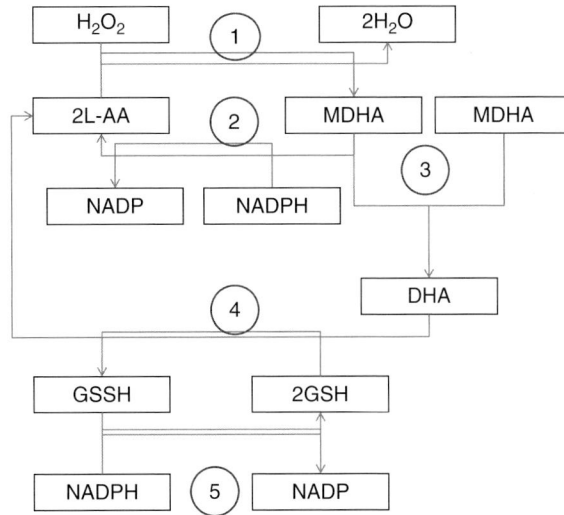

Figure 5.4 Hydrogen peroxide scavenging and regeneration of vitamin C. 1: Ascorbate peroxidase; 2: MDHA reductase; 3: MDHA disproportionation; 4: DHA reductase; 5:Glutathione reductase.

The MDHA formed can be reduced back to ascorbate by two potential mechanisms. First, it can react directly with the photosynthetic electron transport chain and accept an electron. This seems to occur by the MDHA reacting with the ferridoxin in photosystem 1 (PS1). Secondly, the ascorbate can be regenerated through the action of the ascorbate/ glutathione cycle as first described by Foyer and Halliwell (1976) and depicted in Figure 5.4. In this case the MDHA is reduced back to ascorbate by a stromal enzyme – monodehydroascorbate reductase – using the reducing power of NADPH. Any MDHA that is not converted by this mechanism can disproportionate to ascorbate and dehydroascorbate which can then be reduced by the remainder of the ascorbate/glutathione cycle. The DHA is reduced by the action of dehydroascorbate reductase using glutathione as the reductant, the glutathione then being regenerated from the resultant glutathione disulphide by glutathione reductase at the expense of NADPH. The direct reduction of MDHA by interaction with an electron transport chain is thought to be restricted to the chloroplasts as this is thought to be a specific interaction with PS1. This is also likely to be the major route for the regeneration of ascorbate in this organelle. The ascorbate/glutathione cycle is much more widespread across the plant cell and whilst potentially active in the chloroplast, may be of more significance in the protection of mitochondria and peroxisomes from ROS. Another important role for the radical scavenging properties of ascorbate is in the regeneration of other key antioxidant molecules. This may be particularly the case in the regeneration of vitamin E, a role that this vitamin may also perform in animals and will be discussed further in the section on vitamin E.

Another major role of ascorbate in plants is to act as an essential cofactor in several enzyme reactions. The enzymes tend to be either mono- or dioxygenases and the principle role of the ascorbate is to retain the metal ion in the reactive centre of these enzymes in a reduced state. Thus some examples are the enzymes 1-aminocyclopropane-carboxylate oxidase and gibberellin-3-dioxygenase, key enzymes in the biosynthesis of the plant hormones ethylene and gibberellins, respectively. Ascorbate is also thought to play a role in the action of violaxanthin de-epoxidase, an enzyme involved in the synthesis of the xanthopylls, which are phytoprotective pigments. Ascorbate has also been implicated in the biosynthesis of hydroxyproline rich proteins such as extensin that form part of the complex structure of the plant cell wall. Indeed it is thought that apoplastic ascorbate (that exists outside the cell in the plant cell wall) may play a role in regulating the oxido-reduction potential of the cell wall and as such impact, through a variety of potential mechanisms, on cell growth and expansion. It is thus apparent that ascorbate is involved in a diverse range of important metabolic processes in the plant.

Vitamin C manipulation in plants

The nutritional drive for enhancing the endogenous levels of ascorbate in food is not very strong. There are no widespread deficiencies for this vitamin, and evidence linking higher consumption to increased general health is often mixed. Also ascorbate can be synthesised chemically in high volume and at low cost, and as such can be readily used to fortify food as required, for either nutritional or processing benefits. However, high ascorbate levels may be associated with improved postharvest quality in fruit (Barden and Bramlage 1994) and may also be involved in the responses or resistance of plants to a range of biotic and abiotic stresses (Davey et al. 2000). Thus there may be good horticultural or agronomic reasons to enhance the endogenous levels of ascorbate in some food crops.

Ascorbate levels can be influenced by several developmental and environmental factors (Lee and Kader 2000). Thus ascorbate levels can be influenced by light (Smirnoff 2000) and varies during such processes as germination (Pallanca and Smirnoff 2000), fruit ripening (Agius et al. 2003) or senescence. These latter two processes are important in terms of the postharvest storage and marketing of fruit and vegetables. One way to enhance levels of ascorbate, in these food commodities, is to use appropriate postharvest storage conditions. Thus low temperature storage in general delays the loss of ascorbate (Lee and Kader 2000).

Genetic modification could also be used to enhance ascorbate levels in plants (Ishikawa et al. 2006). This approach would be greatly facilitated by an understanding of the molecular genetic factors determining and influencing the ascorbate pool size. Whilst much is known about the biosynthesis of ascorbate, the actual regulatory mechanisms controlling its accumulation are less well understood. There have been three basic approaches to the manipulation of ascorbate levels: enhancing the biosynthetic pathway, modification to the recycling pathway, and influencing catabolism (ascorbate oxidase). These have been reviewed by Ishikawa et al. (2006). Several studies have shown that ascorbate levels in tissues, and changes in levels associated with stress responses, are often associated with changes in the activity or expression of L-galactono-1,4-lactone dehydrogenase. This is the last enzyme in the biosynthetic pathway and as such would be unusual in terms of regulating the pathway. The over-expression of this gene has been achieved in tobacco plants (Gatzek et al. 2002) but with no change in ascorbate levels. In contrast over-expression in tobacco cells in suspension culture did result in around a doubling of the ascorbate (Tokunaga et al. 2005). Over-expression of D-galacturonate reductase, an enzyme potentially involved in the synthesis of ascorbate from galacturonic acid, in *Arabidopsis* resulted in a two- to three-fold enhancement of ascorbate levels in the leaves (Agius et al. 2003). Attempts to modify the recycling of MDHA and DHA have also been successful in increasing ascorbate levels. Thus over-expression of dehydroascorbate reductase in tobacco chloroplasts resulted in a two- to fourfold increase in total ascorbate as well as an increase in the ascorbate/DHA ratio (Chen et al. 2003). Attempts to manipulate ascorbate levels by modification of its catabolism are hampered by the relative lack of understanding of the pathways and the genes involved. However, several groups have modified the activity of the apoplastic ascorbate oxidase (see Ishikawa et al. 2006) with variable effects on total ascorbate. This approach however, does seem to consistently effect the ascorbate/DHA ratio. It has been found that ascorbate levels can also be manipulated by the modification of other, seemingly unrelated, biochemical pathways. Thus Nunes-Nesi et al. (2005) have silenced malate dehydrogenase activity in the mitochondria of tomato. These transgenic plants demonstrated a more than five-fold increase in the levels of ascorbate in their leaves. The reason for this is not clear but probably serves to illustrate the diversity of biochemical pathways with which ascorbate interacts within the cell.

The use of genetic modification to enhance the nutritional value of crops is currently impractical from a commercial point of view, primarily because of strong consumer resistance to this technology in general. Another approach would be to exploit natural variation within crops. One powerful approach is to identify quantitative trait loci (QTL) controlling ascorbate accumulation, which can then be used in marker-assisted breeding programmes. The identification of QTL implicated in ascorbate accumulation has been achieved for fruit, in particular tomato (Rousseaux et al. 2005; Schauer et al. 2006) and apple (Davey et al. 2006).

Absorption and transport of vitamin C in mammals

Since the various forms of vitamin C (ascorbic acid/ascorbate and dehydroascorbic acid) are water soluble and structurally similar to glucose, the mechanism of uptake across the gut and cell membranes is very similar to that of glucose. Both forms of vitamin C are transported across cell membranes via active transport mechanisms, mediated by two distinct classes of membrane protein, the sodium vitamin C co-transporters (SVCT) and glucose transporters (GLUT).

There are two isoforms of SVCT (SVCT1 and SVCT2), which are specific transporters for ascorbic acid (AA). SVCT1 is often referred to as the bulk transporter, having higher transport capacity than SVCT2. However SVCT2 is mainly expressed in the brain and retina and has a higher affinity for AA, and is therefore vital for maintenance of neuronal functions via its effects on the vitamin C status of the cells. SVCT1 is the only transporter expressed in the intestine and is therefore the main mechanism by which vitamin C gets across the gut and into the circulation. However, high levels of AA down-regulate SVCT1 expression, thereby limiting the amount of vitamin C able to get into the blood from the gut. In addition, high levels of vitamin C within the blood are cleared by the kidneys, again limiting the levels achievable in the blood. Once vitamin C has got into the blood, it equilibrates across the various aqueous compartments with transport across membranes achieved via the SVCT or GLUT.

Three different glucose transporters (GLUT1, GLUT3 and GLUT4) have equal affinities for both glucose and the oxidised form of vitamin C, dehydroascorbic acid (DHAA), but no detectable affinity for the reduced (antioxidant) form, AA. Therefore AA is oxidised to DHAA extracellularly, transported into cells via GLUT, where it is then reduced back to AA. Glucose and DHAA therefore act as competitive inhibitors of each other for the GLUT, suggesting that high blood concentrations of vitamin C might induce hyperglycaemia and diabetes. Indeed, translocation of GLUT4 to the cell membrane in muscle and adipose cells is stimulated by insulin and therefore associated with insulin resistance/type 2 diabetes.

Vitamin E: structure and chemistry

Vitamin E (α-, β-, δ- and γ-tocopherols and tocotrienols) is a family of amphiphilic molecules, collectively known as the tocochromanols. Tocochromanols are synthesised in photosynthetic organisms, such as plants and cyanobacteria. Eight homologues exist: α-, β-, δ- and γ-tocopherol; and α-, β-, δ- and γ-tocotrienol. Both tocopherols and tocotrienols contain a chromanol ring, the hydroxyl group of which is crucial for antioxidant activity, and a hydrophobic chain made up of 16 carbon atoms (see Figure 5.5). The presence of three unsaturated bonds in the tocotrienols distinguishes them from the tocopherols, and is indicative of the single difference in their biosynthetic routes.

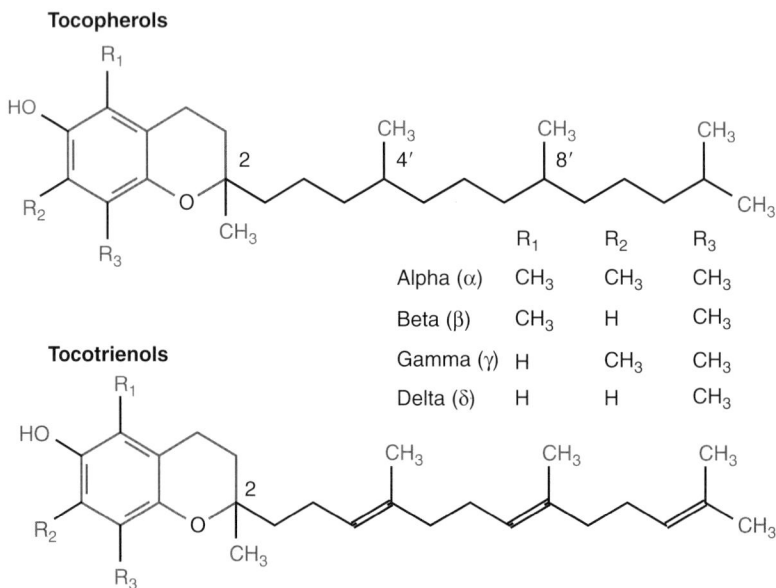

Figure 5.5 Chemical structures of tocochromanols.

In vitro studies that measure the relative antioxidant activity of tocochromanol homologues vary widely depending on the precise composition of the system, the temperature used, the structure of the lipid phase, the presence or absence of pro-oxidants such as transition metal ions, and the concentration of tocochromanols added. It is therefore not surprising that the relative order of tocochromanol antioxidant activity *in vitro*, reported in publications using different experimental conditions and evaluation methods, varies (Gottstein and Grosch 1990; Yoshida et al. 2003).

Predicting antioxidant activity, even based on a detailed understanding of chemical structures, is unreliable. For example, the presence of two methyl groups in the ortho- and para- positions of the chromanol ring of α-tocopherol renders this, in theory, the most potent antioxidant, due to the electron-inducing effect of the methyl groups weakening the OH bond and thus promoting the neutralisation of a free radical species through the donation of a proton. However, this chemical property can also promote undesirable pro-oxidant or co-oxidant (indirect pro-oxidant) reactions, such as the reduction of transition metal cations to more active oxidants, or the decomposition of hydroperoxides to chain-propagating free radical species. Such 'side reactions' can be influenced by tocochromanol concentration, the presence of even low concentrations of transition metals and/or hydroperoxides, temperature, solvents and light. There is therefore a complex interplay between all the chemical and physical parameters of the system that affects the kinetics of antioxidant activity. The order of antioxidant activity of tocochromanol homologues is therefore governed by the balance between anti- and pro-oxidant activities; this balance is determined to a great extent by the chemical and physical natures of the lipid substrate and of the overall system.

In 1996, Kamal-Eldin and Appleqvist published an extensive review entitled 'The chemistry and antioxidant properties of tocopherols and tocotrienols'. Most of the review concentrates on the tocopherols since little work had been done on the tocotrienols. Using a detailed description of the chemistry of each tocochromanol homologue, they explain the differences observed in the order of antioxidant activity (chain breaking unless otherwise stated) *in vivo* (i.e. in the body) and *in vitro* (for example in model systems and food). When their paper was published it was already generally accepted that the order of vitamin E biological activity (α>β>γ>δ) reflects the order of proton-donating power and therefore of antioxidant activity *in vivo*, but there is no consensus on their relative antioxidant activity *in vitro*. For example, a reverse order was observed when the system was a bulk oil or an emulsion (Lea and Ward, 1959; Parkhurst et al. 1968; Chow and Draper, 1974; Koskas et al. 1984; Esterbauer et al. 1989; Gottstein and Grosch 1990; Timmermann von F. 1990) and not a homogenous solution in dichlorobenzene (Burton and Ingold 1981).

The consistent conditions met by tocochromanols *in vivo* and the selective transport of α-tocopherol over the other tocochromanols means that the order of vitamin E activity and antioxidant activity *in vivo* is, to a great extent, predictable, and seems to be influenced by the degree of lipophilicity (increased by increasing the degree of methylation and the length of the phytyl chain), which determines their transport within the body and its retention in biological tissues (Ingold et al. 1986, 1987, 1990).

The lower biopotency (vitamin E activity) of the tocotrienols compared with the corresponding tocopherols is recognised, but in some *in vitro* antioxidant studies using membrane substrates (Serbinova et al. 1991; Suzuki at al. 1993) or bulk oils

(Schroeder et al. 2006) the tocotrienols are more potent. Serbinova and co-workers (1991) suggest that the tocotrienol antioxidant is recycled from the chromanoxyl radical more rapidly and that it is well distributed in membranes where it can exert a disordering effect on the lipids thus promoting its interaction with free radicals. This argument was also presented by Palozza and co-workers (2006) who studied the antioxidant potency of tocotrienols in isolated membranes and intact cells. Other workers have found no difference in the tocopherols and their corresponding tocotrienols in terms of antioxidant activity in homogeneous solutions or in membrane-based systems (Suzuki et al. 1993; Yoshida et al. 2003). On the other hand the inter-membrane antioxidant capacity was higher for α-tocotrienol compared with α-tocopherol; the increased mobility between membranes of the latter over the former seems to explain these results (Yoshida et al. 2003).

A scan of the literature reveals that γ-tocochromanol homologues are the most potent chain-breaking antioxidants *in vitro,* and that this potency can be enhanced with a mix of tocochromanols (Pongracz et al. 1995; Suffield and Dillman 2006). It is not entirely clear why the γ-homologues are often the most active antioxidants *in vitro,* but some researchers suggest that this can be explained by the fact that when this homologue forms dimers through side reactions, it is still an active antioxidant. It is also instructive to note from the work of Yoshida and co-workers (2003) that unlike α-tocopherol, γ-tocopherol does not reduce cupric ions (Cu II) to the more potent pro-oxidant cuprous ions (Cu I). There are, however, several reports that reveal an order of antioxidant activity in line with predicted proton-donating powers (Yanishlieva et al. 2002; Yoshida et al. 2003). This order is often inverted in bulk oil and emulsion stability trials by increasing the antioxidant concentration; α-tocopherol is consumed in side reactions at a disproportionate rate above certain concentrations (Huang et al. 1994; Lampi et al. 1999; Yanishlieva et al. 2002).

It seems therefore that the order of vitamin E activity in tocochromanol homologues is not easily explained simply by chain-breaking antioxidant activity per se. More subtle effects of tocochromanols on membranes/cell signalling and on gene expression have recently come to light that may explain this (Pfluger et al. 2004); nonetheless, it is interesting to note that the order of singlet oxygen-quenching antioxidant activity by tocochromanols reflects the order of vitamin E activity (Foote 1979; Neely et al. 1988; Kaiser et al. 1990).

Tocochromanols are the most efficient lipid antioxidants in nature. At low hydroperoxide concentrations one tocopherol molecule can protect between 10^3 and 10^8 polyunsaturated fatty acids (PUFA) molecules (Patterson 1981). A ratio of 1:500 α-tocopherol/arachidonic acid molecules in erythrocyte membranes seems to be sufficient to protect these membranes beyond the action of front-line intrinsic antioxidant enzymes such as catalase, superoxide dismutase and glutathione peroxidase. The tocochromanol concentration found in nature seems to be optimised and is therefore mimicked in food systems where tocopherol can be added as an antioxidant in the range of $1:10^3$ to $1:10^4$ (Budowski and Sklan 1989). This optimum can be defined as the lowest concentration to give maximum protection of lipids and will depend on the tocochromanol homologue used and on the chemical nature of the substrate. For example, high purity oils, containing only triacylglycerols, seem to require lower concentrations of tocochromanols for protection than 'normal' refined oils (Lampi et al. 1997).

Table 5.2 The relative biological activity[a] of tocochromanols

Name	Relative Biological Activity
d-α-Tocopherol	100
d-β-Tocopherol	50
d-γ-Tocopherol	10
d-δ-Tocopherol	3
d-α-Tocotrienol	30
d-β-Tocotrienol	5
d-γ-Tocotrienol	–
d-δ-Tocopherol	–

[a]Biological Activity was measured using the rat resorption-gestation test.
Source: Data is taken from VERIS (1993).

Dietary sources of vitamin E

Although leaf tissue is very active in synthesising tocopherols, its concentration is at least ten times less than that found in oilseeds (30 μg/g fresh weight compared with 300–1000 μg/g[1] fresh weight). Plant-derived oils are therefore a major source of dietary vitamin E, and are consequently a target for bioenrichment. Recent work in our laboratories and by Goffman and Mollers (2000) has shown that tocochromanols, at least in rapeseed, are lost during seed storage, and that the rate of loss is molecule specific. Losses can also occur during conventional oil extraction and refining using organic solvents. It is perhaps not surprising, therefore, that in the literature, there is a range of values for the concentration of tocochromanols in plant-derived oils. As a general rule, relative to other tocochromanols, α-tocopherol is enriched in the chloroplasts of photosynthetic plant tissue and in the germ of cereal grains, tocotrienols are enriched in the endosperm and bran of cereals, and γ-tocopherol is enriched in oilseeds. Plant oils, such as soy, maize and rapeseed are enriched with g-tocopherol, but sunflower oil is enriched with a-tocopherol. The precise compositional profile of tocochromanols within an oil (some values are shown in Table 5.2) will be influenced by genetic and environmental effects, as well as seed storage history.

The main dietary sources of the tocochromanols are plant oils and fats, although nuts, cereals, dairy products, meat and fish also contribute (see Table 5.3). However the contribution from meat and fish depends upon their fat content and the diet of the animal.

An individual's requirements for vitamin E are variable and dependent upon their dietary fat intake, particularly PUFA, and the amount of exercise taken. An increase in either or both of these variables increases the vitamin E requirements.

Vitamin E: biosynthetic pathways

The pathway for vitamin E biosynthesis is known. For a good review of this topic readers are directed to DellaPenna (2005). Biochemical assays of enzyme activities have located the final enzymes in the pathway from HPT (homogentisate phytyldiphosphate transferase)

Table 5.3   Dietary sources of vitamin E

Food	Tocopherol content (mg/100g)				Vitamin E equivalents (mg/100g)[a]
	α-T	β-T	γ-T	δ-T	
Plant oils					
Sunflower oil	48.70	0	5.10	0.80	49.22
Safflower oil	38.70	0	17.40	24.00	40.70
Palm oil	25.60	0	31.60	7.00	33.10
Rapeseed oil	18.40	0	38.00	1.20	22.20
Olive oil	5.10	0	Tr	0	5.10
Fruit & Nuts					
Almonds	23.77	0.26	0.81	0	23.96
Hazelnuts	24.20	0.80	4.33	0.22	24.98
Peanuts	9.21	0.23	7.91	0.37	10.09
Blackberries	2.05	0	2.90	2.75	2.37
Plums	0.60	0	0.07	0	0.61
Raspberries	0.30	0	1.50	2.70	0.48
Dairy Products					
Margarine (soft, PUFA-rich)	11.59	Tr	7.40	0.54	12.34
Butter	1.82	0.07	0.08	0.02	1.85
Fresh double cream	1.62	0.04	Tr	Tr	1.64
Brie	0.81	0.01	0.01	Tr	0.81
Cheddar cheese	0.43	0.12	0.40	0.06	0.52
Meat & fish dishes					
Prawn curry	2.88	Tr	2.75	0.17	3.16
Chicken curry	1.88	Tr	1.81	0.75	2.12
Meat samosa	0.44	Tr	1.09	0.14	0.55
Cereals					
Egg fried rice	0.76	Tr	1.23	0.08	0.88
Pasta	0.68	0.21	0.53	0.13	0.82
Wholemeal bread	0.19	0.12	0.52	0.02	0.29
White bread	0.10	0.09	0.30	0.05	0.17

[a]Includes contributions from Tocotrienols as appropriate.
Tr Traces found (not measurable).
Source: data obtained from Food Standards Agency (2002).

onwards within chloroplasts (Soll et al. 1980; Lichtenthaler et al. 1981) and chromoplasts (Arango and Heise 1998). Cells within oilseeds do not always contain chloroplasts or chromoplasts. Instead they often contain non-green plastids that, amongst other roles, synthesise fatty acids, some of which are exported to the cytoplasm to be incorporated into triacylglycerol during seed maturation. Despite the obvious importance of oilseeds as a source of vitamin E, no one seems to have studied tocochromanol biosynthesis in isolated oilseed plastids. It is generally accepted that tocochromanols are made in plastids, but other locations where tocochromanols could be synthesised cannot be ruled out.

Newton and Pennock (1971) studied the thallus of *Fucus spiralis* (a brown alga), the fruit of tangerine and tomato and the leaves of french bean. Tissues were macerated and plastids separated; α-tocopherol was enriched in plastids whereas other tocopherols were found in the supernatants. They speculated that all tocopherols are synthesised at separate sites, or that tocopherols other than the α form are synthesised outside plastids and then transported into the plastids for the final methylation, or that all tocopherols are synthesised in one place and then transported to their separate sites of action. A study by Marwede and co-workers (2004) on three oilseed rape populations of double haploid lines showed no correlation between α-tocopherol and γ-tocopherol in the seed, indicating an independent regulation of their syntheses. From this they suggest that these tocochromanols are synthesised at different cellular sites. To back up this point they quote Goffman et al. (1999) where a decrease in γ-tocopherol in favour of α-tocopherol accumulation was observed, suggesting separate sites/controls for synthesis. Horvath and co-workers (2003) also provided evidence that the tocotrienols in rice are synthesised in the cytoplasm of endosperm cells. Work by Sattler and co-workers (2003) states that the necessary level of antioxidant protection within seeds would require tocopherol to be associated with oil bodies. Interestingly, recent work in our laboratories has revealed an apparent tight association between oil bodies (the storage organelles for oil in oilseeds) and tocochromanols (White et al. 2006; Fisk et al. 2006); if this location of tocochromanols is accurate it begs the question how do they get there?

Although tocopherols are ubiquitous within photosynthetic organisms, tocotrienols are not; they tend to be found in cereal grains, palm fruits and coconuts, and the endosperm of some dicots such as coriander and tobacco. Homogentisic acid is imported into plastids and condensed with either a phytyl group (to make 2-methy-6-phytylbenzoquinol [MPBQ], the parent molecule for tocopherols), or a geranylgeranyl group (to make 2-methy-6-phytylbenzoquinol [MGGBQ], the parent molecule for tocotrienols). Geranylgeranyl pyrophosphate (GGPP/GGDP) acts as the source for both isoprenoid groups, with phytyl pyrophosphate resulting from the action of geranylgeranyl reductase (GGR). From MGGBQ and MPBQ a series of cyclisation and methylation reactions gives rise to the four homologues of tocotrienols and tocopherols, respectively. The VTE enzymes used in these reactions seem to be the same for both tocopherol and tocotrienol synthesis.

Recent work by Valentin and co-workers (2006) also implicates the role of recycled phytol from chlorophyll as a source of phytyl for tocopherol synthesis. The relative importance of synthesis of PDP (phytyl pyrophosphate) from GGDP versus that synthesised from free phytol remains open. VTE5 seems to be targeted to the plastids, and phytol monophosphate (PMP) has been identified, therefore there must be a further kinase that converts PMP to PDP; this enzyme has not yet been identified.

Roles of tocochromanols in plants

All the genes required to make tocopherols have been identified in *Arabidopsis* and in the cyanobacterium *Synechocyctis*. This knowledge has been harnessed to transform various plants to study the role of tocopherols *in vivo* (Sattler et al. 2004), to enhance their concentration in seeds (Rippert et al. 2004), and to modify the composition of tocopherols (change the γ:α ratio) in seeds (Van Eenennaam et al. 2003).

Tocochromanols have a wide range of biological functions within plant cells. In addition to acting as a membrane stabiliser and providing protection against oxygen toxicity (Munne-Bosch et al. 2007) they also seem to be involved in intracellular signalling (Munne-Bosch et al. 2007) and cyclic electron transport around photosystem II in chloroplasts (Munne-Bosch and Alegre 2002). An ATCTA element that is present in the promoter of photosynthetically related genes is also present in the genes coding for enzymes involved in tocopherol and carotenoid syntheses. There is some interesting speculation that α-tocopherol may decrease lipid peroxidation and therefore decrease the concentration of jasmonic acid. Jasmonic acid regulates gene expression in the nucleus, affecting photosynthesis and anthocyanin and antioxidant metabolism. Indeed, some evidence suggests that jasmonic acid regulates genes involved in α-tocopherol synthesis (Munne-Bosch et al. 2007).

A *vte2* mutant (without homogentisate phytyltransferase) was chosen to study the role of tocopherols in *Arabidopsis*. This mutant showed reduced seed longevity and severe seedling growth defects during germination, along with high levels of lipid hydroperoxides (Sattler et al. 2004). These workers believe that their data indicate that the primary function of tocopherols in plants is to limit non-enzymic lipid oxidation during seed storage, germination and early seedling development. They also compared the performance of seedlings from the *vte1* and *vte2* mutants; DMPBQ (dimethylphytylbenoquinol; still synthesised in *vte1* mutants and the precursor to γ-tocopherol) is capable of functionally compensating for tocopherol except in the realm of seed longevity. They proposed that tocopherol is required for seed longevity because: (1) tocopherol can donate single electrons (DMPBQ cannot), which may enhance the efficient removal of reactive oxygen species or free radicals; (2) tocopheroxyl radicals can be chemically recycled whereas quinones, like DMPBQ, generally require enzymatic reduction coupled to a cofactor or electron transport chain; (3) the chromanol ring of tocopherol allows singlet oxygen quenching.

Falk and co-workers (2004) studied the distribution of tocochromanols in developing barley grain and used the results to consider their functions *in planta*. Tocotrienol and tocopherol distribution throughout the grain, and their accumulation rates were different. Tocopherols (15% of total tocochromanols) were almost exclusive to germ; tocotrienols were found in the pericarp and endosperm in roughly equal proportions. This distinct spatial arrangement of tocochromanols suggests separate functions, probably related to the separate fates of these tissues, the germ becoming the new plant, and the endosperm and pericarp dying during germination. Some authors have made the assumption that a direct correlation must exist between tocochromanol and lipid concentrations during development for a functional link to be implied; this is perhaps too simplistic given that the demand for tocochromanols may increase during seed desiccation, a physiological process that is associated with a change in the redox status of seeds (Finnie et al. 2002; De Cara et al. 2003).

Manipulation of tocochromanol concentration

Successful attempts to alter the tocochromanol composition of seeds have been made through metabolic engineering (Shintani and DellaPenna 1998; Shewmaker et al. 1999; Tsegaye et al. 2002; Van Eenennaam 2003; 2004; Karunanandaa et al. 2005). The over-expression of HPPD in Arabidopsis seed (Tsegaye et al. 2002) caused an increase in the total tocopherol concentration. In terms of controlling flux it seems that HPPDase alone cannot cause large increases in tocopherol since a tenfold increase in enzyme activity only leads to approx 28% increase in seed tocopherol. It is not unusual for metabolic flux to be controlled by multiple pathway enzymes instead of a single enzyme. Genes identified as critical for tocochromanol pathway engineering in *Synechocystis* were expressed as single genes and in combination in *Arabidopsis*, rapeseed and soybean (Karunanandaa et al. 2005). In the best performing events tocochromanol concentrations increased by 15-fold. This provides evidence that HGA levels normally limit tocopherol levels in seed. This is consistent with work reported by Collakova and DellaPenna (2003) and by Rippert et al. (2004). When an increased flux to HGA in seeds leads to a significant increase in tocochromanol concentration, it is striking that most of this increase above wild-type levels is accounted for by an increase in tocotrienols. Cahoon and co-workers (2003) transformed *Arabidopsis* and corn (maize) with the gene encoding for HGGT in cereal crops. Increases in total tocochromanols of 15-fold and 6-fold, mostly accounted for by increases in tocotrienols, were observed in *Arabidopsis* leaves and maize seeds, respectively.

Gene manipulation has also been used to alter the tocochromanol composition in seeds. For example, *Arabidopsis* was transformed with the *VTE4* gene containing a seed specific promoter; this led to a significant increase (80×) in α-tocopherol concentration (Shintani and DellaPenna 1998). A similar approach was used to improve the vitamin E content of soy oil by increasing the concentration of α-tocopherol (Van Eenennaam et al. 2003). When *VTE3* and *VTE4* were co-expressed in transgenic soybeans, seeds with greater than 95% α-tocopherol were produced. The over-expression of these 'qualitative' genes does not alter the flux into the tocochromanol pathway and so does not result in higher concentrations of tocochromanols.

More conventional breeding trials can also be used to manipulate vitamin E concentrations. Not surprisingly crop trials have revealed the importance of the environment as well as the genotype on tocochromanol biosynthesis in developing oilseeds and grain. Genotype- and environment-induced variation for tocochromanol concentration and composition in commercial hybrids of sunflower seeds has been studied (Valesco et al. 2002). α-Tocopherol, β-tocopherol and total tocopherol concentrations were affected more by genotype than environment: the converse was true for γ-tocopherol concentration. There was also a significant genotype–environment interaction for α-tocopherol, γ-tocopherol and total tocopherol concentrations.

Rapeseed oil tocopherol concentration and composition are affected by genotypic and environmental effects (Marquard 1976), particularly the latter (Goffman and Becker 2002). A significant environmental effect means that heritability of tocopherol concentration and composition is low and that consequently more locations or years are required to evaluate the impact of different genotypes on these markers (Marwede et al. 2004). More recent QTL work has been reported by Marwede and co-workers (2005) who used a double haploid population (very reliable for pulling out genetic influences on markers) for 2 years at two locations in replicated field trials. Genotypic differences occurred for α-tocopherol, γ-tocopherol and total tocopherol concentrations as well as for α:γ tocopherol ratios, but highly significant genotype–environment interactions resulted in low heritabilities. However, even incremental advances in levels or ratios can add up to significant and valuable improvements. Therefore the use of genetic markers (marker-assisted selection) to follow the accumulation of beneficial alleles helps to obtain a reasonable genetic 'signal' in a finished variety.

Absorption and transport of vitamin E in mammals

Since the tocochromanols are fat soluble, the mechanism of uptake across the gut is the same as for all other fat soluble molecules, including fatty acids and fat soluble vitamins. The tocochromanol molecules are released from the food matrix by the actions of pancreatic lipase, digesting the triglycerides (TG) and releasing the free fatty acids and TG-associated molecules, which are emulsified to form micelles by the action of bile salts. The micelles are absorbed across the intestinal wall and taken up by the enterocytes by a combination of passive diffusion and active transport mechanisms (e.g. fatty acid transporters). Once inside the enterocyte, the fatty acids and cholesterol are re-esterified and the various lipid molecules incorporated into existing or newly synthesised chylomicra, which act as a lipid transport system between the gut and the circulation. The lipid molecules are transported to various tissues where the action of lipoprotein lipase again digests the TG, releasing the TG-associated molecules to be taken up by the cells. The remaining chylomicra are taken up by the liver where their contents are either metabolised or incorporated into lipoproteins or, for vitamin E, complexed with hepatic α-tocopherol transfer protein (αTTP) for transport around the body. Indeed, αTTP seems to be one of the main reasons why mammals are particularly dependent upon α-tocopherol rather than the other tocochromanols. Even though there seems to be little difference between the eight vitamers in terms of antioxidant activities (dependent upon the method of measurement), αTTP preferentially binds and transports α-tocopherol and not the other tocochromanols. Hence αTTP is essential for maintaining plasma vitamin E concentrations, with vitamin E deficiency associated with the loss of this protein in both αTTP null mice and humans having a defective αTTP gene (see Traber and Atkinson, 2007). The binding of α-tocopherol to αTTP results in an increased half life, but may also be responsible for the preferential removal of the other tocochromanols by the liver, which results in them being preferentially metabolised and excreted. Hence the specificity of αTTP for α-tocopherol may be one of the main reasons why mammals are particularly dependent upon α-tocopherol and not other tocochromanols.

Antioxidant functions of vitamin E

A number of apparent functions have been described for various tocochromanols, but all seem to be attributed to their antioxidant activities. As described earlier, the hydroxyl group on the benzene ring is responsible for the antioxidant capacity, being able to donate a proton but stabilise the resulting free electron around the ring, particularly when the ring also has methyl side groups as in α-tocopherol. The α-tocopheroxyl radical formed is relatively stable but short lived, being oxidised by other antioxidants, making measurement difficult. The main function of vitamin E is to inhibit/prevent lipid peroxidation, whereby the unsaturated, electron-rich bonds in PUFA are attacked by free radicals. Both the antioxidant activity and the location of a-tocopherol in membranes makes it an important inhibitor of lipid peroxidation, however the evidence supporting this role has until recently been unclear due to the interactive nature of how antioxidants work. Indeed whether there is any phenotypic effect of a vitamin E deficiency is dependent upon whether there is also a deficiency of selenium or vitamin C, with deficiencies of two of these often having lethal consequences. Hence there are strong interactions between vitamin E and both selenium and vitamin C, since antioxidants can be recycled by 'passing on' the free radical to other systems. Indeed, combinations of vitamin E and vitamin C are often incorporated into food products to increase shelf life by specifically preventing wastage due to production of free radicals (e.g. rancidity). The interaction with selenium relates to selenium being essential in the action of the antioxidant selenoprotein enzyme, glutathione peroxidise (GSHPx), which catalyses the release of protons (to neutralise the free radicals) and the formation of a stable disulphide bridge between two glutathione (GSH, a tripeptide glu-gly-cys) molecules:

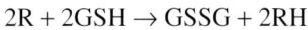

$$2R + 2GSH \rightarrow GSSG + 2RH$$

The antioxidant reactions involving vitamin E, GSHPx and vitamin C can thereby be interlinked to recycle the active forms possessing antioxidant activity, thereby replenishing them even with reduced intake in the diet. In textbooks, vitamin E and C are often shown interacting directly, but vitamin E is in the lipid phase (membrane), whereas vitamin C is water soluble and therefore they are unlikely to interact directly. One form of GSHPx (the lipoprotein form) is normally found at the interphase between lipid and aqueous phases and therefore we would suggest the following interaction is the more likely:

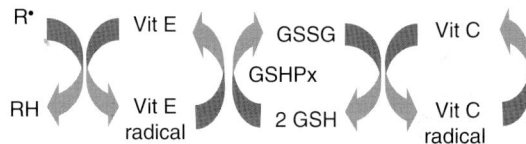

R• ⟶ Vit E ⟶ GSSG ⟶ Vit C
RH ⟵ Vit E radical ⟵ GSHPx / 2 GSH ⟵ Vit C radical

There is increasing evidence that the balance between oxidants and antioxidants (i.e. oxidative stress) has important effects upon cellular functions and metabolism. For example, exposure to low concentrations of hydrogen peroxide induces differentiation of cells, whereas high concentrations induce cell death via apoptosis. These effects can sometimes be modulated by antioxidants and the effects have been shown to be associated with changes in signal transduction molecules, including kinases. In isoforms of vitamin E, the inhibition of lipid peroxidation will affect the fatty acid composition and therefore the fluidity of membranes. Indeed studies indicate that membrane properties play an important role in signalling by membrane-bound receptors, particularly receptors that are associated with lipid rafts. Hence membrane lipid composition can alter the responsiveness of cells to various hormones and growth factors.

Vitamin E can also modulate the signalling by other lipid molecules. The fat-soluble vitamins A and D act as ligands for members of the nuclear receptor superfamily, which act as ligand-dependent transcription factors that bind to consensus sequences in gene promoters and thereby regulate transcription. Whether vitamin E is a specific ligand for any of the numerous nuclear receptors whose ligand is yet to be identified (so called orphan nuclear receptors) is still unclear. However, tocochromanols have been shown to bind to the pregnane X receptor (PXR), which binds and responds to a variety of potentially toxic lipid compounds. In this case, the tocotrienols were more potent than the tocopherols in activating transcription, but this is more likely to reflect mechanisms of metabolising the tocotrienols rather than being a general mechanism for how vitamin E regulates cell functions. In addition, unsaturated fatty acids and metabolites act as ligands for other members of the nuclear receptor superfamily, particularly the peroxisome proliferator activated receptor (PPAR) family. Hence vitamin E, by regulating the fatty acid composition of cells, might thereby modulate the cellular response to fatty acids in terms of changes in gene expression.

There seem to be two main mechanisms for how vitamin E might regulate gene expression, one general and the other more specific, but both relate to its antioxidant capacity. The first mechanism relates to the balance between oxidants and antioxidants altering the activities of signalling molecules, such as kinases and nuclear factor kappa B (NFkB). The other relates to vitamin E specifically regulating the fatty acid composition within cells and thereby altering the response to unsaturated fatty acids and/or membrane bound receptors.

References

Agius, F., Gonzalez-Lamothe, R., Caballero, J.L., Munoz-Blanco, J., Botella, M.A. and Valpuesta, V. (2003) Engineering increased vitamin C levels in plants by overexpression of a D-galacturonic acid reductase. *Nature Biotechnology* **21**, 177–81.

Arango, Y. and Heise, K.P. (1998) Localization of α-tocopherol synthesis in chromoplast envelope membranes of Capsicum annuum L. fruits. *Journal of Experimental Botany* **49**, 1259–62.

Barden, C.L. and Bramlage, W.J. (1994) Accumulation of antioxidants in apple peel as related to preharvest factors and superficial scald susceptibility of the fruit. *Journal of the American Society of Horticultural Sciences* **119**, 264–9.

Bergquist, S.A.M., Gertsson, U.E. and Olsson, M.E. (2006) Influence of growth stage and postharvest storage on ascorbic acid and carotenoid content and visual quality of baby spinach (*Spinacia oleracea* L.). *Journal of the Science of Food and Agriculture* **86**, 346–55.

Borraccino, G., Mastropasqua, L., Leonardis, S. and Dipierro, S. (1994) The role of the ascorbate acid system in delaying the senescence of oat (*Avena sativa* L) leaf segments. *Journal of Plant Physiology* **144**, 161–6.

Budowski, P. and Sklan, D. (1989) Vitamin E and A. In: *The Role of Fats in Human Nutrition* (eds Vergroesen, A.J. and Grawford, M.), pp. 363–406. London: Academic Press.

Burns, J.J. (1960) Ascorbic acid. In *Metabolic Pathways* (ed. D.M. Greenberg), pp. 341–56. New York: Academic Press.

Burton, G.W. and Ingold, K.U. (1981) Autooxidation biological molecules. 1. The antioxidant activity of vitamin e and related chain-breaking phenolic antioxidant *in vitro*. *Journal of the American Chemical Society* **103**, 6472–7.

Cahoon, E.B., Hall, S.E., Ripp, K.G., Ganzke, T.S., Hitz, W.D. and Coughlan, S.J. (2003) Metabolic redesign of vitamin E biosynthesis in plants for tocotrienol production and increased antioxidant content. *Nature Biotechnology* **21**, 1082–7.

Chen, Z., Young, T.E., Ling, J., Chang, S.C. and Gallie, D.R. (2003) Increasing vitamin C content of plants through enhanced ascorbate recycling. *Proceedings of the National Academy of Sciences USA* **100**, 3525–30.

Chow, C.K. and Draper, H.H. (1974) Oxidative stability and activity of the tocopherols in corn and soybean oils. *International Journal of Vitamin and Nutritional. Research* **44**, 396–403.

Collakova, E. and DellaPenna, D. (2003) The role of homogentisate phytyltransfersase and other tocopherol pathway enzymes in the regulation of tocopherol synthesis during abiotic stress. *Plant Physiology* **133**, 930–40.

Conklin, P., Pallanca, J.E., Last, R.L. and Smirnoff, N. (1997) L-ascorbic acid metabolism in the ascorbate-deficient *Arabidopsis* mutant vtc 1. *Plant Physiology* **115**, 1277–85.

Conklin, P.L., Norris, S.R., Wheeler, G.L., Williams, E.H. and Smirnoff, N. (1999) Genetic evidence for the role of GDP-mannose in plant ascorbic acid (vitamin C) biosynthesis. *Proceedings of the National Academy of Sciences USA* **96**, 4198–203.

Conklin, P.L., Sarraco, S.A., Norris, S.R. and Last, R.L. (2000) Identification of ascorbic acid deficient *Arabidopsis thaliana* mutants. *Genetics* **154**, 847–56.

Davey, M.W., Van Montagu, M., Inze, D., Sammartin, M., Kanellis, A., Smirnoff, N., Benzie, I.J.J., Strain, J.J., Favell, D. and Fletcher, J. (2000) Plant L-ascorbic acid: chemistry, function, metabolism, bioavailability and effects of processing. *Journal of the Science of Food and Agriculture* **80**, 825–60.

Davey, M.W., Kenis, K. and Keulemans, J. (2006) Genetic control of fruit vitamin C contents. *Plant Physiology* **142**, 343–51.

DellaPenna, D. (2005) A decade of progress in understanding vitamin E synthesis in plants. *Journal of Plant Physiology* **162**, 729–37.

De Cara, L., de Pinto, M.C., Moliterni, V.M.C. and D'Egidio, M.G. (2003) Redox regulation and storage processes during maturation in kernels of *Triticum durum*. *Journal of Experimental Botany* **54**, 249–58.

Esterbauer, H., Striegl, G., Puhl, H., Oberreither, S., Rothender, M., El-Saadani, M. and Jurgens, G. (1989) The role of vitamin e and carotenoids in preventing the oxidation of low-density lipoproteins. *Annals of the New York Academy of Sciences* **570**, 254–67.

Falk, J., Krahnstover, A., van der Kooji, T.A.W., Schlensog, M. and Krupinska, K. (2004) Tocopherol and tocotrienol accumulation during development of caryopses from barley. *Phytochemistry* **65**, 2977–85.

Finnie, C., Melchior, S., Roepstorff, P. and Svensson, B. (2002) Proteome analysis of grain filling and seed maturation in barley. *Plant Physiology* **129**, 1308–19.

Fisk, I.D., White, D.A., Carvalho, A. and Gray, D.A. (2006) Tocopherol – an intrinsic component of sunflower seed oil bodies. *Journal of the American Oil Chemists Society* **83**, 341–4.

Food Standards Agency (2002) *McCance and Widdowson's the Composition of Foods, Summary edition*, 6th edn. Cambridge: Royal Society of Chemistry.

Foote, C.S. (1979) Quenching of singlet oxygen. In: *Singlet Oxygen* (eds Wasserman, H.H. and Murray, R.W.), pp. 139–71. New York: Academic Press.

Foyer, C.H. and Halliwell, B. (1976) Presence of glutathione and glutathione reductase in chloroplasts: a proposed route in ascorbic acid metabolism. *Planta* **133**, 21–5.

Gatzek, S., Wheeler, G.L. and Smirnoff, N. (2002) Antisense suppression of L-galactose dehydrogenase in *Arabidopsis thaliana* provides evidence for its role in ascorbate biosynthesis and reveals light modulated L-galactose synthesis. *Plant Journal* **30**, 541–53.

Gil, M.I., Ferreres, F. and Tomas-Barberan, F.A. (1999) Effect of postharvest storage and processing on the antioxidant constituents (flavenoids and vitamin C) of fresh cut spinach. *Journal of Agricultural and Food Sciences* **47**, 2213–17.

Gil, M.I., Aguayo, E. and Kader, A.A. (2006) Quality changes and nutrient retention in fresh-cut versus whole fruits during storage. *Journal of Agricultural and Food Chemistry* **54**, 4284–96.

Goffman, F.D., Valesco, L. and Becker, H.C. (1999) Tocopherols accumulation in developing seeds and pods of rapeseed. *Fett-Lipid* **101**, 400–3.

Goffman, F.D. and Mollers, C. (2000) Changes in tocopherol and plastochromanol-8 contents in seeds and oil of oilseed rape (*Brassica napus* L.) during storage as influences by temperature and air oxygen. *Journal of Agricultural and Food Chemistry* **48**, 1605–9.

Goffman, F.D. and Becker, H.C. (2001) Diallel analysis for tocopherol content in seeds of rapeseed. *Crop Science* **41**, 1072–9.

Goffman, F.D. and Becker, H.C. (2002) Genetic variation of tocopherol content in a germplasm collection of *Brassica napus*. *Euphytica* **125**, 189–96.

Gottstein, T. and Grosch, W. (1990) Model study of different antioxidant properties of α- and γ-tocopherol in fats. *Fat Science and Technology* **92**, 139–44.

Green, M.A. and Fry, S.C. (2005) Vitamin C degradation in plant cells via enzymatic hydrolysis of 4-O-oxalyl-L-threonate. *Nature* **433**, 83–7.

Horemans, N., Foyer, C.H. and Asard, H. (2000a) Transport and action of ascorbate at the plant plasma membrane. *Trends in Plant Science* **5**, 263–7.

Horemans, N., Foyer, C., Potters, G. and Asard, H. (2000b) Ascorbate function and associated transport systems in plants. *Plant Physiology and Biochemistry* **38**, 531–40.

Horvath, G., Bigirimana, J., Guisez, Y., Coaubergs, R., Hoffte, M. and Horemans, N. (2003) Indications for a novel tocotrienol (vitamin E) biosynthetic pathway in seeds of cereals. *Joint Symposium Of Lipid and Cereal Sciences in Europe*, Vichy, France, European section of American Oil Chemists Society.

Huang, S.-W., Frankel, E.N. and German, J.B. (1994) Antioxidant activity of α- and γ-tocopherols in bulk oils and in oil-in-water emulsions. *Journal of Agricultural and Food Chemistry* **42**, 2108–14.

Imai, T., Karita, S., Shiratori, G., Hattori, M., Nunome, T., Oba, K. and Hirai, M. (1998) L-galactono-gamma-lactone dehydrogenase from sweet potato: purification and cDNA sequence analysis. *Plant and Cell Physiology* **39**, 1350–8.

Ingold, K.U., Burton, G.W., Foster, D.O., Zuker, M., Hughes, L., Lacelle, S., Lusztyk, E. and Slaby, M. (1986) A new vitamin E analogue more active than α-tocopherol in the rat curative myopathy bioassay. *FEBS Letters* **205**, 117–20.

Ingold, K.U., Burton, G.W., Foster, D. and Hughes, L. (1990) Is methyl-branching in α-tocopherol's 'tail' important for its *in vivo* activity? Rat curative bioassay measurements of the vitamin E activity of three 2RS-*n*-alkyl-2,5,7,8-tetramethyl-6-hydroxychromams. *Free Radical Biology and Medicine* **9**, 205–10.

Ingold, K.U., Webb, A., Witter, D., Burton, G.W., Metacalfe, T.A. and Muller, D.P. (1987) Vitamin E remains the major lipid-soluble, chain-breaking antioxidant in human plasma even in individuals suffering severe vitamin E deficiency. *Archives of Biochemistry and Biophysics* **259**, 224–5.

Ishikawa, T., Dowdle, J. and Smirnoff, N. (2006) Progress in manipulating ascorbic acid biosynthesis and accumulation in plants. *Physiologia Plantarum* **126**, 343–55.

Kaiser, S., DiMascio, P., Murphy, M.E. and Sies, H. (1990) Physical and chemical scavenging of singlet molecular oxygen by the tocopherols. *Archives of Biochemistry and Biophysics* **277**, 101–8.

Kalt, W., Forney, C.F., Martin, A. and Prior, R.L. (1999) Antioxidant capacity, vitamin C, phenolics and anthocyanins after fresh storage of small fruits. *Journal of Agricultural and Food Sciences* **47**, 4638–44.

Kamal-Eldin, A. and Appelqvist, L.A. (1996) The chemistry and antioxidant properties of tocopherols and tocotrienols. *Lipids* **31**, 671–701.

Karunanandaa, B., Qi, Q.G., Hao, M., Baszis, S.R., Jensen, P.K., Wong, Y.H.H., Jiang, J., Venkatramesh, M., Gruys, K.J., Moshiri, F., Post-Beittermiller, D., Weiss, J.D. and Valentin, H.E. (2005) Metabolically engineered oilseed crops with enhanced seed tocopherol. *Metabolic Engineering* **7**, 384–400.

Koskas, J.P., Cillard, J. and Cillard, P. (1984) Autooxidation of linoleic acid and behavior of its hydroperoxides with and without tocopherols. *Journal of American Oil Chemists Society* **61**, 1466–9.

Kostman, T.A., Tarlyn, N.M., Loewus, F.A. and Franceschi, V.R. (2001) Biosynthesis of L-ascorbic acid and conversion of carbons 1 and 2 ofL-ascorbic acid to oxalic acid occurs within individual calcium oxalate idioblasts. *Plant Physiology* **125**, 634–40.

Laing, W.A., Bulley, S., Wright, M., Cooney, J., Jensen, D., Barraclough, D. and MacRae, E. (2004) A highly specific L-galactose-1-phosphate phosphatase on the path to ascorbate biosynthesis. *Proceedings of the National Academy of Sciences USA* **101**, 16976–81.

Laing, W.A., Wright, M.A., Cooney, J. and Bulley, S.M. (2007) The missing step of the L-galactose pathway of ascorbate biosynthesis in plants, an L-galactose quanyltransferase, increases leaf ascorbate. *Proceedings of the National Academy of Sciences USA* **104**, 9534–9.

Lampi, A.-M., Hopia, A. and Piironen, V. (1999) Antioxidant activity of minor amounts of γ-tocopherol in natural triacylglycerols. *Journal of American Oil Chemists Society* **74**, 549–55.

Lampi, A.-M., Kataja, L., Kamal-Eldin, A. and Vieno, P. (1997) Antioxidant activities of α- and γ-tocopherols in the oxidation of rapeseed oil triacylglycerols. *Journal of American Oil Chemists Society* **76**, 749–55.

Lea, C.H. and Ward, R.J. (1959) Relative antioxidant activity of the seven tocopherols. *Journal of the Science of Food and Agriculture* **10**, 537–48.

Lee, S.K. and Kader, A.A. (2000) Preharvest and postharvest factors influencing vitamin C content of horticultural crops. *Postharvest Biology and Technology* **20**, 207–20.

Lichtenthaler, H.K., Prenzel, U., Douce, R. and Joyard, J. (1981) Localization of prenylquinones in the envelope of spinach chloroplasts. *Biochemica et Biophysica Acta* **641**, 99–105.

Logan, B.A., Barker, D.H., Demmig-Adams, B. and Adams, W.W. (1996) Acclimation of leaf carotenoid composition and ascorbate levels to gradients in the light environment within an Australian rainforest. *Plant, Cell and Environment* 19, 1083–90.

Loewus, F.A. (1999) Biosynthesis and metabolism of ascorbic acid in plants and of analogs of ascorbic acid in fungi. *Phytochemistry* **52**, 193–210.

Loewus, F.A. and Loewus, M.W. (1987) Biosynthesis and metabolism of ascorbic acid in plants. *Critical Reviews of Plant Science* **5**, 101–19.

Mapson, L.W. and Isherwood, F.A. (1956) Biological synthesis of ascorbic acid: the conversion of derivatives of D-galacturonic acid into L-ascorbic acid by plant extracts. *Biochemical Journal* **64**, 13–22.

Marquard, R. (1976) Influence of variety, location and individually defined climatic factors on tocopherol content of rapeseed oil. *Fette Seifen Anstrichmittel* **78**, 341–6.

Marwede, V., Schierholt, A., Mollers, C. and Becker, H.C. (2004) GxE interactions and heritability of tocopherol content in canola. *Crop Science* **44**, 728–31.

Marwede, V., Gul, M.K., Becker, H.C. and Ecke, W. (2005) Mapping of QTL controlling tocopherol content in winter oilseed rape. *Plant Breeding* **124**, 20–26.

Munne-Bosche, S. and Alegre, L. (2002) Interplay between ascorbic acid and lipophilic antioxidant defences in chloroplasts of water-stressed *Arabidopsis* plants. *FEBS Letters* **524**, 145–8.

Munne-Bosche, S. and Falk, J. (2004) New insights into the function of tocopherols in plants. *Planta* **218**, 323–6.

Munne-Bosch, S., Weiler, E.W., Alegre, L., Muller, M., Duchting, P. and Falk, J. (2007) Alpha-tocopherol may influence cellular signaling by modulating jasmonic acid levels in plants. *Planta* **225**, 681–91.

Neely, W.C., Martin, J.M. and Baker, S.A. (1988) Products and relative reaction rates of the oxidation of tocopherols with singlet molecular oxygen. *Photochemistry and Photobiology* **48**, 423–8.

Newton, P.P. and Pennock, J.F. (1971) The intracellular distribution of tocopherols in plants. *Phytochemistry* **10**, 2323–8.

Nunes-Nesi, A., Carrari, F., Lytovchenko, A., Smith, A.M.O., Loureiro, M.E., Ratcliffe, R.G., Sweetlove, L.J. and Fernie, A.R. (2005) Enhanced photosynthetic performance and growth as a consequence of decreasing mitochondrial malate dehydrogenase activity in transgenic tomato plants. *Plant Physiology* **137**, 611–22.

Pallanca, J.E. and Smirnoff, N. (2000) The control of ascorbic acid synthesis and turnover in pea seedlings. *Journal of Experimental Botany* **51**, 669–74.

Palozza, P., Verdecchia, S., Avanzi, L., Vertuani, S., Serini, S,. Iannone, A. and Manfredini, S. (2006) Comparative antioxidant activity of tocotrienols and the novel chromanyl-polyisoprenyl molecule FeAox-6 in isolated membranes and intact cells. *Molecular and Cellular Biochemistry* **287**, 21–32.

Parkhurst, R.M., Skinner, W.A. and Strum, P.A. (1968) The effects of various concentrations of tocopherols and tocopherol mixtures on the oxidative stabilities of a sample of lard. *Journal of American Oil Chemists Society* **45**, 641–2.

Patterson, L.K. (1981) Studies of radiation-induced peroxidation in fatty acid micelles. In: *Oxygen and Oxy-radicals in Chemistry and Biology* (eds M.A.J. Rogers and E.L. Powers), pp. 89–95. New York: Academic Press.

Pfluger, P., Kluth, D., Landes, N., Blumke-Vogt, C. and Brigelius-Flohe, R. (2004) Vitamin E: underestimated as an antioxidant. *Redox Report* **9**, 249–54.

Pignocchi, C., Fletcher, J.M., Wilkinson, J.E., Barnes, J.D. and Foyer, C.H. (2003) The function of ascorbate oxidase in tobacco. *Plant Physiology* **132**, 1631–41.

Pongracz, G., Weiser, H. and Matzinger, D. (1995) 'ocopherole – Antioxidantien der Natur. *Fat ScienceTechnology* **97**, 90–104.

Rippert, P., Scimemi, C., Dubald, M. and Matringe, M. (2004) Engineering plant shikimate pathway for the production of tocotrienol and improving herbicide resistance. *Plant Physiology* **134**, 92–100.

Rousseaux, M.C., Jones, C.M., Adams, D., Chetelaqt, R., Bennet, A. and Powell, A. (2005) QTL analysis of fruit antioxidants in tomato using *Lycopersicon pennellii* introgression lines. *Theoretical and Applied Genetics* **111**, 1396–408.

Sato, P. and Udenfriend, S. (1978) Scurvy-prone animals, including man, monkey and guinea pig, do not express the gene for gulonolactone oxidase. *Archives of Biochemistry and Biophysics* **71**, 293–9.

Sattler, S.E., Cahoon, E.B., Coughlan, S.J. and DellaPenna, D. (2003) Characterization of tocopherol cyclases from higher plants and cyanobacteria. Evolutionary implications for tocopherol synthesis and function. *Plant Physiology* **132**, 2184–239.

Sattler, S.E., Gilliland, L.U., Magallanes-Lundback, M., Pollard, M. and DellaPenna, D. (2004) Vitamin E is essential or seed longevity and for preventing lipid peroxidation during germination. *Plant Cell* **16**, 1419–32.

Schauer, N., Semel, Y., Roessner, U., Gur, A., Balbo, I., Carrari, F., Pleban, T., Perez-Melis, A., Bruedigam, C., Kopka, J., Willmitzer, L., Zamir, D. and Fernie, A.R. (2006) Comprehensive metabolic profiling and phenotyping of interspecific introgression lines for tomato improvement. *Nature Biotechnology* **24**, 447–54.

Schroeder, M.T., Becker, E.M. and Skibsted, L.H. (2006) Molecular mechanism of antioxidant synergism of tocotrienols and carotenoids in palm oil. *Journal of Agricultural and Food Chemistry* **54**, 3445–53.

Serbinova. E., Kagan, V., Han, D. and Packer, L. (1991) Free radical recycling and intermembrane mobility in the antioxidation properties of alpha-tocopherol and alpha-tocotrienol. *Free Radical Biology and Medicine* **10**, 263–75.

Shintani, D.K. and DellaPenna, D. (1998) Elevating the vitamin E content of plants through metabolic engineering. *Science* **282**, 2098–100.

Shewmaker, C.K., Sheehy, J.A., Daley, M., Colburn, S. and Ke, D.Y. (1999) Seed-specific overexpression of phytoene synthase: increase in carotenoids and other metabolic effects. *Plant Journal* **20**, 401–12.

Smirnoff, N. (2000) Ascorbate biosynthesis and function in photoprotection. *Philosophical Transactions of the Royal Society of London* **355**, 1455–64.

Soll, J., Kemmerling, M. and Schultz, G. (1980) Tocopherol and plastoquinone synthesis in spinack chloroplasts subfractions. *Archives of Biochemistry and Biophysics* **204**, 544–50.

Suffield, R.M. and Dillman, S.H. (2006) Performance of tocopherols as antioxidants in ABS. *Journal of Vinyl and Additive Technology* **12**, 66–72.

Suzuki, Y.J., Tsuchiya, M., Wassall, S.R., Choo, Y.M., Govil, G., Kagan, V.E. and Parker, L. (1993) Structural and dynamic membrane properties of α-tocopherol and α-tocotrienol: implications to the molecular mechanism of their antioxidant potency. *Biochemistry* **32**, 10692–9.

Timmermann, von F. (1990) Tocopherole-Antioxidative wirkung bei Fetten und Ölen. *Fat Science Technology* **92**, 201–6.

Tokunaga, T., Miyahara, K., Tabata. K. and Esaka, M. (2005) Generation and properties of ascorbic acid over producing transgenic tobacco cells expressing sense RNA for L-galactono-1,4-lactone dehydrogenase. *Planta* **220**, 854–63.

Tsegaye, Y., Shintani, D.K. and DellaPenna, D. (2002) Overexpression of the enzyme p-hydroxyphenolpyruvate dioxygenase in *Arabidopsis* and its relation to tocopherol biosynthesis. *Plant Physiology and Biochemistry* **40**, 913–20.

Valentin, H.E., Lincoln, K., Moshiri, F., Jensen, P.K., Qi, Q.G., Venkatesh, T.V., Karunanandaa, B., Baszis, S.R., Norris, S.R., Savidge, B., Gruys, K.J. and Last, R.L. (2006) The *Arabidopsis* vitamin E pathway gene5-1 mutant reveals a critical role for phytol kinase in seed tocopherol biosynthesis. *Plant Cell* **18**, 212–24.

Valesco, L., Fernandez-Martinez, J.M., Garcia-Ruiz, R. and Dominguez, J. (2002) Genetic and environmental variation for tocopherol content and composition in sunflower commercial hybrids. *Journal of Agricultural Science* **139**, 425–9.

Valesco, L., Perez-Vich, B. and Fernandez-Martinez, J.M. (2004) Novel variation for the tocopherol profile in sunflower created by mutagenesis and recombination. *Plant Breeding* **123**, 490–2.

Van Eenennaam, A.L., Lincoln, K., Durrett, T.P., Valentin, H.E., Shewmaker, C.K., Thorne, G.M., Jiang, J., Baszis, S.R., Levering, C.K., Aasen, E.D., Hao, M., Stein, J.C., Norris, S.R. and Last, R.L. (2003) Engineering vitamin E content: from *Arabidopsis* mutant to soy oil. *Plant Cell* **15**, 3007–19.

Van Eenennaam, A.L., Li, G.F., Venkatramesh, M., Levering, C., Gong, X.S., Jamieson, A.C., Rebar, E.J., Shewmaker, C.K and Case, C.C. (2004) Elevation of seed α-tocopherol levels using plant-based transcription factors targeted to an endogenous location. *Metabolic Engineering* **6**, 101–8.

VERIS (1993) *1993 Vitamin E Abstracts* (ed. M.K. Horwitt). LaGrange, IL: Vitamin E Research and Information Service.

Wheeler, G.L., Jones, M.A. and Smirnoff, N. (1998). The biosynthetic pathway of vitamin C in higher plants. *Nature* **393**, 365–9.

White, D.A., Fisk, I.D. and Gray, D.A. (2006) Characterisation of oat (*Avena sativa* L.) oil bodies and intrinsically associated E-vitamers. *Journal of Cereal Science* **43**, 244–9.

Wolucka, B.A., Persiau, G., Van Doorsselaere, J., Davey, M.W., Demol, H., Vandekerckhove, J., Van Montagu, M., Zabeau, M. and Boerjan, W. (2001) Partial purification and identification of GDP-mannose 3',5'-epimerase of Arabidopsis thaliana, a key enzyme of the palnt vitamin C pathway. *Proceedings of the National Academy of Science USA* **98**, 14843–8.

Yanishlieva, N.V., Kamal-Eldin, A., Marinov, E.M. and Toneva, A.G. (2002) Kinetics of antioxidant action of α- and γ-tocopherols in sunflower and soybean triacylglycerols. *European Journal of Lipid Science and Technology* **104**, 262–70.

Yoshida, Y., Niki, E. and Noguchi, N. (2003) Comparative study on the action of tocopherols and tocotrienols as antioxidant: chemical and physical effects. *Chemistry and Physics of Lipids* **123**, 63–75.

Chapter 6

Folate

Stéphane Ravanel and Fabrice Rébeillé

Introduction

Folate is a water-soluble vitamin (B9) that was first discovered in 1931 by Dr Wills who identified a previously unknown component of yeast that could cure and prevent large-cell anaemia of pregnancy. The 'Wills factor' was then purified from spinach leaves in 1941 and named folic acid, a term which derives from the Latin term folium (leaf). Chemically, folic acid (or pteroylglutamic acid) is a tripartite molecule composed of a pterin, a para-aminobenzoic acid (pABA) and a γ-linked glutamate residue (Figure 6.1). From this chemical architecture, there is a large diversity of related species resulting from the oxidation state of the pterin ring, the differential substitution of single-carbon units on the pterin and/or pABA moieties and/or the length of the glutamyl side chain. Folic acid and its derivatives are commonly grouped under the generic term 'folates'.

Cellular folates occur as dihydro- or tetrahydro- derivatives of pteroylglutamic acid, i.e. dihydrofolates and tetrahydrofolates (THF), but folic acid does not exist in nature to any significant extent. Its occurrence is dependent on the chemical oxidation of reduced folates or on commercial synthesis for use in supplements and in food fortification. Only THF participate in one-carbon (C1) metabolism by accepting and donating C1-units. These C1-groups range in oxidation state from formyl (most oxidised) to methyl (most reduced) and are attached at N-5 of the pterin moiety, N-10 of the pABA moiety, or bridged between the two (Figure 6.1). Also, naturally occurring folates are predominantly polyglutamylated and are therefore termed folylpolyglutamates. The glutamyl side chain of folates (1 to 8 residues) is somewhat unusual in that residues are γ-linked and not α-linked as with proteins. In all organisms, polyglutamylation is known to be essential for three physiological roles (Shane 1989). First, folylpolyglutamates are the preferred coenzymes for most of the enzymes involved in C1 metabolism. Second, the chain enhances folate stability by favouring binding to proteins, bound folates being less sensitive to oxidative degradation. Third, polyglutamylation is the principal means by which folates are retained within cells and subcellular compartments. Chain elongation increases the anionic nature of folate

Phytonutrients, First Edition. Edited by Andrew Salter, Helen Wiseman and Gregory Tucker.
© 2012 Blackwell Publishing Ltd. Published 2012 by Blackwell Publishing Ltd.

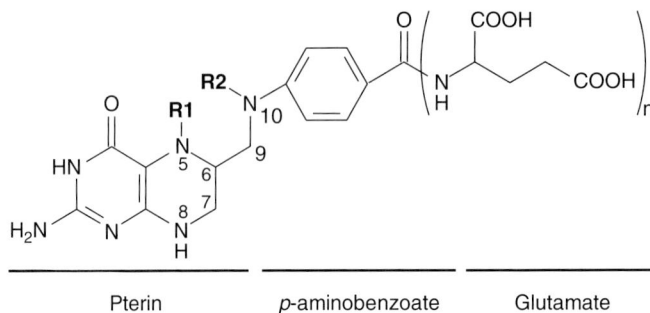

Figure 6.1 Chemical structure of tetrahydrofolate and its C1-substituted derivatives. Cellular folates are substituted at the N-5 and/or N-10 positions by C1-units of different oxidation states and usually contain 5 to 8 glutamate residues. See plate section for colour version of this figure.

Folates	R1	R2
5-formyl-THF	CHO	H
10-formyl-THF	H	CHO
5,10-methenyl-THF	=CH$^+$-	
5,10-methylene-THF	-CH$_2$-	
5-methyl-THF	CH$_3$	H
5-formimino-THF	CH=NH	H

coenzymes by providing α-carboxyl charges and decreases affinity for membrane carriers, thus impairing folate diffusion through hydrophobic barriers.

One-carbon metabolism

The N-5 and N-10 atoms of the THF cofactor are modified with C1-units at the oxidation state of methanol (5-methyl-THF), formaldehyde (5,10-methylene-THF) and formate (10-formyl-THF, 5-formyl-THF and 5,10-methenyl-THF). Serine, glycine and formate are the principal sources for C1 units, the catabolism of these compounds resulting in the synthesis of 5,10-methylene-THF and 10-formyl-THF (Figure 6.2). These folates are then enzymatically interconverted to other derivatives which serve a particular metabolic function: 5-methyl-THF is required for methionine synthesis, 5,10-methylene-THF is required to convert deoxy-uridine monophosphate (dUMP) to deoxy-thymidine monophosphate (dTMP) and to produce pantothenate, whereas 10-formyl-THF supplies C-2 and C-8 for purine ring biosynthesis and contributes to formylmethionyl-tRNA synthesis (Figure 6.2).

The overall organisation of this complex metabolic network is generally conserved between organisms, from microbes to human. However, depending on species, tissues

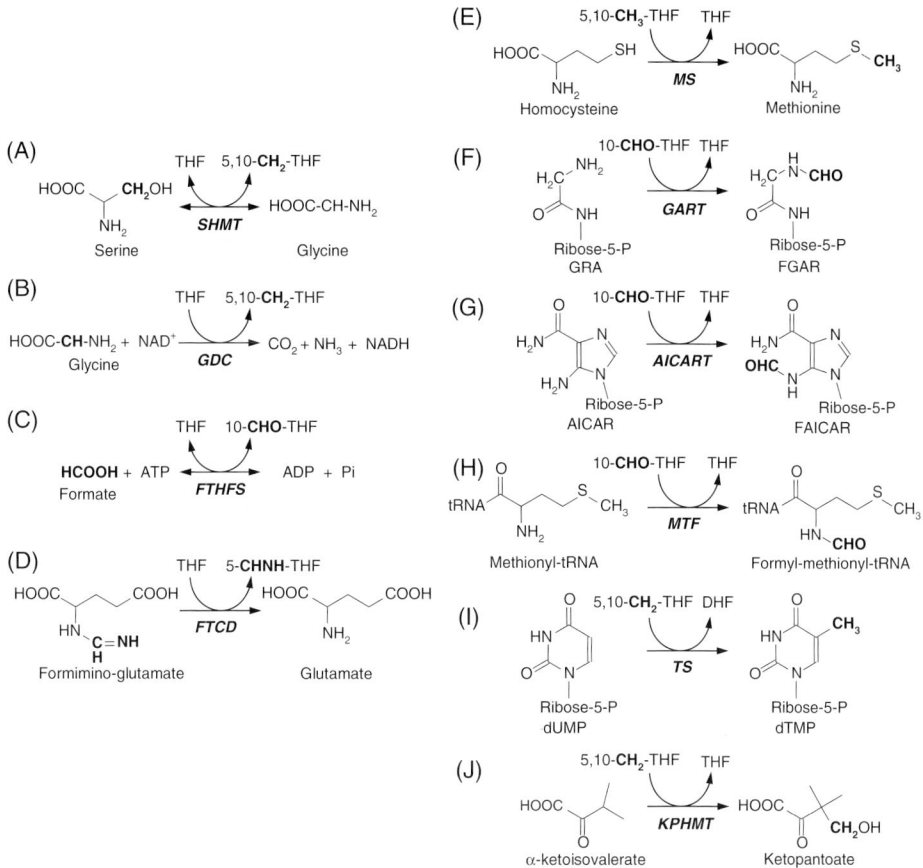

Figure 6.2 Key reactions of C1 metabolism. Reactions involved in the generation of C1-substituted folates are described on the left column and the anabolic reactions utilizing folates on the right. A, serine-glycine interconversion catalyzed by serine hydroxymethyl transferase (SHMT); B, catabolism of glycine catalyzed by the glycine decarboxylase complex (GDC); C, synthesis of 10-formyl-THF by 10-formyl-THF synthetase (FTHFS); D, synthesis of 5-formimino-THF by the formiminotransferase domain of the bifunctional enzyme glutamate formiminotransferase / formimino-THF cyclodeaminase (FTCD); E, methylation of homocysteine to methionine catalyzed by methionine synthase (MS); F and G, purine ring synthesis involves two formylation reactions catalyzed by glycinamide ribonucleotide transformylase (GART) and aminoimidazole carboximide ribonucleide transformylase (AICART); H, formylation of methionyl-tRNA catalyzed by methionyl-tRNA transformylase (MTF); I, methylation of dUMP to dTMP catalyzed by thymidylate synthase (TS), note that this reaction produces dihydrofolate (DHF); J, synthesis of ketopantoate, precursor of pantothenate, from α-ketoisovalerate catalyzed by ketopantoate hydroxymethyl transferase (KPHMT). See plate section for colour version of this figure.

and developmental stages, C1 metabolism has been adapted to meet specific metabolic requirements (Ravanel et al. 2004a; Nzila et al. 2005a,b; Christensen and MacKenzie 2006). The ubiquitous and specific features of C1 metabolism in animals, yeast and plants will be described in the following sections.

Generation and interconversion of C1-units

Serine–glycine metabolism

The conversion of serine into glycine, a reaction catalysed by the pyridoxal-phosphate dependent enzyme serine hydroxymethyl transferase (SHMT) and leading to 5,10-methylene-THF formation, is by far the main source of C1 units in all organisms (Figure 6.2). Although the interconversion of serine and glycine by SHMT is fully reversible, the equilibrium distribution of the substrates indicates that glycine formation is favoured. In eukaryotes, SHMT is present in the cytosol and the organelles, mitochondria and plastids, indicating that serine can act as C1-unit donor in these compartments (Figure 6.3) (Appling 1991; Hanson and Roje 2001; Tibbets and Appling 2010). In mitochondria, the glycine decarboxylase (GDC) activity allows glycine to be used as an alternative C1-unit donor. GDC is a multi-enzyme complex that catalyses the oxidative decarboxylation and deamination of glycine into CO_2 and NH_3 with the concomitant conversion of THF into 5,10-methylene-THF (Figure 6.2) (Douce et al. 2001). Thus, most of the C1 units in animal and yeast mitochondria are derived from serine and glycine through the activities of SHMT and GDC. In mitochondria from photosynthetic tissues, the situation is different because the functions of SHMT and GDC have been adapted to participate in photorespiration, a complex pathway connected to photosynthesis in C3 plants (Douce and Neuburger 1999; Foyer et al. 2009). In leaf mitochondria, almost all 5,10-methylene-THF formed upon glycine oxidation is used in serine synthesis for recycling of ribulose-1,5-bisphosphate, a key intermediate of the Calvin cycle. In mitochondria from non-photosynthetic tissues, the coupled action of GDC and SHMT is also dedicated primarily to serine formation, which is then used as a source of C1 units in the cytosol (Mouillon et al. 1999).

Formate activation

Formate is an alternative source of C1-units in eukaryotes. The synthesis of 10-formyl-THF from formate and THF is catalysed by the ATP-dependent enzyme 10-formyl-THF synthetase (FTHFS). As this reaction is reversible (Figure 6.2), it could be also considered as a route by which formate exits C1 metabolism. The cytosolic and mitochondrial FTHFS isoforms found in yeast and the cytosolic isoform from mammals are associated with two other activities, 5,10-methylene-THF dehydrogenase (MTHFD) and 5,10-methenyl-THF cyclohydrolase (MTHFC), to form a trifunctional enzyme called C1-THF synthase (Appling 1991; Tibbets and Appling 2010). Mammals also have a monofunctional FTHFS and a bifunctional MTHFD-MTHFC in mitochondria, which is similar to the arrangement found in the cytosol, mitochondria and chloroplasts from higher plants (Figure 6.3) (Christensen and MacKenzie 2006; Hanson and Roje 2001). In mammalian and yeast cells, the general consensus is that mitochondria use the FTHFS activity in reverse to produce formate and THF from 10-formyl-THF. After translocation to the cytoplasm, formate is then re-used as an important source of C1 units by the activities of the cytoplasmic C1-THF synthase (Figure 6.3). Thus, C1 flux seems to be in the oxidative direction in mitochondria and in the reductive direction in the cytosol (Christensen and MacKenzie 2006). In plants, most of the formate is degraded to CO_2 via

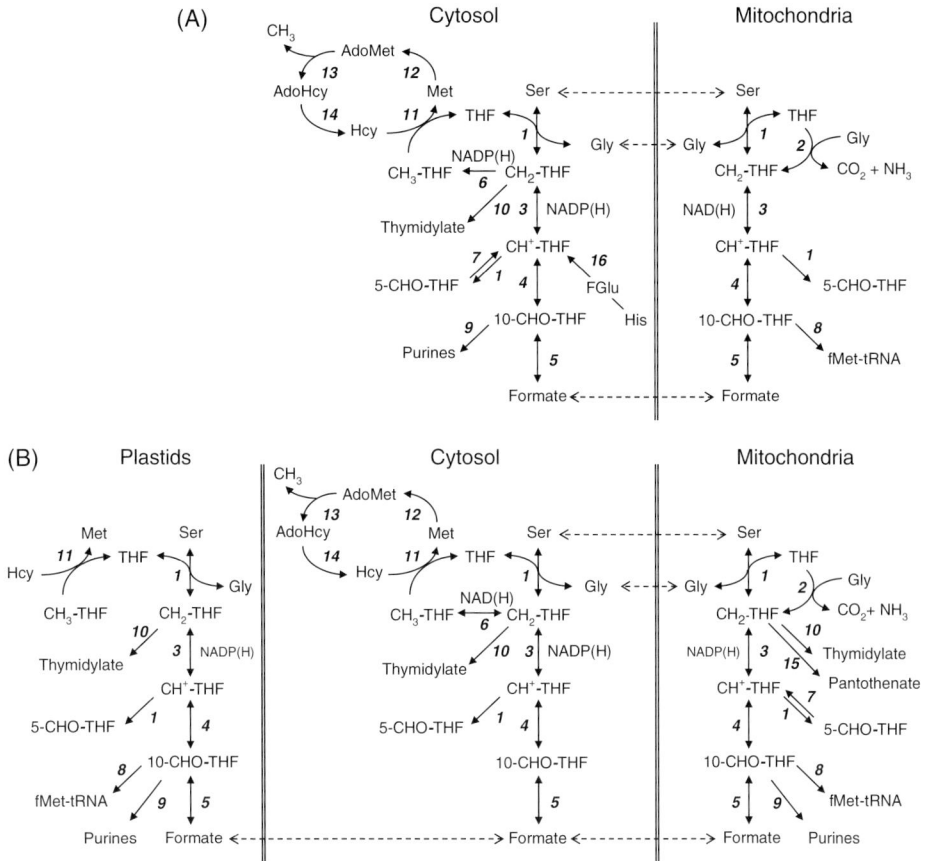

Figure 6.3 Compartmentation of C1 metabolism in mammals (A) and plants (B). *1*: serine hydroxymethyl transferase; *2*: glycine decarboxylase; *3*: 5,10-methylene-THF dehydrogenase; *4*: 5,10-methenyl-THF cyclohydrolase; *5*: 10-formyl-THF synthetase; *6*: 5,10-methylene-THF reductase; *7*: 5-formyl-THF cycloligase; *8*: methionyl-tRNA formyltransferase; *9*: glycinamide ribonucleotide transformylase and aminoimidazole carboximide ribonucleide transformylase; *10*: thymidylate synthase; *11*: methionine synthase; *12*: AdoMet synthetase; *13*: AdoMet-dependent methyltransferase; *14*: AdoHcy hydrolase; *15*: ketopantoate hydroxymethyltransferase; *16*: glutamate formimino transferase and formimino-THF cyclodeaminase. AdoHcy, *S*-adenosylhomocysteine; AdoMet, S-adenosylmethionine; FGlu, N-formiminoglutamate; Gly, glycine; Hcy, homocysteine; His, histidine; Ser, serine.

a mitochondrial formate dehydrogenase but low amounts can serve as a C1 donor (Prabhu et al. 1996; Gout et al. 2000; Li et al. 2003).

Histidine catabolism

In animals and some microorganisms, the catabolism of histidine is linked to folate metabolism through the key intermediate 5-formimino-THF. The bifunctional enzyme glutamate formiminotransferase formimino-THF cyclodeaminase (FTCD) catalyses two consecutive reactions in this pathway. First, the formiminotransferase domain of the protein catalyses the transfer of the formimino group from formimino-glutamate, a product of histidine catabolism, to THF to produce 5-formimino-THF and glutamate (Figure 6.2). The folate coenzyme is then channelled to the deaminase catalytic site where it undergoes cyclisation to produce 5,10-methenyl-THF and ammonia (Mao et al. 2004). FTCD is present in every mammalian cell type either free in the cytosol (Figure 6.3) or tightly bound to the Golgi complex, but is most highly abundant in the liver. In plants, little is known about histidine catabolism and the FTCD activity has never been described.

Interconvertion of C1-substituted folates

5,10-Methylene-THF, 5,10-methenyl-THF and 10-formyl-THF can be interconverted by the enzymes MTHFD and MTHFC. These activities are reversible and are associated with the cytosol, mitochondria and plastids (Figure 6.3) (Hanson and Roje 2001; Christensen and MacKenzie 2006). Thus, the combination of SHMT, MTHFD and MTHFC activities can supply each cell compartment with C1-substituted folates required for nucleotides, formyl-methionyl-tRNA or pantothenate synthesis (Figure 6.3).

Methyl-THF has no other known metabolic fate than methionine synthesis. Methylene-THF reductase (MTHFR) serves a key role in C1 metabolism by converting 5,10-methylene-THF to 5-methyl-THF. The NADPH-dependent MTHFR from yeast and animals irreversibly directs the methyl group of 5-methyl-THF to methylation of homocysteine (Figure 6.3) (Roje et al. 2002a). Because this reaction has the potential to deplete the cytosolic 5,10-methylene-THF pool, the regulation of MTHFR is crucial for C1 metabolism. In yeast and animal cells, methyl group biogenesis is regulated *in vivo* by a feedback loop in which *S*-adenosylmethionine (AdoMet), a derivative of methionine which is used for methylation reactions, inhibits MTHFR (Roje et al. 2002a). Plant MTHFRs are cytosolic enzymes that differ from their yeast and mammalian counterparts because they are NADH-dependent, reversible and not regulated by AdoMet (Figure 6.3) (Roje et al. 1999). The reversibility of the reaction is sufficient to control C1-fluxes into methyl-group biogenesis and does not need a feedback inhibition by AdoMet.

5-Formyl-THF is a ubiquitous member of biological folates but is the only derivative that does not serve as a C1-unit donor (Figure 6.3). It is considered that 5-formyl-THF is a potential regulator of C1 metabolism because it is a potent inhibitor of SHMT and several other folate-utilising enzymes (Stover and Schirch 1993). 5-formyl-THF is formed during the irreversible hydrolysis of 5,10-methenyl-THF catalysed by a side reaction of SHMT in the presence of glycine (Figure 6.3). 5-formyl-THF cycloligase (FCL, also referred to as 5,10-methenyl-THF synthetase) is the only enzyme that uses 5-formyl-THF by catalysing an ATP-dependent conversion to the metabolically active form 5,10-methenyl-THF (Stover and Schirch 1993). FCL is a cytosolic enzyme in yeast and animals whereas it is located in plant mitochondria (Figure 6.3), a compartment where the 5-CHO derivatives represent up to 50–70% of the folate pool (Roje et al. 2002b; Chan and Cossins 2003; Orsomando et al. 2005).

Utilisation of C1-units

Methionine synthesis

The pool of C1-substituted folates forms the core of C1 metabolism, from which single-carbon units are withdrawn by anabolic reactions. The synthesis of methionine using 5-methyl-THF is the largest anabolic flux of C1-units in many physiological situations. Indeed, in addition to protein synthesis, methionine serves as a methyl group donor through conversion to AdoMet, a key biological methylating agent involved in dozens of methyltransferase reactions with a wide variety of acceptor molecules (nucleic acids, proteins and metabolites). In plants, AdoMet is also involved in the biogenesis of biotin (vitamin B8) and the phytohormone ethylene and has a regulatory role in the synthesis of aspartate-derived amino acids (Ravanel et al. 1998; Curien et al. 2009). In all organisms, methionine is produced from homocysteine and 5-methyl-THF through a reaction catalysed by methionine synthase (Figure 6.2). Two types of methionine synthase, whose activities depend or not on the presence of a cobalamin (vitamin B12) cofactor, are known. Cobalamin-dependent enzymes are found in animals, bacteria and algae whereas cobalamin-independent isoforms exist in bacteria, fungi, algae and plants (Drummond and Matthews 1993; Ravanel et al. 2004b; Croft et al. 2005). Methionine synthase, like AdoMet synthetase and *S*-adenosylhomocysteine hydrolase, is present in the cytosol, where it is involved in the regeneration of methionine to ensure a rapid turnover of AdoMet (a set of reactions referred to as the 'activated methyl cycle', see Figure 6.3). Thus, AdoMet is synthesised exclusively in the cytosol and thereafter is transported to other cell compartments to enable numerous methylation reactions or regulatory roles (Marobbio et al. 2003; Agrimi et al. 2004; Bouvier et al. 2006). In vascular plants, methionine synthase activity is also located in plastids to participate in *de novo* synthesis of methionine (Figure 6.3) (Ravanel et al. 2004b).

Purine ring formation

Synthesis of the purine ring is a central metabolic function of all organisms. The products, AMP and GMP, provide purine bases for DNA and RNA, as well as for a number of essential coenzymes (NAD(P), FAD, AdoMet and CoA) and signalling molecules (cAMP). In plants, the nucleotides are also the precursors for purine alkaloids and the hormone cytokinin. The pathways for synthesis and salvage of nucleotides in animals, plants and microorganisms are similar (Smith and Atkins 2002; Boldt and Zrenner 2003). Starting from phosphoribosyl pyrophosphate, *de novo* synthesis of AMP and GMP is a complex 14-step process involving two formylation reactions that depend on 10-formyl-THF (Figure 6.2). The third reaction of the pathway is the formylation of glycinamide ribonucleotide (GAR) into formyl-GAR, a reaction catalysed by GAR transformylase. The bifunctional enzyme aminoimidazole carboxamide ribonucleotide (AICAR) transformylase / inosine monophosphate (IMP) cyclohydrolase is responsible for catalysis of steps 9 and 10 in the purine pathway, with formyl-AICAR as an intermediate. In animal and fungal cells purine ring synthesis is cytosolic whereas in plants it is located in the organelles (Figure 6.3) (Smith and Atkins 2002; Boldt and Zrenner 2003; Christensen and MacKenzie 2006).

Formylation of methionyl-tRNA

In addition to its role in the assembly of the purine ring, 10-formyl-THF plays an essential function as donor of the formyl group during the synthesis of formyl-methionyl-tRNA. Thus, protein synthesis in the organelles, which is initiated by this formylated tRNA, is tightly associated with C1 metabolism. The synthesis of formyl-methionyl-tRNA from methionyl-tRNA and 10-formyl-THF is catalysed by methionyl-tRNA transformylase (Figure 6.2), an enzyme present in both mitochondria and chloroplasts (Figure 6.3) (Appling 1991; Cossins 2000).

Thymidylate synthesis

The synthesis of thymidylate is closely linked to C1 metabolism through the enzyme thymidylate synthase (TS). Because of its essential role in DNA replication, TS from human is the target of several anticancer agents (e.g. 5-fluorouracil) used in colon and breast chemotherapy. TS catalyses the final step in *de novo* synthesis of thymidylate, the reductive methylation of dUMP to dTMP with concomitant conversion of 5,10-methylene-THF to dihydrofolate (Figure 6.2). This is the only reaction in C1 metabolism in which the folate substrate is oxidised during single-unit transfer, with the electrons being used to reduce the C1-unit to the methyl level. It is therefore necessary to regenerate the fully reduced form of folate for a sustained synthesis of DNA. This reduction of dihydrofolate into THF is achieved by dihydrofolate reductase (DHFR), a ubiquitous enzyme which is also involved in *de novo* synthesis of THF in folate-autotrophs (Figure 6.4). TS and DHFR are monofunctional enzymes in most species except protozoa and plants where they exist as a bifunctional enzyme (Nzila et al. 2005a; Rébeillé et al. 2006; Blancquaert et al. 2010). Thymidylate synthesis was thought to be restricted to the cytosol in animals but recent evidence indicates a folate-mediated synthesis of dTMP in the nucleus (Tibbets and Appling 2010). This synthesis may be cell-specific and involves translocation into the nucleus during the S and G2/M phases of TS, DHFR and the cytoplasmic SHMT following modification by sumoylation (Woeller et al. 2007). In plants, the probable existence of bifunctional DHFR-TS isoforms in mitochondria, plastids and the cytosol also suggests a multi-compartmented synthesis of thymidylate (Rébeillé et al. 2006; Blancquaert et al. 2010) (Figure 6.3).

Pantothenate synthesis

Pantothenate is a water-soluble vitamin (B5) that is synthesised *de novo* by plants and micro-organisms but obtained through the diet by animals. Pantothenate is the precursor of the 4′-phosphopantetheine moiety of CoA and acyl-carrier protein, cofactors in energy yielding reactions including carbohydrate metabolism and fatty acid synthesis (Coxon et al. 2005). In plants, CoA is also important in many aspects of secondary metabolism, including lignin biosynthesis. The first reaction in the 4-step pantothenate synthesis pathway involves the transfer of a hydroxymethyl group from 5,10-methylene-THF to α-ketoisovalerate, generating ketopantoate (Figure 6.2). This reaction is catalysed by ketopantoate hydroxymethyltransferase. The folate-dependent enzymes from plants and

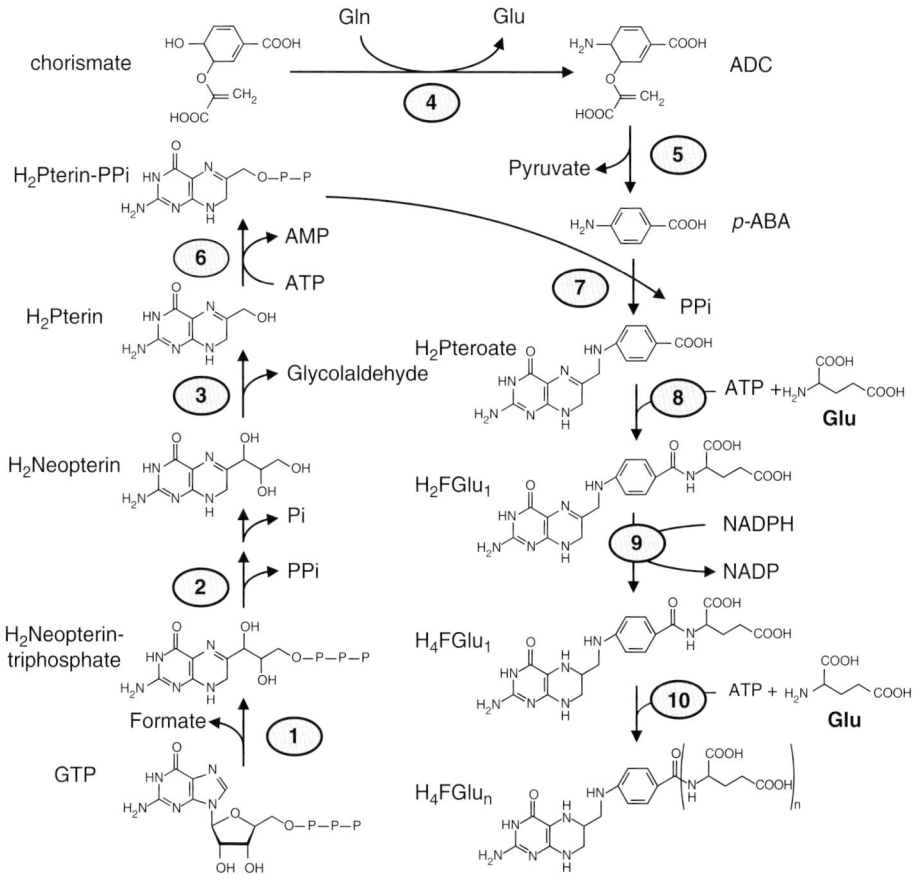

Figure 6.4 Tetrahydrofolate biosynthetic pathway in plants. The enzymes involved in the synthesis of THF polyglutamate are: **1**: GTP cyclohydrolase I; **2**: dihydroneopterin triphosphate pyrophosphatase; **3**: dihydroneopterin aldolase; **4**: aminodeoxychorismate (ADC) synthase; **5**: ADC lyase; **6**: hydroxymethyldihydropterin pyrophosphokinase; **7**: dihydropteroate synthase; **8**: dihydrofolate synthetase; **9**: dihydrofolate reductase; **10**: folylpolyglutamate synthetase. pABA, para-aminobenzoate.

yeast are located in mitochondria (Figure 6.3), whereas the remaining steps of the pathway are most likely present in the cytosol (Ottenhof et al. 2004; Coxon et al. 2005).

Folate synthesis and distribution in plants

Biosynthesis of tetrahydrofolate in plants

Plants, fungi, most micro-organisms and apicomplexan parasites such as *Plasmodium falciparum* have the capacity to synthesise THF *de novo* (Cossins and Chen 1997; Nzila et al. 2005a; Rébeillé et al. 2006; Blancquaert et al. 2010). Humans and animals in general do not have this capacity because seven out of the ten enzymes required for this complex

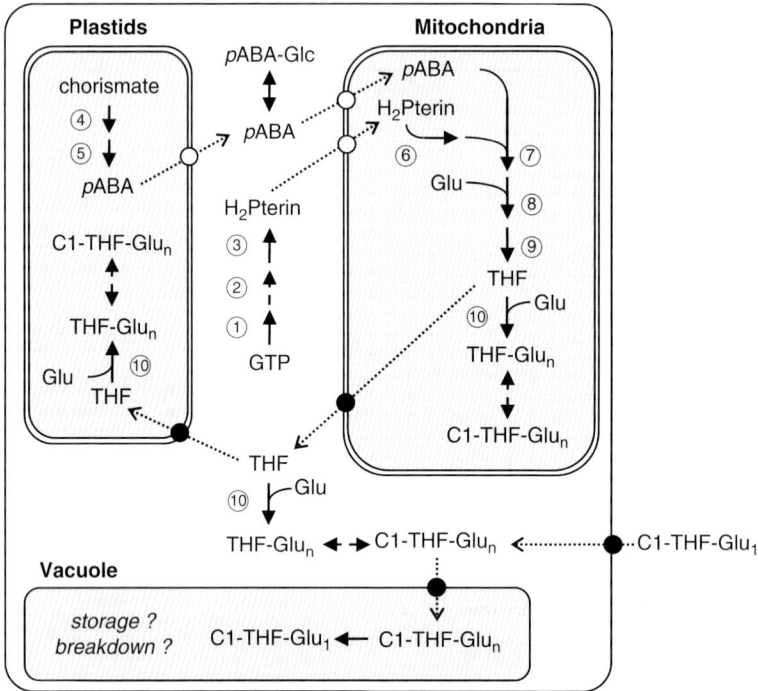

Figure 6.5 Subcellular compartmentation of tetrahydrofolate synthesis and probable transport steps in plant cells. Enzymes involved in THF synthesis are numbered as in Figure 6.3. Probable transport steps of folates and precursors are indicated by black and white circles, respectively. pABA, para-aminobenzoate; H_2Pterin, hydromethyldihydropterin; C1-THF-Glu$_n$, C1 derivative of folylpolyglutamates.

metabolic route are absent. The plant THF biosynthetic pathway is now completely elucidated and is the same as in bacteria (Figure 6.4) (Rébeillé et al. 2006; Blancquaert et al. 2010). The plant enzymes possess unique structural and biochemical properties and present a fascinating spatial organisation in which three subcellular compartments participate (Figure 6.5). The pterin and pABA parts of THF are first synthesised in separate routes originating from GTP and chorismate, respectively. These moieties are then assembled, together with glutamate, to produce dihydrofolate, which is then converted to folylpolyglutamates in two steps.

Pterin branch

The conversion of GTP into 6-hydroxymethyl-7,8-dihydropterin is a three-step process located in the cytosol of plant cells (Figures 6.4 and 6.5). The first reaction is catalysed by GTP-cyclohydrolase I (GTPCHI) to form 7,8-dihydroneopterin (DHN) triphosphate. GTPCHI is present in folate-synthesising organisms and in mammals where it is involved in the synthesis of other pteridines. Indeed, the tetrahydrobiopterin cofactors for aromatic amino acid hydroxylases and NO synthases and other pteridines that have key roles as chromophores or UV protectants derive from DHN triphosphate in animals (Werner-Felmayer et al. 2002). Given that GTPCHI catalyses the first step in the synthesis of pterin derivatives, the enzyme is considered to control fluxes into these pathways (Basset et al. 2002). In support of this proposal, genetic engineering of the GTPCHI step in transgenic *Arabidopsis* and tomato plants led to an important increase in pteridine production (Hossain et al. 2004; Diaz de la Garza et al. 2004). The triphosphate side chain of DHN triphosphate is further removed in two steps to produce DHN. First, DHN triphosphate pyrophosphatase specifically cleaves DHN to produce DHN monophosphate (Klaus et al. 2005a). Second, the remaining phosphate is cleaved from DHN monophosphate by the action of a phosphatase. This enzyme has not yet been identified in plants; it may be non-specific as in *Escherichia coli*. The last step of the pterin branch is catalysed by DHN aldolase that cleaves the trihydroxypropyl side chain of DHN to yield 6-hydroxymethyl-7,8-dihydropterin (Goyer et al. 2004). The plant enzyme is encoded by a small gene family and is monofunctional whereas the fungal activity is part of a trifunctional enzyme (see below; Guldener et al. 2004).

pABA branch

pABA is synthesised from chorismate, a compound that is also involved in the synthesis of aromatic amino acids and their derivatives. The synthesis of pABA from chorismate occurs in two steps located in plastids (Figures 6.4 and 6.5). First, the amination of chorismate yields 4-amino-4-deoxychorismate (ADC), which is subsequently aromatised to pABA with elimination of pyruvate. In bacteria, the synthesis of ADC is catalysed by ADC synthase, a two-component enzyme in which the glutamine amido-transferase protein PabA supplies an amino group to PabB, which catalyses the amination reaction. In plants, both of these reactions are catalysed by a single protein which is a fusion of the PabA and PabB domains (Basset et al. 2004a). Besides its unusual primary structure, plant ADC synthase is inhibited by dihydrofolate and its analogue methotrexate, a feature never reported for the bacterial enzyme (Sahr et al. 2006). These unique features support the view that the plant ADC synthase is a potential regulatory step that can participate in partitioning the flux of chorismate towards folate, tryptophan, tyrosine and phenylalanine syntheses. The second step of pABA synthesis in bacteria and plants is catalysed by the pyridoxal-phosphate dependent enzyme ADC lyase (PabC) (Basset et al. 2004b). The pABA pool in different plant tissues is mainly in an esterified form with glucose (pABA-Glc) that is formed in the cytosol and is largely sequestered in vacuoles (Eudes et al. 2008). The physiological role of pABA-Glc is not yet elucidated, it may be involved in regulating pABA storage or may be the form in which pABA is trafficked within plant cells (Quinlivan et al. 2003).

Assembly of the pterin, pABA and glutamate moieties

The combination of 6-hydroxymethyl-7,8-dihydropterin, pABA and glutamate to produce dihydrofolate involves three reactions that are located within mitochondria (Figures 6.4 and 6.5). First, hydroxymethyl-dihydropterin is activated into its pyrophosphorylated form through the operation of hydroxymethyldihydropterin pyrophosphokinase (HPPK).

Second, dihydropteroate is produced by condensation of pABA with the activated pterin in a reaction catalysed by dihydropteroate synthase (DHPS). In plants, these two reactions are catalysed by a bifunctional enzyme whereas the activities are carried by separate proteins in bacteria (Rébeillé et al. 1997). In plant HPPK-DHPS, the DHPS reaction is feedback inhibited by dihydropteroate, dihydrofolate and THF-Glu$_1$, suggesting that this domain could be a potential regulatory point of the mitochondrial branch of the folate pathway (Mouillon et al. 2002). *Arabidopsis* is unique among higher plants with sequenced genomes in having two genes coding HPPK-DHPS (Storozhenko et al. 2007). The first one encodes the mitochondrial isoform involved in *de novo* synthesis of THF while the second is highly expressed in developing seeds and encodes a cytosolic enzyme whose function remains to be established. The third mitochondrial step is the ATP-dependent attachment of glutamate to the carboxyl moiety of pABA to form dihydrofolate. It is catalysed by a monofunctional dihydrofolate synthetase (Ravanel et al. 2001), an enzyme that is essential for plant development because a mutation of this gene is embryo-lethal in *Arabidopsis* (Ishikawa et al. 2003).

Reduction and polyglutamylation

Before entering C1 metabolism, dihydrofolate is reduced to THF and polyglutamylated by the operation of two enzymes that are present in all kingdoms. Dihydrofolate is reduced to THF-Glu$_1$ by dihydrofolate reductase (DHFR) using NADPH as electron donor (Figure 6.4). In animals, fungi and bacteria, DHFR is a monofunctional enzyme (Cossins and Chen 1997; Schnell et al. 2004). DHFR is inhibited by the dihydrofolate analogue metho-trexate, a molecule that is used as an antifolate in chemotherapy. In higher plants, the activity is catalysed by the third bifunctional enzyme of the folate pathway, which also carries a thymidylate synthase (TS) activity (Rébeillé et al. 2006; Blancquaert et al. 2010). As a result, the DHFR domain of the enzyme has a dual function; it is involved in the reduction of dihydrofolate monoglutamate originating from *de novo* synthesis of folate or dihydrofolate polyglutamate resulting from the oxidation of THF-Glu$_n$ during TS activity (Neuburger et al. 1996).

The polyglutamate tail of THF-Glu$_n$ is formed by the sequential addition of γ-linked glutamate residues to THF-Glu$_1$, a reaction catalysed by folylpolyglutamate synthetase (FPGS). In all eukaryotes studied so far, FPGS isoforms are found in each subcellular compartment containing folylpolyglutamates, indicating that these derivatives cannot cross membranes and must be synthesised *in situ*. In plant cells, FPGS is present as three distinct isoforms located in the cytosol, mitochondria and chloroplasts (Figure 6.5) (Ravanel et al. 2001). Higher plants have two or more gene coding FPGS and in the dicot model *Arabidopsis*, each isoform is encoded by a separate gene. In mammalian and yeast cells, the cytosolic and mitochondrial FPGS isoforms derive from the same gene by the use of alternative translation initiation codons and, in plant genomes sequenced so far, FPGS is present as two copies (Blancquaert et al. 2010). Recently, the functional importance of folate polyglutamylation in C1-metabolism and plant development was assessed through genetic studies (Mehrshahi et al. 2010; Srivastava et al. 2011). Biochemical characterisa-tion of single and double FPGS loss-of-function mutants in *Arabidopsis* established that the glutamylation step is essential for organelle and whole-plant folate homeostasis. Also, these data were consistent with a degree of redundancy in compartmentalised FPGS activity, with targeting of one or more FPGS to multiple organelles, at least in above-ground organs (Mehrshahi et al. 2010). In roots, the plastidial FPGS isoform is essential for quiescent centre organisation, cell division and expansion during primary root development, and none of the other FPGS isoenzymes can fulfil this role (Srivastava et al. 2011).

Catabolism and salvage pathway

In mammals, the breakdown products resulting from folate catabolism are excreted in the urine with rates of approximately 0.5% per day (Gregory and Quinlivan 2002). Plants can have high folate-breakdown rates, up to 10% per day, but recent data indicate that they have the capacity to re-use breakdown products in THF synthesis (Orsomando et al. 2006). Salvage of the pterin aldehyde derivatives consists of their reduction into hydroxymethyldihydropterin and involves a NADPH-dependent reductase, which remains to be identified (Noiriel et al. 2007a, b). Recycling of the pABA moiety is initiated by the hydrolysis of the polyglutamate chain of $pABAGlu_n$ to release free pABA. This is a two-step process involving the enzyme folylpolyglutamate γ-glutamyl hydrolase (FGGH) to cleave the γ-glutamyl peptide bond of $pABAGlu_n$ and a pABAGlu hydrolase, as yet not identified, to produce free pABA (Orsomando et al. 2006). Plant FGGHs share many common features with the enzymes from mammals; they act on both $pABAGlu_n$ and folylpolyglutamates and are located in the vacuole, a lytic compartment that corresponds to the lysosomes in mammalian cells (Orsomando et al. 2005). FGGHs play an important role in governing glutamate tail length *in vivo* and plant folate homeostasis. A threefold over-expression of GGH caused an important deglutamylation of folates and reduced the coenzyme pool by 40% in *Arabidopsis* leaves and tomato fruits (Akhtar et al. 2010). Conversely, an almost complete silencing of GGH expression in *Arabidopsis* led to an increase in both tail length and folates content. Together, these data suggest that folates can enter the vacuole as polyglutamates, accumulate there following binding to hypothetical folate-binding proteins, are hydrolysed by GGH and exit to the cytosol as mono-glutamates (Akhtar et al. 2010).

Compartmentation and transport of folates

Subcellular location of folates

Plant folates are present in different subcellular compartments. The overall distribution of total folates in photosynthetic pea leaves is ~40% in mitochondria, ~10% in chloroplasts, ~20% in vacuoles and ~30% in the cytosol (Chan and Cossins 2003; Jabrin et al. 2003; Orsomando et al. 2005). In the organelles, folates are almost exclusively polyglutamylated, with the penta- and hexa-glutamate species being the most abundant, but folate profiles are different. Mitochondrial folates are dominated by 5-formyl-THF, which is not directly involved in C1 transfer reactions (Figure 6.3) and unsubstituted THF, which probably results from *de novo* synthesis (Chan and Cossins 2003; Orsomando et al. 2005). Chloroplasts are rich in 10-formyl-THF/5,10-methenyl-THF and contain significant amount of 5-methyl-THF (Orsomando et al. 2005), in accordance with the metabolic activity of these organelles for purine and methionine synthesis (Figure 6.3). In pea leaves and in red beet roots, vacuoles contain almost exclusively 5-methyl-THF, of which 50–75% is polyglutamylated (Orsomando et al. 2005). Because methionine synthase is absent from vacuoles, these data suggest that 5-methyl-THF is a potential storage form for folate in plant cells, a situation that is conceivable as this derivative is quite stable to oxidative breakdown and is readily converted to other folates (Figure 6.3).

Folate transporters

The plant folate biosynthetic pathway is split among the cytosol, plastids and mitochondria, whereas it is cytosolic in other organisms (Figure 6.5). This complex organisation, together with the presence of folates in different subcellular compartments, suggests a sophisticated traffic of folate-coenzymes and their biosynthetic intermediates between the organelles via the cytosol. These intracellular transport steps include: pterin uptake into mitochondria; pABA export from plastids and import into mitochondria; folate release from mitochondria and uptake into plastids; and folate influx and efflux into vacuoles (Figure 6.5). In addition, there is evidence that folates, at least 5-formyl-THF and the antifolate methotrexate, can be taken up by plant cells (Prabhu et al. 1998; Loizeau et al. 2007, 2008), thus indicating a folate uptake system at the plasma membrane.

Except for pABA, which is a hydrophobic weak acid possibly transported by simple diffusion (Quinlivan et al. 2003), all these transport steps are probably mediated by specific membrane integral proteins. To date, only three folate carriers have been functionally characterised in plants (Bedhomme et al. 2005; Klaus et al. 2005b; Raichaudhuri et al. 2009). Two of these transporters are located on the envelope of chloroplasts and belong to distinct families. The first system is homologue to the mitochondrial folate transporter formerly characterised in mammals (Bedhomme et al. 2005), whereas the second belongs to the folate-biopterin transporter family originally described in *Leishmania,* a parasitic protist that is heterotrophic for folates and pteridines (Klaus et al. 2005b). Because null mutants for these proteins are not affected in growth and display modest changes in chloroplastic folates, it is likely that these carriers exhibit different specificity/activity towards folate derivatives. In animals, several multidrug resistance-associated proteins (MRP) belonging to the ATP-binding cassette transporter superfamily, catalyse a high-capacity and low-affinity transport of methotrexate and physiological folates (Kruh and Belinsky 2003). In plants, two MRPs located either at the plasmalemma (AtMRP4) or tonoplast (AtMRP1) membranes have been cloned but their physiological role in regulation of folate homeostasis remains to be established (Klein et al. 2006). The vacuolar MRP protein AtMRP1 proved to be competent for folic acid and methotrexate transport *in vitro* and contributed to antifolate tolerance *in planta* (Raichaudhuri et al. 2009). It is suggested therefore that AtMRP1 and its counterparts in other plant species have the potential for importing folates into the vacuole.

Folates distribution in plants

As detailed above, folates are present in the cytosol, mitochondria, chloroplasts and vacuoles of plant cells where the C1-derivatives are not equally distributed. When considering whole plant tissues or organs, folates are largely dominated by the methyl (45–65%) and formyl (30–55%) derivatives, with the unsubstituted and methylene forms representing only 10–15% of the total pool (Cossins 2000). Although the 5-formyl-THF is not directly involved in C1-transfer reaction, it represents 15–40% of the folate pool in photosynthetic leaves and other plant organs, which is about a fivefold higher proportion than in animals and yeasts (Cossins 2000). The metabolic role of 5-formyl-THF is still not well defined in plants, but it could serve as a regulatory factor of photorespiration through the inhibition of mitochondrial SHMT. However, the near-normal growth of mutant *Arabidopsis* plants accumulating high 5-formyl-THF levels suggests that this derivative does not affect fluxes much through SHMT or any other folate-dependent reaction (Goyer et al. 2005). In seeds and quiescent tissues, 5-formyl-THF could act as a storage form of folates, this derivative being the most stable natural folate.

The total folate content greatly varies from one plant to another and with the nature of the organ or tissue. Also, the folate pool fluctuates importantly during the course of plant development, suggesting that folate synthesis and turnover is tightly controlled and modulated as a function of the metabolic requirements (Cossins 2000; Jabrin et al. 2003; Basset et al. 2004a). In developing pea seedlings, it was found that tissues with a reduced metabolic activity such as cotyledons, roots and stems contained a limited amount of folates and expressed folate-synthesising enzymes at low levels (Jabrin et al. 2003; Rébeillé et al. 2006). Similarly, tomato fruits had a low folate content and the pool gradually decreased during ripening (Basset et al. 2004a). This reduction was associated with a collapse in the expression of the enzymes of the pABA and pterin branches of folate synthesis (Basset et al. 2002; Basset et al. 2004a, b).

Folate synthesis and accumulation is important in rapidly dividing tissues. In pea, the germination process is accompanied by an increase in both the levels of folate-synthesising enzymes and folate cofactors in embryos (Jabrin et al. 2003). The rise in folate biogenesis during this period correlates with the transition from a quiescent to an active metabolic state and a resumption of cell cycle activity. Also, meristematic tissues of the root tips contain fivefold more folate than the mature root (Jabrin et al. 2003) and *Arabidopsis* cell suspension cultures, which have a short generation time, show very high folate content (Rébeillé et al. 2006). These observations suggest that proliferating tissues have a high capacity to synthesise and accumulate folate coenzymes to meet the demand for nucleotide synthesis. Green mature leaves are also characterised by a high folate content that is triggered by the acquisition of photosynthesis and thus is related to light (Jabrin et al. 2003). The relationship between folate accumulation in leaves and photosynthesis is not yet fully understood. Photorespiration involves two folate-dependent enzymes, GDC and SHMT (Figure 6.3), that accumulate within the mitochondria during greening (Douce et al. 2001). Part of the folate synthesised in light might contribute to the photorespiratory process, but most folate accumulates in the extra-organelle fraction (cytosol plus vacuoles) as 5-methyl-THF derivatives. Therefore, it is likely that the high folate content in green leaves is associated with an elevated activity of the methyl cycle to ensure a fast turnover of AdoMet (Rébeillé et al. 2006). This assumption is supported by the important decrease (threefold) in chlorophyll synthesis, which depends on an AdoMet-dependent methylation step, in pea seedlings displaying a modest (~25%) shortage of folates (van Wilder et al. 2009).

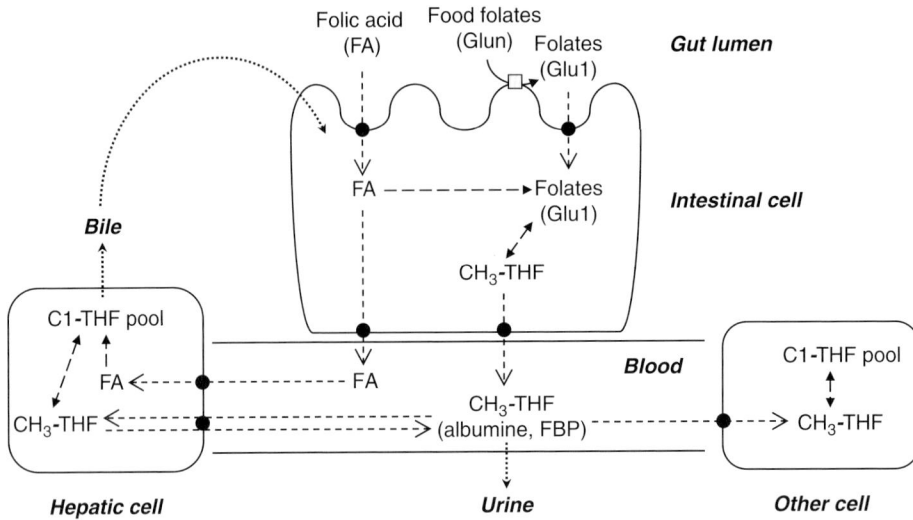

Figure 6.6   Schematic overview of folate absorption and transport in animals. □, folate conjugase associated with the brush border membrane; •, folate transport systems.

Physiology of folate in human health and disease

Absorption

Naturally occurring food folates occur mainly as polyglutamate forms, principally 5-methyl-THF and 10-formyl-THF. These molecules cannot cross cell membranes and must undergo enzymatic removal of the polyglutamate chain, referred to as deconjugation, in the small intestine before absorption. The glutamyl residues are cleaved primarily by a folylpolyglutamate γ-glutamyl hydrolase (FGGH), more commonly called folate conjugase, associated with the jejunal brush border membrane (Figure 6.6) (McNulty and Pentieva 2004). This enzyme is encoded by the glutamate carboxypeptidase II gene and cleaves the terminal γ-glutamate-residue (exopeptidase activity). A second enzyme that cleaves both terminal and internal γ-glutamate linkages (exo- and endopeptidase activities) is found in the lysosomes of intestinal cells (McNulty and Pentieva 2004).

Absorption of monoglutamyl folates by the luminal epithelium of small intestine occurs primarily via a saturable transport process with acidic pH optimum (Sirotnak and Tolner 1999). The affinity of the system for folic acid, folate coenzymes and folate analogues is comparable (influx K_m or K_i of about 2–4 μM). This transport involves a reduced folate carrier encoded by the RFC1 gene, for which the expression is developmentally regulated. A different absorption system, which is pH-independent and non-saturable (passive diffusion), also functions when folate concentrations in intestinal contents are elevated, e.g. when pharmacological doses of folate are consumed (Sirotnak and Tolner 1999).

Transport, storage, catabolism and excretion

The primary form of folate entering human circulation from the intestinal cells is 5-methyl-THF monoglutamate. Prior to entry into the portal vein, dietary folates are converted to 5-methyl-THF while folic acid has to be reduced first to THF by the enzyme dihydrofolate reductase (Figure 6.6). This process has been found to be saturable as supplementation with synthetic folic acid above 200 μg/day results in unaltered folic acid entering the circulation (Gregory 2001). Monoglutamates are taken up by the liver, which is the major site for C1 metabolism and contains the higher folate concentration. Indeed, the total folate content in the human body has been estimated in the range 10–70 mg (average 20–25 mg), of which approximately 50% is in the liver. In hepatic cells, folate is converted to folylpolygluta-mates and stored, or released into the circulation or in the bile (Figure 6.6). Enterohepatic circulation is an important aspect of folate physiology because reabsorption of biliary folate accounts for about 10% of daily folate intake (Gregory and Quinlivan 2002).

The major form of folate in circulation is 5-methyl-THF, most of which originates from the liver. An important fraction of serum folate (>50%) is bound unspecifically and with low affinity to proteins, primarily albumin, forming complexes that dissociate readily. A minor fraction is also specifically and non-covalently attached to high-affinity folate-binding proteins. Folate is taken up by the peripheral tissues using a number of different transport systems, including either plasma membrane carriers or folate-receptor-mediated systems (Antony 1996; Sirotnak and Tolner 1999). Within the cell, monoglutamates are distributed between the cytoplasm and mitochondria through the mitochondrial folate carrier (McCarthy et al. 2004) and converted to folylpolyglutamates to function in single-carbon transfer reactions.

Folate is cleared from the body by the kidneys where it is either reabsorbed from the glomerular filtrate or excreted in the urine. The bulk of the excretion products in humans are pterin and pABA derivatives originating from folate catabolism. Reduced folates are labile compounds that undergo oxidative degradation. *In vivo,* folates are mainly associated with proteins and are less labile under bound form than free in solution. Also, C1 substitution at N-5 or N-10 can alter the reactivity of THF to oxidative degradation, 5-formyl-THF being the most stable derivative. Oxidation can occur by at least two distinct mechanisms that are essentially irreversible. First, the pterin ring of THF can be sequentially oxidised to dihydrofolate and then to folic acid. Second, THF or dihydrofolate can undergo an oxidative scission reaction at the C^9-N^{10} bond (Figure 6.1), giving a pterin aldehyde derivative and *p*-aminobenzoyl(poly)glutamate ($pABAGlu_n$). Such non-enzymatic cleavage is thought to be the main way by which folates break down in all organisms, although proteins, e.g. ferritin, may sometimes facilitate the reaction (Suh et al. 2001). In mammals, the pABA and pterin moieties resulting from folate catabolism are excreted in the urine with breakdown rates of less than 1% per day (Gregory and Quinlivan 2002).

Metabolic and clinical manifestations of folate deficiency

Folate deficiency is one of the most prevalent vitamin deficiencies worldwide. It may be due to several factors including a limited diet, impaired absorption (e.g. coeliac disease) and pharmacological treatments (e.g. folate antagonists, anticonvulsants). Also, pregnant women are at risk of folate deficiency because pregnancy significantly increases the folate requirement, especially during periods of rapid foetal growth. In folate deficiency, all the reactions in C1 metabolism will be compromised to varying degrees, leading to the modification of substrate/product pools that may have negative consequences. Folate attracts considerable interest as it has an established role in the prevention of neural tube defects (NTDs) and possible preventive roles against cardiovascular diseases, certain cancers and neuropsychiatric disorders.

Upon folate deficiency, the inefficient re-methylation of homocysteine to methionine (Figure 6.2) is associated with increased homocysteine levels in blood. Epidemiological evidences indicate that elevated plasma homocysteine concentration ($>14\,\mu mol/L$) is an independent risk factor for cardiovascular disease and stroke (Stover 2004). Increased plasma homocysteine content may also be a risk factor for neurodegenerative disorders, including Alzheimer's and Parkinson's diseases (Mattson and Shea 2003). The impairment of methionine synthesis upon folate deficiency also results in insufficient amounts of AdoMet being available for methylation reactions. These are required for the biosynthesis of many important products and for methylation of DNA and histones, which are important epigenetic determinants in gene expression. DNA hypomethylation is an early and consistent event in carcinogenesis and is associated with genomic instability and increased mutations (Choi and Mason 2000). Another consequence of folate deficiency is a decrease of dTMP synthesis due to a limiting supply of 5,10-methylene-THF to thymidylate synthase. Modification of the intracellular dUMP/dTMP balance results in a higher incorporation of dUTP into DNA, which generates point mutations, single- and double-strand DNA breaks and ultimately chromosomal breakage. These events related to DNA structure, stability and transcriptional regulation are likely to underlie a whole range of cancers. In particular, a relationship between folate status and colorectal, cervical and breast carcinomas has been observed in several studies (Choi and Mason 2000).

In addition to its role in thymidylate synthesis, folate also supports nucleic acid synthesis through the biogenesis of purine rings. Thus, there is general impairment of cell division upon folate deficiency, which is more obvious in tissues with rapid turnover, such as the haematopoietic system. The specific type of anaemia associated with folate deficiency (megaloblastic anaemia) is characterised by the accumulation in the bone marrow of large, abnormal, nucleated precursor cells of erythrocytes. Folate deficiency also affects the intestinal epithelium, where impaired DNA synthesis causes megaloblastosis of enterocytes.

There is general consensus that reduced maternal folate status is associated with an increased risk of NTDs (Geisel 2003). Two of the most common serious birth defects of the brain and spine are spina bifida and anencephaly. Although the mechanism by which adequate folate intake reduces risk during the crucial developmental phase of the embryonic neural tube is unknown, public-health campaigns in many countries recommend periconceptional supplementation of synthetic folic acid to reduce the risk of NTDs.

Diagnosis of folate deficiency

Biochemical assessment of folate nutritional status is most commonly achieved by measuring serum and red cell folate levels. Serum levels are a responsive indicator of folate status which reflect recent intake. Folate concentrations in erythrocytes are a less responsive indicator, but are considered to be the best index of long-term status. It is generally accepted that folate levels below 300–330 nmol/L in red cells are considered to be suggestive of risk and may be symptomatic of folate deficiency. Measurements of plasma concentrations of homocysteine are also used as an indicator of folate status. This criterion is, however, not sufficient to establish folate deficiency because vitamin B12 or vitamin B6 nutritional status, as well as other factors, may also affect homocysteine concentration (Stover 2004).

Folate bioavailability, requirements and food fortification

Bioavailability

Folate bioavailability refers to the proportion of ingested folate that is absorbed and becomes available for metabolic processes or storage. Several studies have shown that the bioavailability of folate in a wide variety of foods is incomplete and highly variable (Gregory 2001). Factors thought to affect folate bioavailability focus on the efficiency of intestinal absorption. They include: the incomplete release from plant cellular structure; the entrapment in the food matrix during digestion; the instability of certain labile folates during digestion; the intestinal deconjugation of folylpolyglutamates, with possible inhibition of this process by other dietary constituents (e.g. organic acids); the presence of certain dietary constituents that may enhance folate stability during digestion (e.g. folate-binding proteins); and the uptake process by the brush border (Gregory 2001; McNulty and Pentieva 2004). Postabsorptive metabolism, i.e. conversion to 5-methyl-THF and release into the circulation can affect bioavailability in certain contexts, but this is mainly relevant to intakes of folic acid at doses that exceed the requirement and the metabolic capacity.

There is general agreement that the bioavailability of folic acid, both supplemental and in fortified foods, is almost always substantially higher than the bioavailability of naturally occurring food folates. However, the extent to which bioavailability of food folates is reduced shows great variation in human studies, depending primarily on the methodological approach used, ranging from 10% to 98% (McNulty and Pentieva 2004). It seems that there is little difference in the absorption of various C1-substituted monoglutamyl folates at low doses (Gregory 2001). There is conflicting evidence, however, as to whether the degree of conjugation of folylpolyglutamates affects bioavailability. This issue is essential since dietary folates comprise about one-third monoglutamate and two-thirds polyglutamate, which are derived mainly from vegetables.

In an effort to place all sources of ingested folate on a comparable basis, the Institute of Medicine of the United States National Academy of Sciences defined the use of dietary folate equivalents (DFE). The DFE is defined as the quantity of naturally occurring food folates (μg) plus 1.7 times the quantity of synthetic folic acid (μg) added in the diet. The reliability of this approach is questionable because of the uncertainties in the relative bioavailability of dietary folates, assumed to be 50% and of folic acid consumed with food (85%) (Gregory 2001; McNulty and Pentieva 2004). The exact relative bioavailability still needs to be determined, in particular for mixed diets in which folate bioavailability is probably not a weighted average of that present in the various foods consumed.

Apart from the incomplete bioavailability of food folates, the poor stability of folates in foods (particularly green vegetables) under typical conditions of harvesting, processing,

Table 6.1 Recommended Dietary Allowances for folate by age group

Group	RDA (mg/day)*
Infants and children	
0–6 / 6–12 months	65/80
1–3 years	150
4–8 years	200
Adolescents	
9–13 years	300
14–18 years	400
Adults (> 19 years)	400
Pregnant women	600
Lactating women	500

*RDAs are expressed as Dietary Folate Equivalents (DFE). 1 µg DFE = 1 µg food folate = 0.6 µg folic acid from supplements and fortified foods.
Source: Data were adapted from the Food and Nutrition Board (1998).

storage and cooking can substantially reduce the amount of vitamin ingested (Scott et al. 2000). Also, genetic polymorphism and pharmacological factors have been associated with impaired absorption of dietary folates (Gregory 2001; McNulty and Pentieva 2004). Thus, a better understanding of folate bioavailability in representative human diets remains a fundamental concern for future research.

Dietary intake recommendations

In 1998, the United States National Academy of Sciences exhaustively reviewed the evidence of folate intake, status and health for all age groups (Food and Nutrition Board 1998). Accordingly, folate requirements have been defined as the intakes required for maintenance of normal C1-transfer reactions, as estimated by measuring red cell folate concentration (Bailey and Gregory 1999). The NAS review led to calculations of an estimated average requirement and a subsequent estimation of the recommended dietary allowances (RDAs; Table 6.1). RDAs were defined as the average level of daily dietary intake sufficient to meet the nutrient requirement of ~98% of the population (healthy individuals in each life-stage and gender group). This definition agrees with the recommended nutrient intakes edited by the Food and Agriculture Organization of the United Nations and the World Health Organization. For male and female adults >19 years of age, the folate RDA is 400 µg DFE/day (Table 6.1). For pregnant women, the RDA is 200 µg higher than for non-pregnant women because of the increased requirements for folate that are associated with the rapid rate of maternal and foetal cellular growth and development during pregnancy.

Dietary sources of folate

Folate contents have been determined for a wide variety of foods, including raw, processed and cooked foodstuffs. Foods particularly rich in folate include liver, yeast, green leafy vegetables, legumes and certain fruits (Table 6.2). As mentioned earlier, the amount of folate in plant foods depends primarily on the species and the nature of the tissue. With

Table 6.2   Amount of folate provided by a range of foods

Food	Folate (µg/100 g)*
Vegetables	
Spinach (raw/cooked)	193/146
Lettuce, different cultivars, raw	29–136
Broccoli (raw/cooked)	62/108
Cauliflower (raw/cooked)	57/44
Carrot (raw/cooked)	19/14
Potatoes (baked)	9
Fruits (raw)	
Avocado	35–88
Oranges (orange juice)	30 (30)
Apples, apricots	3–8
Bananas, melons, strawberries	20–25
Tomatoes	15
Legumes	
Lentils, cooked	181
Beans, snap, green, cooked	33
Beans, mature seeds, cooked	130–172
Cereals	
Barley (raw/cooked)	23/16
Rice, white, cooked (regular/enriched)	97/136
Wheat flour (whole-grain regular/white enriched)	44/300
Bread, French or mixed-grain, regular	165–232
Fortified breakfast cereals, ready-to-eat	550–2600
Dairy products	
Cow's milk, yogurt	5–11
Most cheese varieties	10–40
Ripened soft cheese, e.g. Camembert	60–100
Meats and fishery products	
Meat, beef or chicken, cooked	7–10
Liver, beef or chicken, cooked	260–576
Fish, cooked	2–15
Crustaceans, cooked	43–61
Molluscs, raw	9–16
Others	
Eggs, raw, fresh (whole/yolk/white)	48/145/1
Eggs, whole, cooked	48
Baker's yeast (dried)	2350
Beer, regular or light	6

*The amount of Dietary Folate Equivalents provided by different foods is given per
100 g portion. 1 µg of DFE = 1 µg food folate = 0.6 µg folic acid with meals = 0.5 µg folic
acid on an empty stomach.
Source: Data were adapted from the United States Department of Agriculture National
Nutrient Database for Standard Reference, Release 19, 2006.

the exception of liver, which is the major storage organ for folate, meat, poultry and fish-
ery products generally contain a small amount of folate (5–60 µg/100 g). Also, folate content in dairy products is often low, e.g. total folate in cow's milk is in the range
5–10 µg/100 g. The contribution of different food sources to the total dietary folate intake

is influenced by numerous parameters including bioavailability, stability throughout storage, processing and cooking and dietary habits (Scott et al. 2000). Various dietary surveys in northern America and western European countries indicate that plant foods are by far the main contributors to the folate intake in adults. Thus, about 35–40% of dietary folate is provided by vegetables (including potatoes) and fruits and about one-third by cereal/grain products (Scott et al. 2000). Foods that contain small amounts of folate can contribute significant amounts of folate to an individual's diet if these foods are eaten often or in large amounts. On average, milk and dairy products provide 8–15% of the daily folate intake in many Western countries.

Food fortification

Several national health surveys in rich countries indicated that, even with plentiful calories and apparently balanced and sufficient nutrition, typical folate intakes are suboptimal in the diets of many individuals. For example, the average total intakes of folate among adults ranged from 168 to 326 µg/day in several European countries, i.e. 20–60% below the recommended level of 400 µg/day (De Bree et al. 1997). In 1996, the United States Food and Drug Administration published regulations requiring the addition of synthetic folic acid (fortification) to cereals and grain products (e.g. bread, flour, pasta, rice). The main motivation behind fortification was to decrease the occurrence of NTDs. Beginning in January 1998, enriched cereal-grain products were fortified at the level of 140 µg/100 g of product, on the assumption that this would increase daily uptake by 100 µg/day (Eichholzer et al. 2006). To receive the recommended 400–600 µg/day of folate, women were advised to supplement their folate intake from fortified food with folic acid tablets. Canada in 1998 and Chile in 2000 have opted for mandatory fortification with substantially higher levels of folate (150–220 µg/100 g).

Mandatory folate fortification has clearly improved folate status (Eichholzer et al. 2006). Since cereals and grains are widely consumed in the United States, these products have become a very important contributor of folate to the American diet (≥ 20%). The increase in folate intake was larger than predicted, with an average enhancement of 190–215 µg/day. As a result, several surveys indicated an increase in folate levels by two- to three-fold in serum and by 38% in red blood cells and a decrease in total homocysteine concentration by 7% (Eichholzer et al. 2006). More importantly, the incidence of NTDs in the United States was reduced by 19% since the onset of fortification. However, these changes cannot be definitely attributed solely to fortification because of the gradual decline in NTDs incidence observed even before fortification in the United States and in many western countries without mandatory fortification.

At the end of 2003, 38 countries had introduced or agreed to introduce folate fortification of grain products, but no European country was among them. Depending on the European country, folate fortification is either prohibited or permitted on a voluntary basis. Although bearing in mind the beneficial effects of a fortification approach on folate status, the major concern of European health councils was the possibility of masking vitamin B12 deficiency, principally in older people, allowing neurological complications to progress undiagnosed. Also, even though folate could prevent cancer in healthy people and antifolate treatments inhibit tumour growth in humans, a few studies suggested that supra-physiological doses of folic acid could promote the progression of pre-malignant and malignant lesions (Eichholzer et al. 2006). Given that folic acid is considered generally free of toxicity and that definite adverse effects have not been observed after several year's of supplementation, the safe upper limit has been set at 1 mg folic acid/day. Discussions are currently at an advanced stage regarding the details of a European Union directive on the addition of nutrients, including folate, to foods.

Prospects for plant foods biofortification

Although folate fortification and supplementation programmes have proved reasonably efficient in developed countries, these are probably not the most effective options for many developing countries because of their unstable political and economic situation. In the absence of fortification programmes, alternative strategies are needed to provide folate-rich and enriched-foods for optimal bioavailability, function and health. Enhancement of folate level in crops by biotechnological means (biofortification) provides a rational alternative, or at least complementary solution, in addressing folate malnutrition (Basset et al. 2005; Storozhenko et al. 2005; Rébeillé et al. 2006; Blancquaert et al. 2010). The great variation in folate levels in different plant species and organs (Table 6.2) implies that there is a natural potential for folate enhancement and hence a fairly good chance of success. Conceptually, folate biofortification can be achieved by exploiting the natural variation in folate levels or by metabolic engineering strategies.

Conventional breeding combined with the recent developments in plant molecular genetics and genomics is a powerful tool for the development of plant cultivars with useful traits. A number of quantitative trait loci (QTLs) were identified as responsible for the enhanced content of carotenoids (pro-vitamin A) or tocopherols (vitamin E) in maize, carrot or tomato (Storozhenko et al. 2005). Given the natural variability in folate levels, molecular marker-assisted breeding can be used for the selection of plants with higher levels of the vitamin. To achieve this, several varieties of the crop of interest have to be screened to detect accessions with substantially higher levels of folate. Further, traits responsible for the enhancement can be mapped and eventually used in a breeding programme.

Metabolic engineering consists of molecular and genetic manipulations of a metabolic pathway to increase the production and/or accumulation of useful metabolites. Recent progress in our understanding of folate synthesis, compartmentation and distribution in plants makes such an approach feasible. Conceptually, there are two potential strategies for improving folate content in plants through engineering: (1) over-expressing limiting steps in the pathway (enzymes or transporters) to increase the overall biosynthetic flux; (2) reducing the expression of catabolic enzyme(s) or favouring the synthesis of a stable derivative to decrease chemical and enzymatic breakdown. Engineering of folate catabolism and/or recycling has not yet been reported because knowledge of these routes in plants is recent and only fragmentary (Orsomando et al. 2006). It has been postulated that an increase in the production of 5-formyl-THF, the most stable natural folate, or the production of a folate-binding protein to stabilise folates could enhance plant folate content (Basset et al. 2005; Storozhenko et al. 2005; Rébeillé et al. 2006; Blancquaert et al. 2010).

The most obvious and straightforward approach towards an increase in folate levels is manipulating the folate synthesis pathway. Often, the first committed step(s) regulate(s) the entire flux of metabolites through the pathway and, thus, might be the best choice for engineering. For folate, recent studies indicated that the simultaneous enhancement of both the pterin and pABA branches (Figure 6.4) are required to achieve a high level of folate accumulation. In a first experiment, the GTPCHI gene from *Escherichia coli* under the control of a strong constitutive promoter has been expressed in *Arabidopsis* (Hossain et al. 2004). The transgenic lines exhibited a >1000-fold increase of pteridines and a two- to four-fold enhancement of folate levels in leaves. Using a similar strategy, Diaz de la Garza et al. (2004) expressed a mammalian GTPCHI gene under the control of a fruit specific promoter in transgenic tomato plants. This resulted in a 140-fold increase of pteridines levels in fruits with concomitant increase in folate content of up to twofold. Both reports indicated that GTPCHI is a limiting step in folate synthesis in plants. Evidence that the synthesis of pABA also limits folate accumulation was obtained. The pABA branch was subsequently engineered through the fruit-specific over-expression of ADC synthase from *Arabidopsis* in tomato plants (Diaz de la Garza et al. 2007). The resulting fruits contained about 20-fold more pABA than controls but the level of folates was not improved. In the double GTPCHI/ADC synthase transgenic lines, however, fruits accumulated up to 25-fold more folate than wild-type plants. Thus, these tomatoes contained enough folate ($840\,\mu g/100\,g$) to provide the RDA for a pregnant woman in a standard serving portion (Diaz de la Garza et al. 2007). Although other activities of the THF biosynthetic pathway and/or transporters still constrain folate accumulation in these transgenic fruits, the success of this two-gene engineering strategy opens the door for folate biofortification in a wide range of agricultural crops.

References

Agrimi, G., Di Noia, M.A., Marobbio, C.M., Fiermonte, G., Lasorsa, F.M. and Palmieri, F. (2004) Identification of the human mitochondrial S-adenosylmethionine transporter: bacterial expression, reconstitution, functional characterization and tissue distribution. *Biochem Journal* **379**, 183–90.

Akhtar, T.A., Orsomando, G., Mehrshahi, P., Lara-Nunez, A., Bennett, M.J., Gregory, J.F., 3rd and Hanson, A.D. (2010) A central role for gamma-glutamyl hydrolases in plant folate homeostasis. *Plant Journal* **64**, 256–66.

Antony, A.C. (1996) Folate receptors. *Annual Review of Nutrition* **16**, 501–21.

Appling, D.R. (1991) Compartmentation of folate-mediated one-carbon metabolism in eukaryotes. *FASEB Journal* **5**, 2645–51.

Bailey, L.B. and Gregory, J.F., 3rd. (1999) Folate metabolism and requirements. *Journal of Nutrition* **129**, 779–82.

Basset, G.J., Ravanel, S., Quinlivan, E.P., White, R., Giovannoni, J.J., Rébeillé, F., Nichols, B.P., Shinozaki, K., Seki, M., Gregory, J.F., 3rd and Hanson, A.D. (2004b) Folate synthesis in plants: the last step of the p-aminobenzoate branch is catalysed by a plastidial aminodeoxychorismate lyase. *Plant Journal* **40**, 453–61.

Basset, G.J., Quinlivan, E.P., Gregory, J.F., 3rd and Hanson, A.D. (2005) Folate synthesis and metabolism in plants and prospects for biofortification. *Crop Science* **45**, 449–53.

Basset, G.J., Quinlivan, E.P., Ravanel, S., Rébeillé, F., Nichols, B.P., Shinozaki, K., Seki, M., Adams-Phillips, L.C., Giovannoni, J.J., Gregory, J.F., 3rd and Hanson, A.D. (2004a) Folate synthesis in plants: the p-aminobenzoate branch is initiated by a bifunctional PabA-PabB protein that is targeted to plastids. *Proceedings of the National Academy of Sciences USA* **101**, 1496–501.

Basset, G., Quinlivan, E.P., Ziemak, M.J., Diaz De La Garza, R., Fischer, M., Schiffmann, S., Bacher, A., Gregory, J.F., 3rd and Hanson, A.D. (2002) Folate synthesis in plants: the first step of the pterin branch is mediated by a unique bimodular GTP cyclohydrolase I. *Proceedings of the National Academy of Sciences USA* **99**, 12489–94.

Bedhomme, M., Hoffmann, M., McCarthy, E.A., Gambonnet, B., Moran, R.G., Rébeillé, F. and Ravanel, S. (2005) Folate metabolism in plants: an Arabidopsis homolog of the mammalian mitochondrial folate transporter mediates folate import into chloroplasts. *Journal of Biological Chemistry* **280**, 34823–31.

Blancquaert, D., Storozhenko, S., Loizeau, K., De Steur, H., De Brouwer, V., Viaene, J., Ravanel, S., Rebeille, F., Lambert, W. and Van Der Straeten, D. (2010) Folates and Folic Acid: From Fundamental Research Toward Sustainable Health. *Critical Reviews in Plant Science* **29**, 14–35.

Boldt, R. and Zrenner, R. (2003) Purine and pyrimidine biosynthesis in higher plants. *Physiologia Plantarum* **117**, 297–304.

Bouvier, F., Linka, N., Isner, J.C., Mutterer, J., Weber, A.P. and Camara, B. (2006) Arabidopsis SAMT1 defines a plastid transporter regulating plastid biogenesis and plant development. *Plant Cell* **18**, 3088–105.

Chan, S.Y. and Cossins, E.A. (2003) The intracellular distribution of folate derivatives in pea leaves. *Pteridines* **14**, 17–26.

Choi, S.W. and Mason, J.B. (2000) Folate and carcinogenesis: an integrated scheme. *Journal of Nutrition* **130**, 129–32.

Christensen, K.E. and MacKenzie, R.E. (2006) Mitochondrial one-carbon metabolism is adapted to the specific needs of yeast, plants and mammals. *Bioessays* **28**, 595–605.

Cossins, E.A. (2000) The fascinating world of folate and one-carbon metabolism. *Canadian Journal of Botany* **78**, 691–708.

Cossins, E.A. and Chen, L. (1997) Folates and one-carbon metabolism in plants and fungi. *Phytochemistry* **45**, 437–52.

Coxon, K.M., Chakauya, E., Ottenhof, H.H., Whitney, H.M., Blundell, T.L., Abell, C. and Smith, A.G. (2005) Pantothenate biosynthesis in higher plants. *Biochemical Society Transactions* **33**, 743–6.

Croft, M.T., Lawrence, A.D., Raux-Deery, E., Warren, M.J. and Smith, A.G. (2005) Algae acquire vitamin B12 through a symbiotic relationship with bacteria. *Nature* **438**, 90–3.

Curien, G., Bastien, O., Robert-Genthon, M., Cornish-Bowden, A., Cardenas, M.L. and Dumas, R. (2009) Understanding the regulation of aspartate metabolism using a model based on measured kinetic parameters. *Molecular Systems Biology* **5**, 271.

De Bree, A., van Dusseldorp, M., Brouwer, I.A., van het Hof, K.H. and Steegers-Theunissen, R.P. (1997) Folate intake in Europe: recommended, actual and desired intake. *European Journal of Clinical Nutrition* **51**, 643–60.

Diaz de la Garza, R.I., Gregory, J.F., 3rd and Hanson, A.D. (2007) Folate biofortification of tomato fruit. *Proceedings of the National Academy of Sciences USA* **104**, 4218–22.

Diaz de la Garza, R., Quinlivan, E.P., Klaus, S.M., Basset, G.J., Gregory, J.F., 3rd and Hanson, A.D. (2004) Folate biofortification in tomatoes by engineering the pteridine branch of folate synthesis. *Proceedings of the National Academy of Sciences USA* **101**, 13720–5.

Douce, R., Bourguignon, J., Neuburger, M. and Rébeillé, F. (2001) The glycine decarboxylase system: a fascinating complex. *Trends in Plant Science* **6**, 167–76.

Douce, R. and Neuburger, M. (1999) Biochemical dissection of photorespiration. *Current Opinion in Plant Biology* **2**, 214–22.

Drummond, J.T. and Matthews, R.G. (1993) Cobalamin-dependent and cobalamin-independent methionine synthases in *Escherichia coli*: two solutions to the same chemical problem. *Advances in Experimental Medicine and Biology* **338**, 687–92.

Eichholzer, M., Tonz, T. and Zimmermann, R. (2006) Folic acid: a public-health challenge. *Lancet* **367**, 1352–61.

Eudes, A., Bozzo, G.G., Waller, J.C., Naponelli, V., Lim, E.K., Bowles, D.J., Gregory, J.F., 3rd and Hanson, A.D. (2008) Metabolism of the folate precursor p-aminobenzoate in plants: glucose ester formation and vacuolar storage. *Journal of Biological Chemistry* **283**, 15451–59.

Food and Nutrition Board (1998) *Dietary Reference Intakes for Thiamin, Riboflavin, Niacin, Vitamin B6, Folate, Vitamin B12, Pantothenic Acid, Biotin and Choline*. Institute of Medicine. Washington, DC: National Academies Press.

Foyer, C.H., Bloom, A.J., Queval, G. and Noctor, G. (2009) Photorespiratory metabolism: genes, mutants, energetics and redox signaling. *Annual Review of Plant Biology* **60**, 455–84.

Geisel, J. (2003) Folic acid and neural tube defects in pregnancy: a review. *Journal of Perinatal and Neonatal Nursing* **17**, 268–79.

Gout, E., Aubert, S., Bligny, R., Rébeillé, F., Nonomura, A.R., Benson, A.A. and Douce, R. (2000) Metabolism of methanol in plant cells. Carbon-13 nuclear magnetic resonance studies. *Plant Physiology* **123**, 287–96.

Goyer, A., Collakova, E., Diaz de la Garza, R., Quinlivan, E.P., Williamson, J., Gregory, J.F., 3rd, Shachar-Hill, Y. and Hanson, A.D. (2005) 5-Formyltetrahydrofolate is an inhibitory but well tolerated metabolite in Arabidopsis leaves. *Journal of Biological Chemistry* **280**, 26137–42.

Goyer, A., Illarionova, V., Roje, S., Fischer, M., Bacher, A. and Hanson, A.D. (2004) Folate biosynthesis in higher plants. cDNA cloning, heterologous expression and characterization of dihydroneopterin aldolases. *Plant Physiology* **135**, 103–11.

Gregory, J.F., 3rd. (2001) Case study: folate bioavailability. *Journal of Nutrition* **131**, 1376S–1382S.

Gregory, J.F., 3rd and Quinlivan, E.P. (2002) In vivo kinetics of folate metabolism. *Annual Review of Nutrition* **22**, 199–220.

Guldener, U., Koehler, G.J., Haussmann, C., Bacher, A., Kricke, J., Becher, D. and Hegemann, J.H. (2004) Characterization of the *Saccharomyces cerevisiae* Fol1 protein: starvation for C1 carrier induces pseudohyphal growth. *Molecular Biology of the Cell* **15**, 3811–28.

Hanson, A.D. and Roje, S. (2001) One-carbon metabolism in higher plants. *Annual Review of Plant Biology* **52**, 119–37.

Hossain, T., Rosenberg, I., Selhub, J., Kishore, G., Beachy, R. and Schubert, K. (2004) Enhancement of folates in plants through metabolic engineering. *Proceedings of the National Academy of Sciences USA* **101**, 5158–63.

Ishikawa, T., Machida, C., Yoshioka, Y., Kitano, H. and Machida, Y. (2003) The GLOBULAR ARREST1 gene, which is involved in the biosynthesis of folates, is essential for embryogenesis in *Arabidopsis thaliana*. *Plant Journal* **33**, 235–44.

Jabrin, S., Ravanel, S., Gambonnet, B., Douce, R. and Rébeillé, F. (2003) One-carbon metabolism in plants. Regulation of tetrahydrofolate synthesis during germination and seedling development. *Plant Physiology* **131**, 1431–9.

Klaus, S.M., Kunji, E.R., Bozzo, G.G., Noiriel, A., de la Garza, R.D., Basset, G.J., Ravanel, S., Rébeillé, F., Gregory, J.F., 3rd and Hanson, A.D. (2005b) Higher plant plastids and cyanobacteria have folate carriers related to those of trypanosomatids. *Journal of Biological Chemistry* **280**, 38457–63.

Klaus, S.M., Wegkamp, A., Sybesma, W., Hugenholtz, J., Gregory, J.F., 3rd and Hanson, A.D. (2005a) A nudix enzyme removes pyrophosphate from dihydroneopterin triphosphate in the folate synthesis pathway of bacteria and plants. *Journal of Biological Chemistry* **280**, 5274–80.

Klein, M., Burla, B. and Martinoia, E. (2006) The multidrug resistance-associated protein (MRP/ABCC) subfamily of ATP-binding cassette transporters in plants. *FEBS Letters* **580**, 1112–22.

Kruh, G.D. and Belinsky, M.G. (2003) The MRP family of drug efflux pumps. *Oncogene* **22**, 7537–52.

Li, R., Moore, M. and King, J. (2003) Investigating the regulation of one-carbon metabolism in *Arabidopsis thaliana*. *Plant Cell Physiology* **44**, 233–41.

Loizeau, K., De Brouwer, V., Gambonnet, B., Yu, A., Renou, J.P., Van Der Straeten, D., Lambert, W.E., Rebeille, F. and Ravanel, S. (2008) A genome-wide and metabolic analysis determined the adaptive response of Arabidopsis cells to folate depletion induced by methotrexate. *Plant Physiology* **148**, 2083–95.

Loizeau, K., Gambonnet, B., Zhang, G.F., Curien, G., Jabrin, S., Van Der Straeten, D., Lambert, W.E., Rebeille, F. and Ravanel, S. (2007) Regulation of one-carbon metabolism in Arabidopsis: the N-terminal regulatory domain of cystathionine gamma-synthase is cleaved in response to folate starvation. *Plant Physiology* **145**, 491–503.

McCarthy, E.A., Titus, S.A., Taylor, S.M., Jackson-Cook, C. and Moran, R.G. (2004) A mutation inactivating the mitochondrial inner membrane folate transporter creates a glycine requirement for survival of chinese hamster cells. *Journal of Biological Chemistry* **279**, 33829–36.

McNulty, H. and Pentieva, K. (2004) Folate bioavailability. *Proceedings of the Nutrition Society* **63**, 529–36.

Mao, Y., Vyas, N.K., Vyas, M.N., Chen, D.H., Ludtke, S.J., Chiu, W. and Quiocho, F.A. (2004) Structure of the bifunctional and Golgi-associated formiminotransferase cyclodeaminase octamer. *EMBO Journal* **23**, 2963–71.

Marobbio, C.M., Agrimi, G., Lasorsa, F.M. and Palmieri, F. (2003) Identification and functional reconstitution of yeast mitochondrial carrier for S-adenosylmethionine. *EMBO Journal* **22**, 5975–82.

Mattson, M.P. and Shea, T.B. (2003) Folate and homocysteine metabolism in neural plasticity and neurodegenerative disorders. *Trends Neuroscience* **26**, 137–46.

Mehrshahi, P., Gonzalez-Jorge, S., Akhtar, T.A., Ward, J.L., Santoyo-Castelazo, A., Marcus, S.E., Lara-Nunez, A., Ravanel, S., Hawkins, N.D., Beale, M.H., Barrett, D.A., Knox, J.P., Gregory, J.F., 3rd, Hanson, A.D., Bennett, M.J. and Dellapenna, D. (2010) Functional analysis of folate polyglutamylation and its essential role in plant metabolism and development. *Plant Journal* **64**, 267–79.

Mouillon, J.M., Aubert, S., Bourguignon, J., Gout, E., Douce, R. and Rébeillé, F. (1999) Glycine and serine catabolism in non-photosynthetic higher plant cells: their role in C1 metabolism. *Plant Journal* **20**, 197–205.

Mouillon, J.M., Ravanel, S., Douce, R. and Rébeillé, F. (2002) Folate synthesis in higher-plant mitochondria: coupling between the dihydropterin pyrophosphokinase and the dihydropteroate synthase activities. *Biochemical Journal* **363**, 313–19.

Neuburger, M., Rebeille, F., Jourdain, A., Nakamura, S. and Douce, R. (1996) Mitochondria are a major site for folate and thymidylate synthesis in plants. *Journal of Biological Chemistry* **271**, 9466–72.

Noiriel, A., Naponelli, V., Bozzo, G.G., Gregory, J.F., 3rd and Hanson, A.D. (2007a) Folate salvage in plants: pterin aldehyde reduction is mediated by multiple non-specific aldehyde reductases. *Plant Journal* **51**, 378–89.

Noiriel, A., Naponelli, V., Gregory, J.F., 3rd and Hanson, A.D. (2007b) Pterin and folate salvage. Plants and *Escherichia coli* lack capacity to reduce oxidized pterins. *Plant Physiology* **143**, 1101–9.

Nzila, A., Ward, S.A., Marsh, K., Sims, P.F.G. and Hyde, J.E. (2005a) Comparative folate metabolism in humans and malaria parasites (part I): pointers for malaria treatment from cancer chemotherapy. *Trends in Parasitology* **21**, 292–8.

Nzila, A., Ward, S.A., Marsh, K., Sims, P.F.G. and Hyde, J.E. (2005b) Comparative folate metabolism in humans and malaria parasites (part II): activities as yet untargeted or specific to Plasmodium. *Trends in Parasitology* **21**, 334–9.

Orsomando, G., Bozzo, G.G., de la Garza, R.D., Basset, G.J., Quinlivan, E.P., Naponelli, V., Rébeillé, F., Ravanel, S., Gregory, J.F., 3rd and Hanson, A.D. (2006) Evidence for folate-salvage reactions in plants. *Plant Journal* **46**, 426–35.

Orsomando, G., de la Garza, R.D., Green, B.J., Peng, M., Rea, P.A., Ryan, T.J., Gregory, J.F., 3rd and Hanson, A.D. (2005) Plant gamma-glutamyl hydrolases and folate polyglutamates: characterization, compartmentation and co-occurrence in vacuoles. *Journal of Biological Chemistry* **280**, 28877–84.

Ottenhof, H.H., Ashurst, J.L., Whitney, H.M., Saldanha, S.A., Schmitzberger, F., Gweon, H.S., Blundell, T.L., Abell, C. and Smith, A.G. (2004) Organisation of the pantothenate (vitamin B5) biosynthesis pathway in higher plants. *Plant Journal* **37**, 61–72.

Prabhu, V., Chatson, K.B., Abrams, G.D. and King, J. (1996) 13C nuclear magnetic resonance detection of interactions of serine hydroxymethyltransferase with C1-tetrahydrofolate synthase and glycine decarboxylase complex activities in *Arabidopsis. Plant Physiology* **112**, 207–16.

Prabhu, V., Chatson, K.B., Lui, H., Abrams, G.D. and King, J. (1998) Effects of sulfanilamide and methotrexate on 13C fluxes through the glycine decarboxylase/serine hydroxymethyltransferase enzyme system in arabidopsis. *Plant Physiology* **116**, 137–44.

Quinlivan, E.P., Roje, S., Basset, G., Shachar-Hill, Y., Gregory, J.F., 3rd and Hanson, A.D. (2003) The folate precursor p-aminobenzoate is reversibly converted to its glucose ester in the plant cytosol. *Journal of Biological Chemistry* **278**, 20731–7.

Raichaudhuri, A., Peng, M., Naponelli, V., Chen, S., Sanchez-Fernandez, R., Gu, H., Gregory, J.F., 3rd, Hanson, A.D. and Rea, P.A. (2009) Plant vacuolar ATP-binding cassette transporters that translocate folates and antifolates *in vitro* and contribute to antifolate tolerance *in vivo. Journal of Biological Chemistry* **284**, 8449–60.

Ravanel, S., Block, M.A., Rippert, P., Jabrin, S., Curien, G., Rébeillé, F. and Douce, R. (2004b) Methionine metabolism in plants: chloroplasts are autonomous for de novo methionine synthesis and can import S-adenosylmethionine from the cytosol. *Journal of Biological Chemistry* **279**, 22548–57.

Ravanel, S., Cherest, H., Jabrin, S., Grunwald, D., Surdin-Kerjan, Y., Douce, R. and Rébeillé, F. (2001) Tetrahydrofolate biosynthesis in plants: molecular and functional characterization of dihydrofolate synthetase and three isoforms of folylpolyglutamate synthetase in Arabidopsis thaliana. *Proceedings of the National Academy of Sciences USA* **98**, 15360–65.

Ravanel, S., Douce, R. and Rébeillé, F. (2004a) The uniqueness of tetrahydrofolate synthesis and one-carbon metabolism in plants. In: *Advances in Photosynthesis and Respiration. Plant Mitochondria, from Genome to Function* (eds D.A. Day, A.H. Millar and J. Whelan), pp. 277–292. The Netherlands: Kluwer Academic.

Ravanel, S., Gakiere, B., Job, D. and Douce, R. (1998) The specific features of methionine biosynthesis and metabolism in plants. *Proceedings of the National Academy of Sciences USA* **95**, 7805–12.

Rébeillé, F., Macherel, D., Mouillon, J.M., Garin, J. and Douce, R. (1997) Folate biosynthesis in higher plants: purification and molecular cloning of a bifunctional 6-hydroxymethyl-7,

8-dihydropterin pyrophosphokinase/7,8-dihydropteroate synthase localized in mitochondria. *EMBO Journal* **16**, 947–57.

Rébeillé, F., Ravanel, S., Jabrin, S., Douce, R., Storozhenko, S. and Van Der Straeten, D. (2006) Folates in plants: biosynthesis, distribution and enhancement. *Physiologia Plantarum* **126**, 330–42.

Roje, S., Chan, S.Y., Kaplan, F., Raymond, R.K., Horne, D.W., Appling, D.R. and Hanson, A.D. (2002a) Metabolic engineering in yeast demonstrates that S-adenosylmethionine controls flux through the methylenetetrahydrofolate reductase reaction *in vivo*. *Journal of Biological Chemistry* **277**, 4056–61.

Roje, S., Janave, M.T., Ziemak, M.J. and Hanson, A.D. (2002b) Cloning and characterization of mitochondrial 5-formyltetrahydrofolate cycloligase from higher plants. *Journal of Biological Chemistry* **274**, 42748–54.

Roje, S., Wang, H., McNeil, S.D., Raymond, R.K., Appling, D.R., Shachar-Hill, Y., Bohnert, H.J. and Hanson, A.D. (1999) Isolation, characterization and functional expression of cDNAs encoding NADH-dependent methylenetetrahydrofolate reductase from higher plants. *Journal of Biological Chemistry* **274**, 36089–96.

Sahr, T., Ravanel, S., Basset, G., Nichols, B.P., Hanson, A.D. and Rebeille, F. (2006) Folate synthesis in plants: purification, kinetic properties and inhibition of aminodeoxychorismate synthase. *Biochemical Journal* **396**, 157–62.

Schnell, J.R., Dyson, H.J. and Wright, P.E. (2004) Structure, dynamics and catalytic function of dihydrofolate reductase. *Annual Review of Biophysics and Biomolecular Structure* **33**, 119–40.

Scott, J., Rébeillé, F. and Fletcher, J. (2000) Folic acid and folates: the feasibility for nutritionnal enhancement in plant foods. *Journal of the Science of Food and Agriculture* **80**, 795–824.

Shane, B. (1989) Folylpolyglutamate synthesis and role in the regulation of one-carbon metabolism. *Vitamins and Hormones* **45**, 263–335.

Sirotnak, F.M. and Tolner, B. (1999) Carrier-mediated membrane transport of folates in mammalian cells. *Annual Review of Nutrition* **19**, 91–122.

Smith, P.M. and Atkins, C.A. (2002) Purine biosynthesis. Big in cell division, even bigger in nitrogen assimilation. *Plant Physiology* **128**, 793–802.

Srivastava, A.C., Ramos-Parra, P.A., Bedair, M., Robledo-Hernandez, A.L., Tang, Y., Sumner, L.W., Diaz de la Garza, R.I. and Blancaflor, E.B. (2011) The folylpolyglutamate synthetase plastidial isoform is required for postembryonic root development in *Arabidopsis*. *Plant Physiology* **155**, 1237–51.

Storozhenko, S., Navarrete, O., Ravanel, S., De Brouwer, V., Chaerle, P., Zhang, G.F., Bastien, O., Lambert, W., Rebeille, F. and Van Der Straeten, D. (2007) Cytosolic hydroxymethyldihydropterin pyrophosphokinase/dihydropteroate synthase from *Arabidopsis thaliana*: a specific role in early development and stress response. *Journal of Biological Chemistry* **282**, 10749–61.

Storozhenko, S., Ravanel, S., Zhang, G.-F., Rébeillé, F., Lambert, W. and Van der Straeten, D. (2005) Folate enhancement in staple crops by metabolic engineering. *Trends in Food Science and Technology* **16**, 271–81.

Stover, P. and Schirch, V. (1993) The metabolic role of leucovorin. *Trends in Biochemical Science* **18**, 102–6.

Stover, P.J. (2004) Physiology of folate and vitamin B-12 in health and disease. *Nutrition Reviews* **62**, S3–12.

Suh, J.R., Herbig, A.K. and Stover, P.J. (2001) New perspectives on folate catabolism. *Annual Review of Nutrition* **21**, 255–82.

Tibbetts, A.S. and Appling, D.R. (2010) Compartmentalization of mammalian folate-mediated one-carbon metabolism. *Annual Review of Nutrition* **30**, 57–81.

Van Wilder, V., De Brouwer, V., Loizeau, K., Gambonnet, B., Albrieux, C., Van Der Straeten, D., Lambert, W.E., Douce, R., Block, M.A., Rebeille, F. and Ravanel, S. (2009) C1 metabolism and chlorophyll synthesis: the Mg-protoporphyrin IX methyltransferase activity is dependent on the folate status. *New Phytologist* **182**, 137–45.

Werner-Felmayer, G., Golderer, G. and Werner, E.R. (2002) Tetrahydrobiopterin biosynthesis, utilization and pharmacological effects. *Current Drug Metabolism* **3**, 159–73.

Woeller, C.F., Anderson, D.D., Szebenyi, D.M. and Stover, P.J. (2007) Evidence for small ubiquitin-like modifier-dependent nuclear import of the thymidylate biosynthesis pathway. *Journal of Biological Chemistry* **282**, 17623–31.

Chapter 7

Phytoestrogens

Helen Wiseman

Introduction

Phytoestrogens are plant-derived non-steroidal oestrogen mimics, and include the isoflavonoids such as the soya isoflavones genistein and daidzein, lignans such as secoisolariciresinol, coumestans such as coumestrol and prenylflavonoids such as 8-prenylnaringenin (see Figure 7.1), Phytoestrogens, in particular the isoflavonoids, are being extensively investigated to determine their biological significance especially in the protection of human health and accordingly the main focus of this chapter is on the soya isoflavones (Barnes 1998; Bingham et al. 1998; Wiseman 1999, 2000a,b; Cornwell et al. 2004; Dixon 2004; Wiseman 2005, 2006; Messina 2010; Wiseman 2012).

Biosynthesis of phytoestrogens

Introduction

Phytoestrogens are plant secondary metabolites that have roles in plant defence mechanisms including antimicrobial properties and involvement in hypersensitivity reactions. Generally, in their resemblance of 17β-oestradiol they have at least one phenolic ring and are mostly biphenolic flavonoid related compounds (except the lignans which consist of two units of coniferyl alcohol). One sub-unit of a flavonoid is derived from shikimate and the other aromatic ring is of polyketide origin; 4-coumaroyl-CoA and 3 molecules of malonyl-CoA condense together to form naringenin chalcone. The production of naringenin chalcone is catalyzed by chalcone synthase (CHS) and the subsequent conversion to naringenin by chalcone isomerase (CHI).

Isoflavonoids

Isoflavonoids are formed by a branch of the flavonoid biosynthetic pathway. They originate from central flavanone intermediates: naringenin (4′,5,7-trihydroxyflavanone) in genistein biosynthesis and liquirtigenin (4′,7-dihydroxyflavanone) in daidzein biosynthesis.

Phytonutrients, First Edition. Edited by Andrew Salter, Helen Wiseman and Gregory Tucker.
© 2012 Blackwell Publishing Ltd. Published 2012 by Blackwell Publishing Ltd.

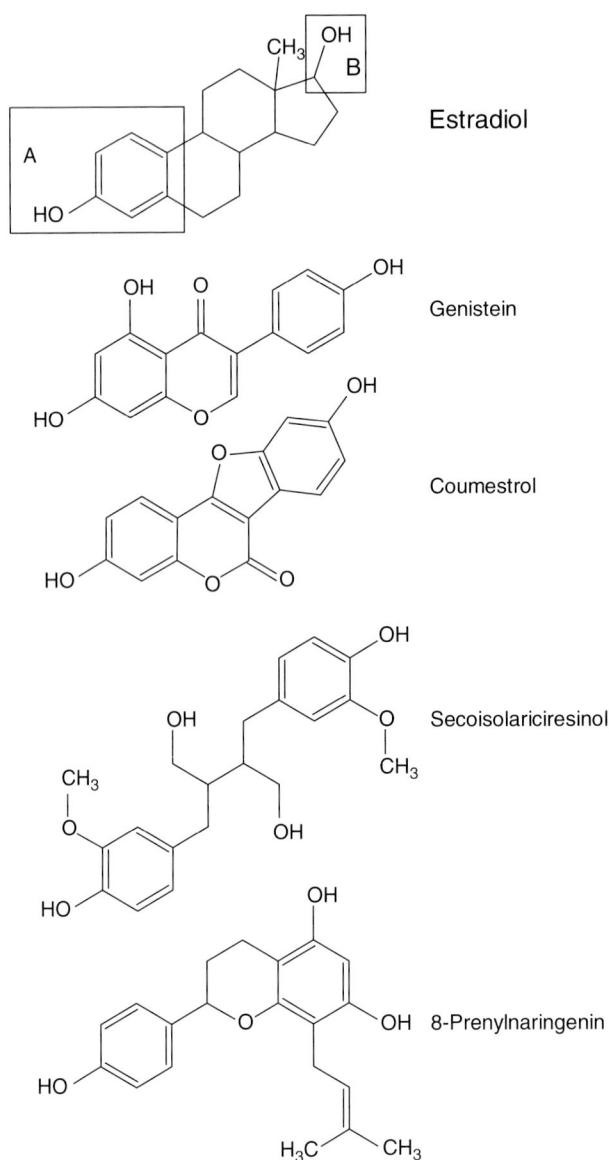

Figure 7.1 The structural relationship between phytoestrogens and 17β-oestradiol.

On the flavonone molecules abstraction of a hydrogen molecule at C-3 is followed by B-ring migration from C-2 to C-3 and hydroxylation of the resulting C-2 radical. The reaction is dependent upon reduced nicotinamide adenine dinucleotide phosphate (NADPH) and also requires molecular oxygen. The reaction is catalyzed by isoflavone synthase (IFS), a microsomal cytochrome P450 enzyme (2-hydroxyisoflavanone synthase) which is stereospecific. The 2-hydroxyisoflavanones which result from the reaction are unstable and undergo dehydration to give genistein or daidzein at acidic pH (Dixon 2004).

Prenylated flavonoids

The prenylation reaction of xanthohumol, a prenyl chalcone, uses dimethylallypyrophosphate (DMAPP) as the prenyl group donor. Any 8-prenylnaringenin is likely to be formed by non-enzymatic cyclisation of prenylated naringenin as the enzyme chalcone isomerase produces only the (–)-flavanone and the compound when extracted from hops is a racemic mixture of both (+) and (–) enantiomers. It is also possible for the direct prenylation of naringenin to occur in plants, for example during the biosyntheis of sophoroflavanone G (8-lavanduly-2′-hydroxynaringenin) in *Sophora flavescens* (Yamamoto et al. 2000).

Stilbenes

The synthesis of stilbenes is related to that of flavonoids as the enzyme stilbene synthase (SS) is a polyketide synthase which is evolutionarily related to the chalcone synthase of flavonoid biosynthesis. The condensation of one molecule of 4-coumaroyl CoA and three molecules of malonyl CoA, forms the same polyketide intermediate as CHS, but with SS the final cyclisation is accompanied by a decarboxylation reaction to produce resveratrol (trans-3,5,4′-trihydroxystilbene) (Dixon 2004).

Lignans

Coniferyl alcohol, a monolignol is the principle unit of the dimeric lignans as it is also of the polymeric lignins. The mechanism for the production of lignans involves stereospecific free radical coupling (Dixon 2004). The dimerisation is initiated by single electron oxidation catalyzed by an oxidase such as a laccase or peroxidase. It is the additional presence of a non-catalytic dirigent protein that enables the formation of stereospecific lignans. In flaxseed the product of stereoselective monolignol coupling is (–)-pinoresinol. This is subsequently converted to secoisolariciresinol via a two-step reduction, pinoresinol/lariciresinol reductase being a member of a large gene family that includes isoflavone reductases from legumes (Gang et al. 1999).

Genetic engineering

As many of the biosynthetic pathways involved in phytoestrogen synthesis have been described and the enzymes involved characterised and cloned, there is great potential for the development of plants with enhanced levels of phytoestrogens for nutritional and or medicinal purposes. Indeed phytoestrogens seem to be prime targets for plant genetic engineering to deliver clear benefits to the consumer, that is as opposed to the producer benefiting as is the case with crops engineered for herbicide resistance. Potential health benefits could then in time overcome the reluctance of the public to embrace plant genetic engineering.

Examples of genetic engineering that try to produce greater quantities of phytoestrogens in plants include the over-expression of isoflavone synthase in alfalfa (Deavours and Dixon 2005) and the expression of the maize phenylpropanoid pathway-activating transcription factors C1 and R in soybean (Yu et al. 2003). The transgenic soybean seed showed a twofold increase in total isoflavones. The additional down-regulation of flavanone 3-hydroxylase, which suppressed the flavonol synthesis pathway (the alternative to isoflavone synthesis), allowed higher levels of isoflavone to accumulate (Yu et al. 2003).

Apple has been engineered to produce resveratrol (Ruhmann et al. 2006), by transformation with a stilbene synthase gene. This shows how phytoestrogens may become widely available in a variety of fruit and vegetables not just the types they are currently found in.

The potential of genetic engineering also extends to improvement/modification of the enzymes involved in the biosynthesis of phytoestrogens. For example, a bifunctional isoflavone synthase/chalcone isomerase has been created by in-frame gene fusion and expressed in yeast and tobacco (Tian and Dixon 2006). The construction of bifunctional enzymes should simplify the transformation of plants with multiple biosynthetic pathways.

Isoflavonoids

Introduction

Isoflavones are complex molecules with multiple biological activities. Many biological actions for isoflavones have been suggested. Isoflavones affect oestrogen and oestrogen receptor function in several ways possessing both agonist and antagonist effects on oestrogen receptors in addition to functioning as natural selective oestrogen receptor modulators. Other actions of isoflavones include antioxidant action, inhibition of DNA topoisomerases, inhibition of cell cycle progression, inhibition of angiogenesis, tumour invasiveness, and inhibition of enzymes involved in oestrogen biosynthesis effects on the expression of DNA transcription factors c-fos and c-jun and on transforming growth factor-β (TGF-β).

Dietary sources and intakes

Isoflavonoids include the isoflavones genistein and daidzein, which occur mainly as the glycosides genistin and daidzin, respectively in soybeans and consequently in a wide range of soya-derived foods and to a lesser extent in other legumes (Reinli and Block 1996; Wiseman et al. 2002). Traditional soya foods are made from soybeans and include both fermented and non-fermented foods. Non-fermented soya foods contain isoflavones mostly present as β-glucosides, some of which are esterified with malonic acid or acetic acid. Fermented soya foods such as miso or tempeh contain mostly unconjugated isoflavones (Coward et al. 1993). Some alcoholic beverages such as beer contain significant amounts of isoflavones (Lapcik et al. 1998). The isoflavone aglycone and glucoconjugate content of high- and low-soya UK foods used in nutritional studies has been reported (Wiseman et al. 2002). Soybeans (774mg/kg isoflavones) and soybean-containing foods had the highest isoflavone content of the foods examined. The low-soya foods all contained very low concentrations (<8mg/kg) of the isoflavone aglycones and glucoconjugates (Wiseman et al. 2002).

Dietary exposure estimate of isoflavones have been made from the 1998 UK Total Diet Study (Clarke and Lloyd 2004). Each Total Diet Study group consisted of composite samples, one for each of the 20 designated food groups. The composite samples were taken to represent the average consumption of all the individual food elements in each group, processed in the form that they were consumed in. In the Total Diet Survey, individual composites of the bread, processed meat and fish food groups contained >5 mg/kg of the individual isoflavones, daidzein, genistein and glycitein. In addition, individual composites from the groups, miscellaneous cereals, other vegetables, fruit products and nuts contained >1 mg/kg of isoflavones. The Total Diet Survey sample collection model for the average adult consumer, following weighting for average consumption of food from each Total Diet Survey group, gave an estimated daily intake of 3 mg/day of combined isoflavone aglycones (Clarke and Lloyd 2004). This indicates that the UK dietary intake of isoflavone phytoestrogens is higher than previously estimated and this is probably partly because of the extensive use of soya products in processed foods (Clarke and Lloyd 2004). An investigation into the intake of dietary phytoestrogens by Dutch women indicates that pea, nuts, grain products, coffee, tea and soya products were the main sources of isoflavones (Boker et al. 2002). The main sources of lignans were grain products, fruit and alcoholic beverages, and in this population the phytoestrogen intake consisted largely of lignans. In the diets of Europeans generally, food sources of lignans are more widely consumed than those of isoflavones, and lignans may be the more important dietary source of phytoestrogens (Fletcher 2003).

When the reliability and validity of an assessment of usual phytoestrogen consumption in the United States, using a food-frequency questionnaire and database, was investigated, it was found that compared to urinary phytoestrogen concentrations, validity correlations ranged from 0.41 to 0.55 for isoflavones and from 0.16 to 0.21 for lignans (Horn-Ross et al. 2006). This suggests that although the isoflavone assessment was valid and reproducible, providing a useful tool for evaluating the relationship between isoflavone consumption and disease risk in a non-Asian population, further work is needed before lignan consumption can be accurately assessed using these tools (Horn-Ross et al. 2006).

Estimating dietary intakes of isoflavone phytoestrogens can be difficult because of inadequate information regarding the phytoestrogen contents of foods. The validation of a newly constructed UK phytoestrogen database has shown that the 24-h urinary excretion and timed plasma concentrations of genistein and daidzein can be used as biomarkers of intake (Ritchie et al. 2004). This newly constructed and validated isoflavone database for the assessment of total genistein and daidzein intake contains values for approximately 6000 foods and has been used to estimate isoflavone intake in omnivores and vegetarians (Ritchie et al. 2006). The mean intake for the omnivorous group was 1.2 mg/day and the main food sources included soya yogurts, wholemeal bread and rolls, and white bread and rolls, whereas the mean intake for the vegetarian group was 7.4 mg/day and the main food sources included soya milk (plain), meat-substitute foods containing textured vegetable protein and soya protein isolate, soya mince, wholemeal bread and rolls, and white bread and rolls (Ritchie et al. 2006). However, it should be noted that considerable variation has been found in the isoflavone content of isolated soya proteins used in food manufacture and in commercial milks and this exposes the limitations of using food databases for estimating daily isoflavone intakes (Setchell and Cole 2003).

In a UK population cohort study (EPIC-Norfolk), average daily isoflavone intakes for both men and women were less than 1 mg, compared to soya-consumers where average daily intakes were higher at 8.6 mg for women and 7.5 mg for men (Mulligan et al. 2007). Interestingly, bread (62%) and bread rolls (53%) made the highest contribution to isoflavone intakes in both men and women. However, in soya-consumers, milks and vegetable dishes were the main contributors providing 39% and 25% of daily isoflavone intake in men and 26% and 39% in women, respectively. Although isoflavone intake seems to be rather low in the UK, this may be partly the result of underestimation of the amounts of soya added to commercial products. Further analysis of the isoflavone and lignan content of commonly consumed commercial items and basic food ingredients is still required, to allow better estimates of phytoestrogen intake to be determined (Mulligan et al. 2007).

Phytoestrogen intake and plasma concentration has been investigated in South Asian and native British women resident in England. The median daily intakes of isoflavones and lignans were significantly lower in South Asian than in native British women (Bhakta et al. 2006). There were no significant differences in mean plasma isoflavone levels but plasma enterolactone concentrations were significantly lower in the South Asian women. The main sources of phytoestrogens in both groups were bread and vegetables (Bhakta et al. 2006).

Metabolism and bioavailability

The metabolism and bioavailability of isoflavonoids is likely to be of crucial importance to their ability to help protect against disease (Wiseman 1999; Setchell et al. 2002; Rowland et al. 2003). Many studies have been published on the metabolism and bioavailability of isoflavones in adults (Watanabe et al. 1998; Rowland et al. 2000; Setchell et al. 2003a, b). The metabolism of isoflavones is of particular interest because the potency of isoflavone metabolites differs from that of the parent compounds (Markiewicz et al. 1993). The daidzein metabolite equol was three times as potent as is daidzein in an endometrial tumour line. Equol is also a more potent antioxidant *in vitro* (Hodgson et al. 1996; Arora et al. 1998; Mitchell et al. 1998; Wiseman et al. 1998; O'Reilly et al. 2000) and the clinical significance of the ability to form equol has been considered in depth (Setchell et al. 2002).

Daidzin and genistin (and to a lesser extent glycitin) and their glucoconjugates are the predominant isoflavone forms in soya foods (Wiseman et al. 2002). After ingestion, isoflavones are hydrolysed by mammalian lactase phlorizin hydrolase (Rowland et al. 2003), which releases the aglycones, daidzein, genistein and glycitein. These may be absorbed or further metabolised by the gut microflora to metabolites, including the conversion of daidzein to the isoflavan equol and/or *O*-desmethylangolensin, and of genistein to *p*-ethyl phenol. More recently, 4-hydroxyphenyl-2-propionic acid was identified from the metabolism of genistein in rats (Coldham et al. 2002). Studies have shown that particular bacterial groups are involved in the metabolism of the isoflavone glycosides (Hur et al. 2000).

Unconjugated isoflavones are absorbed quickly from the upper small intestine in rats (Sfakianos et al. 1997), whereas the glycoside conjugates are absorbed more slowly, which is consistent with their hydrolysis at more distal sites in the intestine to the unconjugated isoflavones (King and Bursill 1998). Isoflavonoids, once absorbed, are rapidly converted to their β-glucuronides (Sfakianos et al. 1997) and sulfate ester conjugates (Yasuda et al. 1996). These biological conjugates circulate in the plasma and are excreted in the urine and faeces. Indeed, intact sulphate and glucuronide isoflavone conjugates have been measured in human urine, following soya consumption (Clarke et al. 2002). Concentrations of the free aglycones of up to 22% of genistein and 18% of daidzein were observed, and the average pattern of daidzein conjugates was 54% 7-glucuronide, 25%

4′-glucuronide, 13% monosulphates, 7% free daidzein, 0.9% sulphoglucuronides, 0.4% diglucuronide, and < 0.1% disulphate (Clarke et al. 2002).

Plasma isoflavonoid levels in Japanese and Finnish men have been measured and the means of the total daidzein, genistein, *O*-desmethylangolensin, and equol levels were approximately 17-fold, 44-fold, 33-fold, and 55-fold higher for the Japanese subjects compared to the Finnish ones (Adlercreutz et al. 1993). In postmenopausal Australian women following consumption of soya flour, mean plasma levels of daidzein and equol of 68 ng/ml and 31 ng/ml, respectively were observed (Morton et al. 1994). Interestingly only 33% of subjects were able to metabolise daidzein to equol (Morton et al. 1994). Increased concentrations of both genistein and daidzein were observed in male subjects following ingestion of a cake containing soya flour and cracked linseed, within 30 min of consumption, with maximum concentrations reached by 5.5–8.5 h (Morton et al. 1997).

Plasma phytoestrogen concentrations, assessed in vegans and vegetarians in 16 geographical regions in 9 European countries, has been found to vary substantially among subjects from the different regions (Peeters et al. 2007). Excluding subjects from Oxford UK, the highest concentrations of isoflavones were in subjects from the Netherlands and Cambridge UK, whereas subjects from Denmark had the highest lignan concentrations. Variations in isoflavone concentrations were 8- to 13-fold compared to 4-fold for lignans. Concentrations of isoflavones in the vegetarian/vegan cohort of Oxford were 5- to 50-fold higher than in non-vegetarians regions (Peeters et al. 2007).

The importance of the gut microflora in the metabolism of isoflavones has been demonstrated. Antibiotic administration blocks isoflavone metabolism and germfree animals do not excrete metabolites (Setchell and Cassidy 1999). Moreover, only germfree rats colonised with microflora from a good equol producer excrete equol when fed soya (Bowey et al. 2003).

Interindividual variation in the ability to metabolise daidzein to equol (more oestrogenic and a more potent antioxidant than daidzein) could thus influence the potential health protective effects of soya isoflavones (Setchell et al. 2002). The extent of gut microflora metabolism in humans is variable, approximately 35% of a Western population can produce equol (Morton et al. 1994; Lampe et al. 1998; Rowland et al. 2000).

A variable metabolic response to isoflavones has been shown for subjects following consumption of soya flour; urinary excretion concentrations of genistein, daidzein, equol and *O*-desmethylangolensin were increased 8-fold, 4-fold, 45-fold and 66-fold, respectively, compared to baseline (Kelly et al. 1995). Considerable interindividual variation in metabolic response was reported with the peak levels of equol showing the most variation (Kelly et al. 1995).

In healthy young adults, when diets high or low in isoflavones (textured soya protein product containing 56 mg/day or 2 mg/day) were each consumed for 14 days separated by a 25-day washout period, considerable interindividual variation in metabolic response was found (Rowland et al. 2000). In addition, the good equol excretors (36% of subjects) consumed significantly less fat and more carbohydrate (also greater amounts of non-starch polysaccharide: NSP) compared to the poor equol excretors (Rowland et al. 2000). Female equol excretors have been reported to consume a higher percentage of energy as carbohydrate and also greater amounts of plant protein and NSP than non-equol excretors (Lampe et al. 1998).

Dietary modification, such as feeding wheat bran or soya protein has been unsuccessful at changing equol-producing capability (Lampe et al. 2001), which indicates that the intestinal microflora of an individual is relatively stable and resistant to change.

The bioavailability of soya isoflavones has been shown to depend on the gut microflora (Xu et al. 1995). Metabolism by the gut microflora is an important factor influencing the disposition of chemicals in the gut and can result in activation of substances to more biologically active products. The presence of different populations of microflora in the human gut may influence the bioavailability of isoflavones. The identification of the bacterial species involved in the conversion of daidzein to equol is of considerable importance and very challenging given the large number of bacteria present in the colon and the small intestine. In a study that identified equol producers by culturing faecal flora from healthy Japanese adults after they consumed 70 g of tofu, three strains of bacteria were reported to convert pure daidzein to equol *in vitro*: the gram-negative *Bacteroides ovatus* spp., the gram-positive *Streptococcus intermedius* spp. and *Ruminococcus productus* spp. (Ueno and Uchiyama 2001).

Chronic consumption of a high soya diet (104 mg isoflavones/day) has recently been compared with a low soy diet (0.54 mg/day) in 76 healthy young adults. After the 10-week diet period, concentrations of the isoflavonoids in plasma, urine and faeces were significantly higher in the high-soya group than in the low-soya group (Wiseman et al. 2004). Although interindividual variation in isoflavone metabolism was high (34% of subjects were good equol producers), intraindividual variation (assessed by comparing midpoint with endpoint results) in metabolism was low. Only concentrations of *O*-DMA in plasma and urine seemed to be influenced by sex, with men having significantly higher concentrations than women (Wiseman et al. 2004). Other studies suggested that men and women respond differently to chronic exposure to isoflavones (Lu et al. 1995, 1996, 1998), although there are considerable inconsistencies in the data. Furthermore, chronic soy isoflavone consumption did not seem to induce many significant changes to the gut metabolism of isoflavones, other than effects on β-glucosidase activity (this was significantly higher in subjects who consumed the high soya diet than in those who consumed the low-soya diet), suggesting that the gut bacteria and enzymes responsible for equol or *O*-DMA production are not inducible (Wiseman et al. 2004).

The influence of age, gender and the food matrix on the bioavailability of both the aglycone and glucoside forms of isoflavones found in soya milk, textured soya protein and tempeh have been investigated in a randomised crossover study in premenopausal women, postmenopausal women and men (Cassidy et al. 2006). The main findings were that absorption was faster and peak levels of isoflavones were achieved earlier from soya milk than from other soya foods and that tempeh, which contains mainly isoflavone aglycones, resulted in higher serum peak levels of both daidzein and genistein and the associated area under the curve compared with textured soya protein, which contains predominantly isoflavone glycosides (Cassidy et al. 2006). In addition, higher peak concentrations of daidzein were attained in women and 30% of the subjects were equol producers and no differences in equol production with gender or age were observed. When isoflavones were added at a level of 50 mg to three different foods juice, chocolate bars and cookies and consumed to determine the effects of the food matrix and processing on isoflavone absorption, peak genistein concentrations were attained in serum earlier following the consumption of juice (liquid matrix) rather than the other two foods (solid matrix) (de Pascual-Teresa et al. 2006). However, there was a lower total urinary recovery of genistein following ingestion of juice compared to the other two foods (de Pascual-Teresa et al. 2006).

Differences in the equol-producer phenotype have been reported between populations. A higher prevalence of the equol-producer phenotype has been reported for soya-consuming Asian populations than in Western populations. Indeed, in one study, comparing Korean American to Caucasian American women and girls, not only was the prevalence of the equol-producer phenotype higher (51% compared to 36%) but also the *O*-DMA-producer phenotype was lower (84% compared to 92%), suggesting differing general patterns of daidzein metabolism (Song et al. 2006).

In addition to the possible contribution that soya isoflavonoids may make to adult human health, the possible health consequences of early life soya exposure are also attracting attention (Badger et al. 2002; Mendez et al. 2002). Although there have been many studies on the metabolism and bioavailability of isoflavonoids in adults (see above), there is little information available for infants and children. The gut microflora in early childhood is very different to that found in adulthood, therefore it is important to characterise developmental changes in isoflavone metabolism in early life. The development of the microflora occurs gradually and it can take several years before an adult-type flora is established. This has important implications for isoflavone metabolism.

The urinary excretion of isoflavonoids has been investigated in 60 infants and children (aged 4 months to 7 years, divided into four age groups). The study compared infants and children who had been fed soya-based formulas in early infancy, with control (cows'-milk formula-fed) infants and children (Hoey et al. 2004). Infants aged 4–6 months, fed soya-based infant formulas (but not those fed cows'-milk formulas) were found to excrete considerable amounts of genistein, daidzein and glycitein in urine, indicating that these compounds are well absorbed and that the required glucosidase activity has developed (Hoey et al. 2004). The majority of the soya-based infant formula-fed infants and about one half of the cows'-milk formula-fed group (after a soya challenge) were capable of converting daidzein to *O*-DMA. However conversion of daidzein to equol was observed in very few children, even in the oldest age group (3–7 years). These findings, indicate that there seems to be no lasting effect of early-life isoflavone exposure on isoflavone metabolism and they have important developmental implications for isoflavonoid bioavailability (Hoey et al. 2004).

Isoflavonoids and cancer prevention

Hormone-dependent cancer prevention by isoflavonoids

The possible role of isoflavonoids in the prevention of cancer and in particular hormone-dependent cancers such as breast and prostate cancer is currently being extensively investigated (see reviews by Adlercreutz 2002; Magee and Rowland 2004; Dixon 2004; Cornwell et al. 2004; Greenwald 2004; Holzbeierlein et al. 2005). In addition, consumption of soya foods rich in isoflavones has been weakly associated with reduced colon cancer (Adlercreutz 2002; Guo et al. 2004). Colon cancer risk is influenced by oestrogen exposure and although the mechanism of action has not been fully elucidated, studies with ERα knockout mice indicate that it may be independent of ERα (Guo et al. 2004). Breast and prostate cancer is much less prevalent in Far Eastern countries, where there is an abundance of soya phytoestrogens in the diet, compared to Western ones. Emigration of people from Pacific Rim countries to the USA has been shown to increase their risk of breast and prostate cancer. The increase in prostate cancer risk in men occurs in the same generation, whereas for women the increase in breast cancer risk is observed in the next generation (Shimizu et al. 1991). These changes in breast and prostate cancer risk have been mostly attributed to changes in diet, in particular the switch to a low soya Western diet: in countries such as Japan, Korea, China and Taiwan, the mean daily intake of soya products has been estimated to be in the range 10–50 g compared to only 1–3 g in the USA (Messina et al. 1994). Increased soya intake has been associated with a lowered risk of breast cancer in two out of four epidemiological studies that examined a wide range of dietary components in relation to breast cancer risk: no significant effect was observed in the other two studies (Messina et al. 1994; Barnes 1998).

Not only is the incidence of breast cancer lower but survival is longer in Asian women living in China, Japan or the Philippines compared to Caucasian women living in the USA and phytoestrogen intake has been investigated as a possible explanation for these differences in breast cancer incidence and survival (Lyons-Wall et al. 2006). When the association between phytoestrogen intake prior to diagnosis of breast cancer and indicators of breast cancer prognosis was examined, higher intakes of phytoestrogens were associated with favourable indicators of breast cancer, including a reduction in the odds of being diagnosed with any stage of cancer other than stage 1, a reduction in the odds of being diagnosed with positive lymphovascular invasion and an increase in the odds of being diagnosed with a positive progesterone receptor thus phytoestrogen intake prior to diagnosis my improve breast cancer prognosis (Ha et al. 2006).

High urinary excretion of both equol and enterolactone (mammalian metabolite of plant lignans) has been found to be associated with a significant decrease in breast cancer risk, in an epidemiological case-control study in breast cancer patients (Ingram et al. 1997). Although this could suggest the possible importance of isoflavonoid and lignan metabolism in decreased breast cancer risk, the phytoestrogen excretion observed may just be a marker of dietary differences (Barnes 1998).

Plasma phytoestrogen concentrations and subsequent breast cancer risk have been investigated using a prospective approach by performing a nested case-control study within the Prospect cohort, one of the two Dutch cohorts participating in the European Prospective Investigation into Cancer and Nutrition (Verheus et al. 2007). High circulating concentrations of genistein were associated with reduced breast cancer risk and similar protective effects were observed for other isoflavones, although these were not statistically significant. In contrast, plasma lignan concentrations did not seem to be related to breast cancer risk. Furthermore the results were the same in postmenopausal women and in pre- or perimenopausal women (Verheus et al. 2007).

The possible protective effect of isoflavonoids against prostate cancer has been reviewed (Holbeierlein et al. 2004) and it is of particular interest that in rat studies equol may be a novel antiandrogen that inhibits prostate growth and hormone feedback (Lund et al. 2004). Furthermore, when prospective phytoestrogen exposure was assessed (in British men recruited into the Norfolk arm of the European Prospective Investigation into Cancer and

Nutrition who subsequently developed prostate cancer compared to healthy men), although no evidence was found that phytoestrogens alter prostate cancer risk, the C allele for the PvuII polymorphism in the CYP19 gene may be associated with increased risk (Low et al. 2006). The role of isoflavonoids in the prevention of breast cancer is the main focus of the next section of this chapter.

Oestrogens and risk of breast cancer

Breast cancer is still a major cause of death for women in Western countries (Wiseman, 1994). Breast cancer is thought to have a multifactorial causation ranging from gene profile to diet and lifestyle, and mutations in particular tumour suppressor genes such as BRCA1, BRCA2 and p53 are likely to be of particular importance. A ribonucleotide reductase gene (*p53R2*) has been shown to be directly involved in the p53-dependent cell cycle checkpoint for DNA damage, thus clarifying the relationship between a ribonucleotide reductase activity involved in repair of damaged DNA and tumour suppression by p53 (Tanaka et al. 2000). Furthermore, the structural basis has been established for the recognition and repair by 8-hydroxyguanine DNA glycosylase of the oxidative DNA base damage product (and endogenous mutagen) 8-hydroxyguanine (Bruner et al. 2000).

The role of endogenous oestrogens in breast cancer risk is widely recognised. Different forms of oestrogen metabolism result in the formation of mitogenic endogenous oestrogens or the metabolic activation of oestrogens that can result in carcinogenic free-radical-mediated DNA damage. Pregnancy seems to be important in breast cancer risk: nulliparous women have the greatest risk of breast cancer but for parous women, multipregnancies are of no greater benefit than a single pregnancy and an earlier pregnancy is more protective than a later one. This is because of the differentiation of breast epithelial cells into milk-producing cells that occurs in the breast during pregnancy and the apoptosis of breast cells that occurs in the breast following pregnancy thus providing a chance for elimination of mutated epithelial cells (Barnes 1998).

It is of related interest that the effects of soya isoflavones on normal mammary gland morphogenesis and gene expression profile have been investigated in the murine mammary gland by adding isoflavones to the diet throughout either the lactation period or the post-weaning period, or administering 17β-oestradiol orally during the lactation period (Thomsen et al. 2006). A significant increase in branching morphogenesis was observed at postnatal day 28 in all treated groups, especially after 17β-oestradiol exposure and at postnatal day 42–43, the post-weaning isoflavone and the 17β-oestradiol groups showed a transient reduction in the number of terminal end buds. The similar response after isoflavone 17β-oestradiol exposure was reflected in the changes in gene expression, which all correlated with changes in the cellular composition of the mammary gland (more and larger ducts and terminal end buds) indicating an oestrogenic response of isoflavones on mammary gland development resembling that induced by puberty (Thomsen et al. 2006).

Oestrogen receptor-mediated events

Oestrogens play a vital role in the growth, development and homeostasis of oestrogen responsive tissues. Oestrogen receptors mediate the biological activity of oestrogens and are ligand-inducible nuclear transcription factors that belong to the nuclear hormone receptor superfamily. Oestrogen binds to the ligand-binding domain of oestrogen receptors resulting in either the activation or repression of target genes (Katzenellenbogen et al. 1996; Brosens and Parker 2003; Koehler et al. 2005; Dahlman-Wright et al. 2006). Oestrogen receptors are the only steroid receptor able to additionally interact with a large number of non-steroidal compounds, which frequently show a structural similarity to the steroid nucleus of oestrogen, including phytoestrogens, and drug and environmental xenoestrogens such a dioxins (Brosens and Parker 2003). In particular a phenolic ring analogous to ring A in oestradiol is required and these structural features enable them to bind to oestrogen receptors to elicit responses ranging from agonism to antagonism of the endogenous hormone-ligand (Miksicek 1995).

Originally it was accepted that only one oestrogen receptor existed. This is in contrast to other members of the nuclear receptor superfamily where multiple forms have been found. The first oestrogen receptor was identified as a receptor molecule that could bind 17 β-oestradiol in the late 1950s and was cloned in 1986 (Greene et al. 1986), and a second oestrogen receptor was reported in 1996 (Kuiper et al. 1996). Today these two oestrogen receptors are known as ERα and ERβ (Koehler et al. 2005; Dahlman-Wright et al. 2006). The amino acid sequence identity between ERα and ERβ is very high (~97%) in the DNA-binding domain, lower (~56%) in the ligand-binding domain and poor (~24%) in the N terminus (Koehler et al. 2005; Dahlman-Wright et al. 2006).

The selective oestrogen receptor antagonist raloxifene, structurally related to the anticancer drug tamoxifen (Wiseman 1994), can inhibit the mitogenic effects of oestrogen in reproductive tissues, while maintaining the beneficial effects of oestrogen in other tissues. The crystal structures of the ligand-binding domain of human ERα complexed to either 17β-oestradiol or to raloxifene have been reported (Brzozowski et al. 1997) thus providing structural evidence for the mechanisms of oestrogen receptor agonism and antagonism. A combination of specific polar and non-polar interactions enables ERα to selectively recognise and bind 17β-oestradiol with great affinity. Two distinct activation functions (the constitutively active AF-1 located in the receptor protein N-terminal domain and the ligand-dependent AF-2 located in the C-terminal domain) mediate transcriptional activation by ERα. In contrast to this, ERβ seems to have a weaker corresponding AF-1 function and depends more on the ligand-dependent AF-2 for its transcriptional activation function (Dahlman-Wright et al. 2006).

ERβ was identified in cDNA libraries from rat prostate and ovary tissues (Kuiper et al. 1996) and it is of considerable interest that ERβ shows a different tissue distribution to ERα. ERβ was first reported to be strongly expressed in ovary, uterus, brain, bladder, testis, prostate and lung (Kuiper et al. 1997). Evidence has since been found, using reverse-transcription-PCR (polymerase chain reaction), for the presence of ERβ in normal human breast tissue (Crandall et al. 1998) and ERβ has been shown to be highly expressed in rat breast tissue using specific antibodies (Saji et al. 2000). Normal and cancerous breast tissues display distinct ERα and ERβ profiles, some data shows regulation of ERβ by promoter methylation (frequently observed in cancer) and indicates that the ERβ transcript is down-regulated in breast tumours consequently it has been suggested that ERβ is a possible tumour suppressor gene. However, ERβ is expressed in the majority of breast tumours and a similar percentage of tumours express ERβ as ERα (Dahlman-Wright et al. 2006). ERβ has been shown to be expressed in the cardiovascular system (Makela et al. 1999) where results from oestrogen receptor knockout mice indicate that ERα is important in the pathophysiology of the vessel wall, whereas ERβ knockout mice display abnormalities in ion channel function and an age-related hypertension (Dahlman-Wright et al. 2006). Expression of ERβ seems to occur at different sites in the brain from ERα (Kuiper et al. 1997), in rodents ERα is mostly found in regions involved in control of reproductive function such as the hypothalamus, whereas ERβ is more widely distributed including in the hippocampus and cortex. ERβ has also been found to be expressed in bone (Arts et al. 1997; Onoe et al. 1997; Stossi et al. 2004) where studies of female ERβ knockout mice show that ERβ is responsible for repression of the ERα-mediated growth stimulating effect of oestrogen on bone (Dahlman-Wright et al. 2006).

Although genistein is a much better ligand for ERβ than for the ERα (~30-fold higher binding affinity) (Kuiper et al. 1997; Koehler et al. 2005), it can also act as an oestrogen agonist via both ERα and ERβ in some test systems (Kuiper et al. 1998; Mueller et al. 2004). However, genistein also behaves as a partial oestrogen agonist in human kidney cells transiently expressing ERβ, suggesting that it may be a partial oestrogen antagonist in some cells expressing ERβ (Barkhem et al. 1998). Furthermore, although genistein binds to the ligand-binding domain of ERβ in a manner similar to that observed for17β-oestradiol, in the ERβ–genistein complex, the AF-2 helix (H12) does not adopt the normal agonist type position, but instead takes up a similar orientation to that induced by ER antagonists such as raloxifene (Pike et al. 1999). This suboptimal alignment of the transactivation helix is in keeping with the reported partial agonist activity of genistein in ERβ (Barkhem et al. 1998).

The agonist action of genistein for ERβ is thought to predominantly mediate the health benefits of genistein particularly in the cardiovascular system, in bone metabolism and in possible protection against breast and prostate cancer (McCarty 2006).

Several polymorphisms of the ERα gene have been identified producing isoforms such as ER A908G, first identified in premalignant breast lesions, and ERα46, detected in several cell types such as osteoblasts and endothelial cells where it can act as an inhibitor of ERα function (where AF-1 is critical for activity) (Dahlman-Wright et al. 2006). ERβ isoforms include the human variant ERβcx which does not bind any ligands tested and has been reported to inhibit ligand-induced transactivation and DNA binding by ERα but does not affect that of ERβ. ERβcx expression is increased in prostate, breast and ovarian cancer. ERβins acts as a dominant-negative regulator of ERα and ERβ (Dahlman-Wright et al. 2006). Indeed ERβ1 is the only full-function isoform and it prefers to heterodimerise with ERβ isoforms (particularly ERβ 4 and β5) under the stimulation of oestrogens (to enhance ERβ1-induced transactivation in a ligand-dependent manner) but excluding phytoestrogens (Leung et al. 2006).

Animal models

Studies using animal models provided the initial experimental evidence that soya can prevent breast cancer (Messina et al. 1994; Barnes 1998). Results from 26 animal studies of experimental carcinogenesis have shown that in 17 of these studies (65%) protective effects were reported: the risk of cancer (incidence, latency or tumour number) was greatly reduced, and no studies reported that soya intake increased tumour development

(Messina et al. 1994). In a rat model of breast cancer (7,12-dimethylbenz[a]anthracene (DMBA) induced), genistein administered in high doses by injection to young animals suppressed the number of mammary tumours observed over a 6-month period by 50% and delayed the appearance of the tumours (Lamartiniere et al. 1995) indicating the probable importance of the timing of exposure to the protective components of soya. In later studies, similar levels of protection were achieved by adding genistein to the feed (0.25 g/kg) given to the mother such that the offspring were exposed to dietary genistein from conception to day 21 postpartum (Fritz et al. 1998). By contrast, when pregnant female rats were treated daily with subcutaneous injections of genistein (doses given were either 20, 100 or 300 μg/day) between days 15 and 20 of gestation, this *in utero* exposure was found to dose-dependently increase the incidence of DMBA-induced mammary tumours in female offspring (Hilakivi-Clarke et al. 1999a). However, when prepubertal rats were treated with 20 μg of genistein (approximately 1 mg/kg body weight) between postnatal days 7 and 20, this greatly reduced the multiplicity but not the incidence of DMBA-induced mammary tumours and 60% of the tumours that did occur were not malignant offspring (Hilakivi-Clarke et al. 1999b). Furthermore, injection of prepubertal rats with genistein (500 μg/g body weight) or oestradiol benzoate (500 ng/g body weight) on days 16, 18 and 20 showed that both treatments resulted in significantly increased mammary gland terminal end buds and increased ductal branching compared to controls, indicating an ER-dependent action of genistein in mammary gland proliferation and differentiation, which could be protective against mammary cancer (Cotroneo et al. 2002). Overall, these results indicate that genistein has very complex effects on carcinogen-induced mammary cancer in the rat model and great care is required in interpreting these results and drawing parallels with human breast cancer.

Biochanin A, found in certain subterranean clovers and converted to genistein by demethylation in the liver in addition to in the breast, was a good anticancer agent when administered following the carcinogen (Gotoh et al. 1998a), suggesting the benefits of isoflavones other than genistein may not be solely restricted to early life exposure. The fermented soya food miso (which contains mostly unconjugated isoflavones) and tamoxifen acted together to cause an additive reduction in the number of mammary tumours in the rat model (Gotoh et al. 1998b) and this may be of considerable importance for women on standard tamoxifen therapy (Wiseman 1994).

In the mouse model of breast cancer (tamoxifen is oestrogenic in this model), maternal genistein exposure (pregnant mice injected with 20 μg/day between days 15 and 20 of gestation) resulted in similar effects to that of oestrogen on mammary gland development (Hilakiviv-Clarke et al. 1998) and further studies are needed to determine whether these oestrogenic changes could lead to an increased risk of breast tumours. In addition, when human breast cancer cells (MCF-7) are grown orthotopically in ovariectomised rats, addition of genistein to their diets resulted in an increase in the growth of the cancer cells (Hsieh et al. 1998). This could have important implications (in relation to tumour reoccurrence) for the consumption of phytoestrogens including isoflavonoids by women who have had their ovaries removed following a diagnosis of breast cancer. But as the removal of the ovaries will greatly reduce the growth of breast cancer cells, then any increase in risk caused by dietary phytoestrogens would probably be less than if the ovaries remained intact (Barnes 1998).

Mechanisms of anticancer action of isoflavonoids

Genistein is a potent and specific *in vitro* inhibitor of tyrosine kinase action in the autophosphorylation of the epidermal growth factor (EGF) receptor (Akiyama et al. 1987) and is thus frequently used as a pharmacological tool. The EGF receptor is over-expressed in many cancers, in particular those with the greatest ability for metastasis (Kim et al. 1996) and it has therefore often been assumed that some of the anticancer effects of genistein are mediated *via* inhibition of tyrosine kinase activity; however, this is likely to be an oversimplification of the true *in vivo* situation (Barnes 1998).

Isoflavonoids have biphasic effects on the proliferation of breast cancer cells in culture, at concentrations greater than 5 μM, genistein exhibits a concentration-dependent ability to inhibit both growth factor-stimulated and oestrogen-stimulated (reversed by 17β-oestradiol) cell proliferation (So et al. 1997). Genistein at low concentrations can, in the absence of any oestrogens, stimulate the growth of oestrogen receptor-positive MCF-7 cells, (Wang and Kurzer, 1997; Zava and Duwe 1997). Genistein does not, however, stimulate the growth of oestrogen receptor-negative breast cancer cells (Peterson and Barnes 1991; Wang et al. 1996), it only inhibits cell proliferation in these cell lines (Peterson and Barnes 1991). Equol is a much more potent stimulator than daidzein of the expression of oestrogen-specific genes (Sathyamoorthy and Wang 1997). It is of great interest that phytoestrogen-responsive genes (PE-13.1 and pRDA-D) have been identified and characterised from MCF-7 cells and it may be possible to use these as molecular markers in elucidating the role phytoestrogens, including isoflavonoids, play in cancer prevention (Ramanathan and Gray 2003).

Mechanisms other than those involving oestrogen receptors are also likely to be involved in the inhibition of cell proliferation by genistein. This is because genistein inhibits both the EGF-stimulated as well as the 17β-oestradiol-stimulated growth of MCF-7 cells (Akiyama et al. 1987). It has been suggested that the inhibitory action of genistein on cell proliferation involved effects on the autophosphorylation of the EGF receptor in membranes isolated from cells (Akiyama et al. 1987). Although studies have shown that exposure to genistein can reduce the tyrosine phosphorylation of cell proteins in whole cell lysates, studies using cultured human breast and prostate cancer cells have not, however, confirmed that genistein has a direct effect on the autophosphorylation of the EGF receptor (Peterson and Barnes 1996). Furthermore, *in vivo* studies in male rats have shown that genistein decreases the amount of EGF receptor present in the prostate indicating that the observed decrease in tyrosine phosphorylation may be only a secondary effect of the influence of genistein on the expression or turnover of EGF receptor (Barnes 1998; Dalu et al. 1998).

Many other mechanisms of action for isoflavonoids and genistein in particular have been suggested. These include, inhibition of DNA topoisomerases (Kondo et al. 1991), inhibition of cell cycle progression (Kim et al. 1998), inhibition of angiogenesis (Fotsis et al. 1993; Kruse et al. 1997), tumour invasiveness (Yan and Han 1998), inhibition of enzymes involved in oestrogen biosynthesis (Makela et al. 1998), effects on the expression of DNA transcription factors c-fos and c-jun (Wei et al. 1995) and on TGF-β (Kim et al. 1998; Sathyamoorthy et al. 1998), the promotion of p38/mitogen-activated protein kinase phosphorylation and activation of a proapoptotic cascade (Totta et al. 2005). Additionally, the intracellular genistein metabolite 5,7,3′,4′-tetrahydroxyisoflavone has been shown to mediate G2-M cell cycle arrest in cancer cells via modulation of the p38 cell signalling pathway (Nguyen et al. 2006).

Gene expression profiles have indicated that genistein is able to regulate genes critical for the control of cellular proliferation, cell cycle, apoptosis, oncogenesis, transcription regulation and cell signal transduction pathways. Genistein has also been reported to induce apoptosis and inhibit activation of both the AKt and NF-κB signalling pathways. These pathways have been found to play an important role in maintaining a balance between cell survival and apoptosis. Genistein can also increase the sensitivity of cancer cells to apoptosis induced by chemotherapeutic agents such as cisplatin, via inactivation of NF-κB and these properties have been found to be enhanced in structurally modified synthetic derivatives of isoflavone (Sarkar et al. 2006). These synthetic structurally modified isoflavone derivatives and also genistein itself, may be important in the future for cancer prevention and therapy (Sarkar et al. 2006).

Oxidative damage is associated with and may contribute to major age-related diseases including cancer and cardiovascular disease, and the protective effects of dietary phytochemicals such as flavonoids is often attributed to antioxidant action (see reviews by Halliwell and Whiteman 2004; Halliwell et al. 2005). Effects of isoflavones have also been reported on reactive oxygen species (Wei et al. 1995; Mitchell et al. 1998), oxidative membrane damage (Wiseman et al. 1998), membrane-rigidity (Tsuchiya et al. 2002: similar to those found previously to contribute to the antioxidant action of tamoxifen: Wiseman et al. 1990, 1993, Wiseman 1994), and oxidative damage *in vivo* (Wiseman et al. 2000). Although isoflavones and metabolites possess antioxidant action *in vitro,* for example they can scavenge a wide range of radical species such as the superoxide radical anion and the hydroxyl and lipid peroxyl radicals, inhibit lipid peroxidation in membrane model systems and increase the resistance of low density lipoproteins (LDL) against *ex vivo* oxidation, they are relatively poor antioxidants compared to flavonoids such as the flavanol quercetin (Mitchell et al. 1998; Arora et al. 1998; Wiseman et al. 1998; O'Reilly et al. 2000; Rimbach et al. 2003; Rufer and Kulling 2006). However, the oxidative metabolites of genistein, daidzein have increased antioxidant action than the parent compounds (Rufer and Kulling 2006). Equol, a gut microflora metabolite of daidzein, was a more effective antioxidant than genistein or the parent compound daidzein, in model membrane systems (Wiseman et al. 1998) and in other *in vitro* assays (Rufer and Kulling 2006) and shows structural similarity to the tocopherols (Barnes 1998). Daidzein and genistein showed antioxidant action in primary and cancer lymphocytes (Jurkat cells), both isoflavones increased DNA protection against oxidative damage and decreased lipid peroxidation (Foti et al. 2005). Moreover, a protective effect was achieved at concentrations that can be achieved in plasma following soya consumption. Genistein protects prostate cancer cells against hydrogen peroxide-induced DNA damage (as determined by the comet assay) and induces expression of genes involved in the defence against oxidative stress, namely glutathione reductase (2.7-fold induction), microsomal glutathione-S-transferase 1 (1.9-fold induction) and metallothionein 1X (6.3-fold induction) (Raschke et al. 2006). Genistein may thus counteract the age-related decline of these important antioxidant defences, which play an important role in maintaining DNA integrity (Raschke et al. 2006).

The extensively studied aglycone forms of isoflavones (e.g. genistein and daidzein) do not circulate in appreciable amounts because they are metabolised in the gut (mucosa of the small intestine) and liver, e.g. conjugation with sulphuric acid to form sulphated metabolites. These sulphated metabolites were less potent antioxidants than the parent compounds in ESR and spin trapping studies and studies on LDL oxidation *ex vivo* because of blocking of the radical scavenging phenolic hydroxyl groups (Turner et al. 2004; Rimbach et al. 2004). This suggests deconjugation is required for the isoflavones to be effective antioxidants *in vivo*.

An important aspect of cancer risk is the involvement of the inflammatory response, which entails the production of cytokines and proinflammatory oxidants such as the hypochlorous acid produced by neutrophils and peroxynitrite by macrophages that react with phenolic tyrosine residues on proteins to form chloro- and nitrotyrosine (D'Alessandro et al. 2003) It has been reported that neutrophil myleloperoxidase chlorinates and nitrates isoflavones and enhances their antioxidant properties, thus soya isoflavones may have potentially protective benefits at sites of inflammation (Boersma et al. 2003; D'Alessandro et al. 2003). Antioxidant action could also contribute to anticancer ability because reactive oxygen species could initiate signal transduction through the mitogen activated protein (MAP) kinases (Wiseman and Halliwell 1996; Barnes 1998).

Angiogenesis, the formation of new blood vessels, is normally an important process involved in productive function, development and wound repair. Disease states, however, often involve persistent and unregulated angiogenesis. The growth and metastasis of tumours is dependent on angiogenesis. Genistein is a potent inhibitor of angiogenesis *in vitro* (Fotsis et al. 1993) and thus could have therapeutic applications in the treatment of chronic neovascular diseases including solid tumour growth (Fotsis et al. 1995) and inhibition of neovascularisation of the eye by genistein has been reported (Kruse et al. 1997). Recently, novel molecular targets for the inhibition of angiogenesis by genistein have been discovered including tissue factor, endostatin and angiostatin (Su et al. 2005).

Genistein may enhance the action of TGF-β (Kim et al. 1998; Sathyamoorthy et al. 1998). This action may be a link between the effects of genistein in a variety of chronic diseases (Barnes 1998) including atherosclerosis and hereditary haemorrhagic telangiectasia (the Osler-Weber-Rendu syndrome) in which defects in TGF-β have been characterised (Johnson et al. 1996).

Clinical studies

Only a few studies have reported on the use of phytoestrogens as preventative agents for breast cancer. In one study, an isolated soya protein beverage (42 mg genistein and 27 mg daidzein) was administered daily for 6 months to healthy pre- and postmenopausal women and breast cancer risk factors were measured in nipple aspirate fluid (NAF) (Petrakis et al. 1996). Although no change in NAF was observed in postmenopausal women, premenopausal women, showed an increase in NAF volume, which persisted even after treatment ended and indicates the isoflavones were having an undesirable oestrogenic effect in the premenopausal women (Petrakis et al. 1996). This provides some cause for concern that risk of premenopausal breast cancer may actually be enhanced by phytoestrogens (Barnes 1998), although further studies are needed. Furthermore, in a study of 84 normal premenopausal women, consumption of a soya supplement (60 g soy, 45 mg total isoflavones) for 14 days resulted in a weak oestrogenic response in the breast: nipple aspirate levels of apolipoprotein D were significantly lowered and pS2 levels were significantly raised (Hargreaves et al. 1999).

Mammographic breast density has been consistently associated with risk for breast cancer. A review of case-control studies showed odds ratios for breast cancer in women with the highest versus the lowest mammographic breast density ranged from 2.1 to 6.0 (Boyd et al. 1998). Although the reasons for this are not fully understood it is possible that breast density acts as a biomarker for the past and current reproductive and hormonal events that influence breast cancer risk (Boyd et al. 2001). Mammographic breast density can thus also be used as biomarker of oestrogenic or antioestrogenic effects of a particular treatment on breast tissue (Atkinson and Bingham 2002). Consumption of a dietary supplement that provided red clover-derived isoflavones (26 mg biochanin A, 16 mg formononetin, 1 mg genistein and 0.5 mg daidzein) for 12 months, did not increase mammographic breast density in postmenopausal women, suggesting neither oestrogenic nor antioestrogenic effects on the breast of this supplement at the dose given (Atkinson et al. 2004c).

Protection by isoflavonoids against cardiovascular disease

Cholesterol-lowering and isoflavonoids

Oestrogen administration in postmenopausal women has been observed to produce cardioprotective benefits. The exact biomolecular mechanisms for this cardioprotection are unclear but it is likely that actions mediated both through the oestrogen receptors, such as the beneficial alteration in lipid profiles and up-regulation of the LDL receptor, and independently of the oestrogen receptors, such as antioxidant action, contribute to the observed cardioprotective effects of oestrogens.

Lower incidence of heart disease has also been reported in populations consuming large amounts of soya products. Cholesterol-lowering is probably the best-documented cardioprotective effect of soya (Sirtori and Lovati 2001; Clarkson 2002). Soya protein incorporated into a low fat diet can reduce cholesterol and LDL-cholesterol concentrations and the soya isoflavones have been considered to contribute to these effects (Anderson et al. 1995).

Consumption of soya protein (40 g/day providing either 56 mg isoflavones/day or 90 mg isoflavones/day) or caesin and non-fat dry milk (40 g/day) by postmenopausal women for 6 months, showed a significant decrease in non-HDL cholesterol and a significant increase in mononuclear cell LDL receptor mRNA and in HDL cholesterol in both of the soya isoflavone groups compared to the control group (Potter et al. 1998). Indeed, consumption of soya protein (20 g/day containing 80 mg isoflavones/day for 5 weeks) in high risk middle-aged men (45–59 years of age) in Scotland, significantly decreased non-HDL cholesterol and blood pressure, compared to the control treatment (Sagara et al. 2004). In healthy young men, soya protein regardless of isoflavone content was found to beneficially modulate serum lipid ratios (McVeigh et al. 2006).

However, studies in hypercholesterolemic subjects, using soya protein depleted of isoflavones have shown that soya protein independently of isoflavones can favourably affect LDL size, LDL particle distribution was shifted to a less atherogenic pattern, (Desroches et al. 2004) and can decrease triglyceride concentrations, triglyceride fatty acid fractional synthesis rate and cholesterol concentrations (Wang et al. 2004).

A meta-analysis of eight randomised controlled trials of soya protein consumption in humans has found that with identical soya protein intake, high isoflavone intake led to significantly greater decreases in serum LDL cholesterol than low isoflavone intake, suggesting that isoflavones have LDL-cholesterol-lowering effects that are independent of the soya protein (Zhuo et al. 2004).

By contrast, a meta-analysis of randomised controlled trials, indicate that consumption of isolated isoflavones did not seem to have any significant effect on serum cholesterol, suggesting further studies investigating possible interactions of isoflavones with other components of soya protein are needed (Yeung et al. 2003). Indeed, a 12-month intervention with red clover-derived isoflavones (43.5 mg/day) administered in the form of a dietary supplement found only modest protective benefits (decreases in triglycerides and plasminogen activator inhibitor type 1) in perimenopausal women (Atkinson et al. 2004b). This could, however, relate to the use of isolated isoflavones consumed as a dietary supplement rather than in soya protein. ApoE is an important factor influencing blood lipid profiles and the women were genotyped for polymorphisms in the gene encoding apoE to determine potential gene–treatment interactions (Atkinson et al. 2004b). This study also found interactions between the apolipoprotein E genotype and treatment tended to be significant for changes in total and LDL cholesterol in 49- to 65-year-old women, with isoflavone treatment being potentially beneficial (Atkinson et al. 2004b).

The postprandial production of triglyceride-rich remnants has been suggested to contribute to the development of atherosclerosis. The ability of soya (39 g soya, 85 mg isoflavone aglycones) compared to milk protein (40 g protein, 0 mg isoflavone aglycones, control) in combination with a high-fat feeding challenge to modify postprandial atherogenic-associated events and biomarkers for oxidative stress, inflammation and thrombosis has been investigated in 15 young healthy men (Campbell et al. 2006). However, there were no significant differences between soya and control for serum C-reactive protein, serum interleukin-6, serum fibrinogen *ex vivo* copper-induced LDL oxidation or plasma lipids (total cholesterol, HDL, LDL, triglycerides), suggesting that soya or milk protein consumption with a high-fat meal does not alter acutely postprandial oxidative stress, inflammation or plasma lipids in young healthy men (Campbell et al. 2006).

Although soya isoflavone-enriched foods had no effect on lipid or other metabolic biomarkers of cardiovascular disease risk in 117 European postmenopausal women, they may increase HDL cholesterol concentrations in an ERβ gene-polymorphic subgroup (ERβ (cx) Tsp509I genotype AA but not GG or GA) (Hall et al. 2006). There were no effects of isoflavones on glucose metabolism in this study, however beneficial effects on glucose metabolism including improving insulin resistance and on obesity in animal and human studies have been previously reported (reviewed by Usui 2006). In this study of 117 postmenopausal women, isoflavones were found to have beneficial effects on C-reactive protein concentrations but not on other inflammatory biomarkers of cardiovascular disease risk; however, they may improve vascular cell adhesion molecule 1 (VCAM-1) in an ERβ gene-polymorphic subgroup (ERβ AluI genotype) (Hall et al. 2005).

A cross-sectional study in 301 postmenopausal women (60–75 years of age) living in the Netherlands, where habitual isoflavone and lignan intakes were assessed with a food frequency questionnaire covering habitual diet during the year prior to the study, reported that high intakes of isoflavones were associated with lower levels of the atherogenic lipoprotein Lp(a) but had little effect on plasma lipids (total cholesterol, LDL and HDL cholesterol and triglycerides), suggesting that at low levels of intake dietary isoflavones have a limited effect on plasma lipids (Kreijkamp-Kaspers et al. 2005). However, following habitual soya isoflavone consumption, higher blood daidzein levels have been reported to be associated with beneficial lipoprotein levels and most interestingly this association was most evident in a study subgroup of women with low blood oestrogen levels, regardless of age (Bairey Merz et al. 2006). This suggests a possible explanation for the previous variable lipoprotein results in randomised controlled studies (Bairey Merz et al. 2006).

These studies indicate the importance of identifying subgroups of subjects who may preferentially benefit from isoflavone treatment. Particularly, as the American Heart Association has recently concluded that although earlier research suggested that soya protein has clinically important beneficial effects on LDL cholesterol and other cardiovascular risk markers, this has not been confirmed by many studies indicating that the direct cardiovascular health benefit of soya protein or isoflavone supplements is rather minimal (Sacks et al. 2006).

Antioxidant action

Antioxidant action is one of the mechanisms which may contribute to the cardiovascular protective effects of soya and soya isoflavones. Antioxidant properties have been reported for isoflavones both *in vitro* and *in vivo* (see earlier section 'Mechanisms of anticancer action of isoflavonoids').

The oxidation hypothesis of atherosclerosis states that the oxidative modification of LDL (or other lipoproteins) is important and possibly obligatory in the pathogenesis of the atherosclerotic lesion; thus it has been suggested that inhibiting the oxidation of LDL will decrease or prevent atherosclerosis and clinical sequelae (see review by Witzum 1994). LDL oxidation also has important implications for vascular health function. High concentrations of LDL may inhibit arterial function in terms of the release of nitric oxide from the endothelium and many of these effects are mediated by lipid oxidation products (Bruckdorfer 1996). Furthermore, oxidised LDL inhibits endothelium-dependent nitric oxide-mediated relaxations in isolated rabbit coronary arteries (Buckley et al. 1996). Oxidised LDL induces apoptosis in vascular cells including macrophages and this is prevented by nitric oxide (Heinloth et al. 2002).

Isoprostanes are a class of lipids produced *in vivo* principally by a free radical-catalysed peroxidation of polyunsaturated fatty acids (see review by Pratico et al. 2001; Fam and Morrow 2003; Halliwell and Whiteman 2004). Isoprostanes are isomers of the conventional enzymatically derived prostaglandins. F_2-isoprostanes are the most studied species and are isomers of the enzyme-derived prostaglandin $F_{2\alpha}$. F_2-isoprostanes are considered to provide a reliable biomarker for oxidative stress and resultant oxidative lipid damage *in vivo* because of their mechanism of formation, chemical stability and specific structural features that enable them to be distinguished from other free radical-generated products. Increased concentrations of F_2-isoprostanes have been consistently reported in association with cardiovascular risk factors such as chronic cigarette smoking, diabetes mellitus and hypercholesterolemia. Furthermore, some F_2-isoprostanes possess potent biological activities indicating that they may also act as mediators of the cellular effects of oxidative stress. Oxidative stress may also lead to raised blood pressure, another cardiovascular risk factor, possibly via effects on arterial function.

Cellular actions of isoflavones may contribute to the possible cardioprotective effects associated with soya consumption. Protection by genistein and daidzein against oxidative stress-induced endothelial damage has been investigated. Genistein but not daidzein was found to protect endothelial cells from damage induced by oxidative stress and this protection was associated by decreases in intracellular glutathione concentrations (Hernandez-Montes et al. 2006). It has been suggested that the genistein-induced protective effect was primarily related to the activation of glutathione peroxidase mediated by Nrf1 activation (Hernandez-Montes et al. 2006).

There are a number of studies that have attempted to determine whether isoflavones exert antioxidant effects *in vivo*. The effect of dietary soya isoflavones on the F_2-isoprostane, 8-*epi*-prostaglandin $F_{2\alpha}$ (8-*epi*-PGF$_{2\alpha}$) and on resistance of LDL to oxidation has been reported (Wiseman et al. 2000). In a randomised crossover study in 24 young healthy male and female subjects, consuming diets that were rich in soya that was high (56 mg isoflavones/day: 35 mg genistein and 21 mg daidzein) or low in isoflavones (2 mg isoflavones/day), each for 2 weeks, resulted in plasma concentrations of the F_2-isoprostane, 8-*epi*-PGF$_{2\alpha}$ that were significantly lower after the high-isoflavone dietary treatment than after the low-isoflavone dietary treatment (326 ± 32 and 405 ± 50 ng/L, respectively $P = 0.028$). The lag time for copper-ion-induced LDL oxidation was longer (48 ± 2.4 and 44 ± 1.9 min, respectively, $P = 0.017$).

The increased resistance of LDL to oxidation is in agreement with the findings of a number of studies with dietary soya, including the increase in lag time in a study in six young healthy male and female subjects who consumed 3 soya bars/day (providing 57 mg total isoflavones/day: 36 mg genistein and 21 mg daidzein) for 2 weeks (Tikkanen et al. 1998). Increased resistance to LDL oxidation has also been reported in a 12-week single open-group dietary intervention with soya foods (60 mg isoflavones/day) in 42 normal postmenopausal women (Scheiber et al. 2001). Furthermore, consumption of soya protein (110 mg isoflavones/day for 4 weeks) decreased plasma peroxide concentrations and increased total antioxidant status but did not affect a biomarker of oxidative DNA damage (urinary 8-hydroxy-2-deoxyguanosine concentrations: 8-OHdG) (Bazzoli et al. 2002).

The findings of these studies are in contrast to a randomised crossover study in 32 young healthy male and female subjects, consuming diets that were high in flavonoids (131 mg flavonoids/day 89.7 mg quercetin as an onion cake and tea) and low in flavonoids each for 2 weeks, which found no effect of the high flavonoid diet on 8-*epi*-PGF$_{2\alpha}$ or on LDL oxidation resistance *ex vivo* (O'Reilly et al. 2000, 2001). This is of particular interest as quercetin is a much more potent antioxidant *in vitro* than the soya isoflavones and their metabolites. Indeed, when added to LDL isolated from postmenopausal women, daidzein and genistein exhibited a weak antioxidant activity compared to quercetin (Arteaga et al. 2004). However, it has recently been suggested that flavonoids may exert direct protective antioxidant effects within the gastrointestinal tract, because of the high concentrations present and this is supported by measurements of flavonoids and other phenols in human faecal water (Halliwell et al. 2005).

These studies also measured resistance of LDL to *ex vivo* oxidation, which can be difficult to interpret because phytochemicals such as flavonoids and their metabolites could washout from the LDL during the isolation procedures. Although esterified isoflavones can also be incorporated into LDL *ex vivo* (Meng et al. 1999), it has not yet been shown that isoflavones can be esterified to LDL *in vivo*. Measurement of changes in the lag time to LDL oxidation *ex vivo* requires great care to avoid misinterpreting the data due to effects such as seasonal variation (Halliwell et al. 2005).

It is of considerable interest that widely differing effects are frequently reported for isoflavones consumed within the food matrix in soya foods, compared to isoflavone-rich extracts consumed in capsule or tablet form as dietary supplements. For example consumption of a soya isoflavone supplement (50 mg isoflavones, twice a day for 3 weeks) decreased a biomarker of DNA oxidative damage (white cell 5-hydroxymethyl-2′-deoxyuridine concentrations) but did not alter plasma 8-*epi*-PGF$_{2\alpha}$ concentrations (Djuric et al. 2001) and consumption of a soya extract (55 mg for 8 weeks) had no effect on urinary 8-*epi*-PGF$_{2\alpha}$ concentrations (Hodgson et al. 1999).

Two studies that used a soya protein concentrate or a soya protein isolate to incorporate isoflavones into foods, to investigate the antioxidant action of soya protein and phytate, respectively, in addition to that of isoflavones, found no effects on urinary 8-*epi*-PGF$_{2\alpha}$ and plasma total antioxidant capacity (Vega-Lopez et al. 2005) or on plasma 8-*epi*-PGF$_{2\alpha}$ or LDL oxidation (Engelman et al. 2005). Additionally, soya protein with and without isoflavones, consumed on an acute basis, did not significantly increase postprandial serum antioxidant capacity (Heneman et al. 2007). However, consumption of a soya milk supplement (113–207 mg/day total isoflavones) decreased urinary 8-*epi*-PGF$_{2\alpha}$ in an age-dependent manner in premenopausal women with greater effects in older women and with lower doses of isoflavones (Nhan et al. 2005).

An evaluation of the antioxidant and immune function effects of isoflavones both in soya milk and in supplement form in healthy postmenopausal women found that both soya milk and supplemental isoflavones increased lymphocyte B cell populations and decreased plasma concentrations of a biomarker of oxidative DNA damage, 8-hydroxy-2-deoxy-guanosine (Ryan-Borchers et al. 2006). This suggests modulation of immune function and protection against oxidative DNA damage by both food and supplemental isoflavones (Ryan-Borchers et al. 2006).

To try and understand further how the food matrix may influence the ability of isoflavones to protect human health through antioxidant action, we have carried out a randomised crossover study in healthy young women, comparing the effect of isoflavones within the food matrix compared with those in supplements, on biomarkers of oxidative stress. We found that the baseline antioxidant status of the subjects was of importance to response to isoflavones and there was considerable interindividual variation. However, there was, for example, a similar decrease in plasma 8-*epi*-PGF$_{2\alpha}$ after both soya foods and the soya supplement (H. Wiseman et al., unpublished results).

We have also taken a proteomic approach to investigate putative protein biomarkers of isoflavone consumption in soya foods and elucidate further pathways of antioxidant and other biological actions of isoflavones, using 2-D gel electrophoresis with peptide mass fingerprinting using LC-MS/MS to identify changes in serum protein profiles (Wong et al. 2008). In particular concentrations of apolipoprotein E and caeruloplasmin were found to be significantly increased, while alpha-1-acid glycoprotein was found to be significantly decreased after 2 weeks of soya food consumption by healthy young women (Wong et al. 2008). The increase in caeruloplasmin concentration may contribute to improved antioxidant capacity, while the increase in apolipoprotein E may favourably alter the lipid profile. The decrease in alpha-1-acid glycoprotein concentration may indicate a role for soya isoflavones in immunomodulation. These findings suggest that soya food consumption alters protein expression, particularly in relation to oxidative stress and lipid metabolism (Wong et al. 2008).

Arterial function

Arterial function is vital to the prevention of ischaemic changes in the organs that the arteries deliver blood to, and is particularly relevant to ischaemic heart disease. A recent population-based study (the Rotterdam study), has shown arterial stiffness (or compliance) to be strongly associated with atherosclerosis at various sites in the vasculature (aorta and carotid artery) (van Popele et al. 2001). Mechanisms of soy-mediated vascular protection may include effects on arterial function, including flow-mediated endothelium-dependent vasodilation (reflecting endothelial function) and systemic arterial compliance (reflecting arterial elasticity) and these have been measured in a number of studies. A randomised double blind study administering either soya protein isolate (118 mg isoflavones/day) or caesin placebo for 3 months to 213 healthy male and postmenopausal subjects (50–75 years of age) showed a significant improvement in peripheral pulse wave velocity (reflecting peripheral vascular resistance and one component, together with systemic arterial compliance, of vascular function) but worsened flow-mediated vasodilation in the men and had no significant effect on the flow-mediated vasodilation in the postmenopausal women (Teede et al. 2001). Furthermore, consumption of soy protein with isoflavones (107 mg isoflavones/day for 6 weeks) in a randomised, crossover study had favourable effects on the endothelium (postocclusion peak flow velocity of the brachial artery was significantly lower, consistent with a vasodilatory response) in healthy menopausal women (Steinberg et al. 2003).

In a placebo-controlled, randomised, crossover study with 21 peri- and postmenopausal women treated for 5 weeks with a supplement delivering 80 mg total soya isoflavones/day, a significant improvement was reported in systemic arterial compliance, but had no effect on flow-mediated vasodilation (Nestel et al. 1997). This lack of an effect on flow-mediated vasodilation is in agreement with a study of similar design, in 20 postmenopausal women and again using a supplement to provide 80 mg total soya isoflavones/day (Simons et al. 2000).

It is noteworthy that a cross-sectional study in 301 postmenopausal women (60–75 years of age) in the Netherlands, where isoflavone and lignan intakes were assessed with a food frequency questionnaire covering habitual diet during the year prior to the study, reported no associations between isoflavone intake and vascular function, including endothelial function, blood pressure and hypertension, and this is in contrast to the observed protective effect of dietary lignan intake on blood pressure and hypertension (Kreijkamp-Kaspers et al. 2004).

Cellular effects

Vascular protection could also be conferred by the ability of genistein to inhibit proliferation of vascular endothelial cells and smooth muscle cells and to increase levels of growth factors (Raines and Ross 1995) including the cytokine TGF-β. Phytoestrogens including the soya isoflavones genistein and daidzein and the daidzein metabolite equol have all been reported to inhibit growth and MAP kinase activity in human aortic smooth muscle cells (Dubey et al. 1999) and thus may confer protective effects on the cardiovascular system by inhibiting vascular remodelling and neointima formation. TGF-β helps maintain normal vessel wall structure and promotes smooth muscle cell differentiation, while preventing their migration and proliferation. Genistein has been shown to increase TGF-β secretion by cells in culture (see review by Kim et al. 2001) and, as previously suggested for tamoxifen (see review by Grainger and Metcalf 1996) increased TGF-β production may be a mediator of the some of the cardioprotective effects of soya (see review by Kim et al. 2001). However, we have recently found no effect on plasma TGF-β concentrations following consumption of soya either high (56 mg/day) or low (2 mg/day) in isoflavones for 2 weeks in a randomised crossover study in young healthy subjects (Sanders et al. 2002).

Protection by isoflavonoids against osteoporosis, cognitive decline and menopausal symptoms?

Osteoporosis

Osteoporosis is a chronic disease in which the bones become brittle and break more easily. Postmenopausal women may suffer hip fractures caused by osteoporosis, which develops primarily as a consequence of the low oestrogen levels that occur after the menopause. Premenopausal women are therefore, protected by their oestrogen levels against osteoporosis. Although calcium supplementation is important before the menopause, on its own it cannot stop bone loss in perimenopausal and postmenopausal women. Hormone replacement therapy (HRT) can be very effective; 0.625 mg/day of conjugated oestrogens has been reported to prevent bone loss (Thorneycroft 1989) and HRT is osteoprotective if taken postmenopausally for more than 24 months (Fentiman et al. 1994). The drug ipriflavone (a synthetic isoflavone derivative) at a dose of 600 mg/day can prevent the increase in bone turnover and the decrease in bone density in postmenopausal women (Gambacciaini et al. 1997). The protective effects of HRT together with the finding that ERβ is highly expressed in bone and seems to mediate a distinct mechanism of oestrogen action (Arts et al. 1997; Onoe et al. 1997). This suggests that phytoestrogens may thus protect women against postmenopausal bone loss (Anderson and Garner 1998) and the potential skeletal benefits of soya isoflavones has been reviewed (Messina et al. 2004; Reinwald and Weaver 2006). Perimenopausal and early menopausal women may benefit more from the therapeutic effects of isoflavones on bone, prior to the loss of oestrogen receptors (including ERβ) that occurs in the later postmenopausal years (Reinwald and Weaver 2006).

Consumption by postmenopausal women (6-month parallel-group design) of soya protein (40 g/day providing either 56 mg isoflavones/day or 90 mg isoflavones/day) compared to caesin and non-fat dry milk (40 g/day) produced significant increases in bone mineral content and density in the lumbar spine (but not in any other parts of the body) but only in the higher isoflavone (90 mg/day) group compared to the control group (Potter et al. 1998).

Daily intake for 2 years of two glasses of soya milk containing 76 mg of isoflavones has been reported to prevent lumbar spine bone loss in postmenopausal women (Lydeking-Olsen et al. 2004). Consumption daily for 12 months of a soya beverage containing 83 mg isoflavones (45.6 mg genistein, 31.7 mg daidzein aglycone units) resulted in a modest benefit in preserving spine but not hip bone mineral density in older women (Newton et al. 2006). It is of related interest that habitual consumption of the fermented soybean food natto (which contains large amounts of menaqunone-7) by postmenopausal Japanese women was found in the Japanese Population-based Osteoporosis (JPOS) study to be associated with reduced bone loss (Ikeda et al. 2006).

Moreover, consumption of a red clover-derived isoflavone supplement (43.5 mg/day isoflavones) for 1 year significantly decreased loss of lumbar spine bone mineral content and bone mineral density and increased concentrations of the bone formation markers (Atkinson et al. 2004a). Similarly, consumption of a soya isoflavone supplement (80 mg/day isoflavones) for 1 year was found to have a beneficial effect on hip bone mineral content in postmenopausal Chinese women with a low initial bone mass (Chen et al. 2003).

Consumption of soya foods (providing 60 mg/day isoflavones) for 12 weeks by postmenopausal women has been found to significantly decrease clinical risk factors for osteoporosis (short-term markers of bone turnover) including decreased urinary N-telopeptide excretion (bone resorption marker) and increased serum osteocalcin (bone formation marker) (Scheiber et al. 2001). Furthermore, consumption of a soya isoflavone supplement containing 61.8 mg of isoflavones for 4 weeks by postmenopausal Japanese women significantly decreased excretion of bone resorption markers (Uesugi et al. 2002). A study in 500 Australian women (aged 40–80 years) has shown that higher isoflavone intakes are associated with higher concentrations of bone alkaline phosphatase, a short-term marker of bone formation and turnover (Hanna et al. 2004).

Menopausal symptoms and cognitive decline

The oestrogenic properties of phytoestrogens may also help with menopausal symptoms such as hot flushes and vaginitis (Eden 1998). An improvement in hot flushes with dietary supplementation with 45 g of raw soya flour/day, has been reported; however, an improvement was also seen with white wheat flour (which contains very little phytoestrogen) (Murkies et al. 1995). Furthermore, consumption of a red clover-derived isoflavone supplement (80 mg/day isoflavones) has been reported to significantly decrease menopausal hot flush symptoms compared with placebo (van de Weijer and Barensten 2002). However, three systematic reviews have reached differing conclusions: while the first review concludes that there is some evidence to support the efficacy of soya and soya isoflavone preparation for perimenopausal symptoms (Huntley and Ernst 2004), the second concludes that isoflavone phytoestrogens available as soya foods, soya extracts and red clover extracts do not improve hot flushes or other menopausal symptoms (Krebs et al. 2004) and the third concludes that frequency of hot flushes was not reduced by red clover isoflavone extracts and that the results were mixed for soy isoflavone extracts (Nelson et al. 2006), suggesting that further studies are needed.

Oxidative stress, in addition to lack of oestrogen, may contribute to menopausal symptoms and it has been suggested that these may be improved by boosting antioxidant defences by the consumption of a wide range of dietary antioxidants including antioxidant vitamins and soya isoflavones (Miquel et al. 2006).

Similar to oestrogens, dietary phytoestrogens seem to affect certain aspects of cognitive function, although the mechanisms are as yet unclear (see reviews by Lephart et al. 2004; Macready et al. 2005). Consumption of soya foods for 10 weeks (100 mg/day isoflavones) has been reported to improve human memory in young healthy adults (File et al. 2001, 2002) and consumption of a soya isoflavone supplement for 12 weeks (60 mg/day isoflavones) to improve cognitive function in postmenopausal women (Duffy et al. 2003; File et al. 2005). These results are supported by the findings of the SOPHIA study (SOy and Postmenopausal Health in Aging) (Kritz-Silverstein et al. 2003) and a study in postmenopausal women in Italy (Casini et al. 2006).

By contrast, consumption of soya protein (99 mg isoflavones/day) for 12 months failed to improve cognitive function in postmenopausal women (Kreijkamp-Kaspers et al. 2004), suggesting further clinical trials are required to fully determine the possible beneficial effects of isoflavones against cognitive decline.

It is of related interest that grape seed extract, which is a dietary supplement rich in proanthocyanidins and consumed for its antioxidant properties, has similar protective effects to soya and blueberry derived polyphenol-enriched preparations in protecting against age-related cognitive defects (Kim et al. 2006). Ingestion of grape seed extract has been shown by proteomics technology to have neuroprotective activity by affecting specific proteins. Indeed, the direction of change for the majority of the proteins in adult rat brain was opposite to the direction the proteins were changed in either Alzheimer's disease or in transgenic mouse models of dementia (Kim et al. 2006).

Isoflavonoids: potential risks

Phytoestrogens can cause infertility in some animals and thus concerns have been raised over their consumption by human infants. The isoflavones found in a subterranean clover species (in Western Australia) have been identified as the agents responsible for an infertility syndrome in sheep (Adams 1995). Soya isoflavones in the diets of cheetahs in captivity has been shown to lead to their infertility (Setchell et al. 1987). Most animals that are bred commercially and domestic animals, however, are fed diets containing soya (up to 20% by weight) without any apparent reproductive problems (Barnes 1998). No reproductive abnormalities have been found in people living in countries where soya consumption is high. Indeed, the finding that dietary isoflavones are excreted into breast milk by soya-consuming mothers suggests that in cultures where consumption of soya products is the norm, breast-fed infants are exposed to high levels, again without any adverse effects (Franke et al. 1999). Isoflavone exposure shortly after birth at a critical developmental period through breastfeeding may protect against cancer and may be more important to the observation of lower cancer rates in populations in the Far East than adult dietary exposure to isoflavones (Franke et al. 1999).

There have been some concerns expressed regarding the possible health consequences in adulthood (endocrinological and reproductive outcomes) of early-life isoflavone exposure from soya-based infant formula (Strom et al. 2001). The daily exposure of infants to isoflavones in soya-based infant formulas is 6- to 11-fold higher on a body weight basis than the dose that has hormonal effects in adults consuming soya foods (Setchell et al. 1997). However, evidence from adult and infant populations indicates that dietary isoflavones in soya-based infant formulas do not adversely affect human growth, development or reproduction (Mendez et al. 2002; Badger et al. 2002; Giampietro et al. 2004; Merritt and Jenks 2004).

Although toxicity from isoflavones may arise from their action as alternative substrates for the enzyme thyroid peroxidase (Divi et al. 1997) and people in south-east Asia would be protected by the dietary inclusion of iodine-rich seaweed products, a recent study has shown that isoflavone supplements do not affect thyroid function in iodine-replete postmenopausal women (Bruce et al. 2003). Furthermore, a recent review of the literature suggests that there is little evidence that in euthyroid, iodine-replete individuals, soya foods or isoflavones adversely affect thyroid function (Messina and Redmond 2006). However, in hypothyroid patients there is some evidence that soya foods may, by inhibiting absorption, increase the dose of thyroid hormone required by these patients (Messina and Redmond 2006). It is also a possible concern that consumption of soya foods by individuals with compromised thyroid function and/or marginal iodine intake, may increase the risk of clinical hypothyroidism. It would thus seem to be important that an adequate iodine intake is maintained by soya food consumers (Messina and Redmond 2006).

There have also been concerns relating to the possible adverse effects of isoflavones on haematological parameters because the synthetic isoflavone ipriflavone can cause lymphocytopenia in postmenopausal women (Soung do et al. 2006). However, in a study of 87 postmenopausal women, daily consumption of 25 g of soya protein containing 60 mg of isoflavones for 1 year did not cause lymphocytopenia (Soung do et al. 2006).

Considerations of the safety of soya isoflavones is an area of great interest in relation to their potential benefits to human health and has been comprehensively reviewed (Munro et al. 2003). Indeed, as the most likely beneficial health effect of soya and its isoflavones is in prevention of chronic disease, it has been suggested that there may well be long-term health benefits from early-life consumption of soya foods or even soya formula (Setchell 2006).

Lignans

Introduction

Lignans in terms of research output may be secondary to the isoflavones, but in the Western diet they may actually account for the majority of total phytoestrogen exposure. This is because lignans are found in the outer layers of cereals and grains, particularly rye and flaxseed. Lignans are a common, structurally diverse class of phytoestrogen, widely distributed throughout the plant kingdom. They are dimeric phenylpropanoid compounds (C_6–C_3), mostly linked 8–8' (Dixon 2004).

Lignans are found in the plant as glycosides which are subsequently converted to thebioactive forms found in mammals by intestinal bacteria. The glycosides of secoisolariciresinol and matairesinol are converted to enterodiol and enterolactone, which are often refered to as 'mammalian lignans'.

Evidence for the health benefits of lignan consumption comes from epidemiological and intervention studies and, as with the isoflavones, health benefits are thought to be wide, ranging from the prevention of cardiovascular disease and cancer, to cognitive ability.

Production of mammalian lignans

Recent work on the conversion of secoisolariciresinol diglucoside to enterolignans (Clavel et al. 2006) has shown the bacterial strain *Clostridium* sp. SDG-Mt85-3Db to have the highest initial rate of deglycosylation. This, however, was detected in the dominant microbiota of only 10% of faecal samples. *Peptostreptococcus productus* was found to demethylate the lignans pinoresinol, lariciresinol and matairesinol in addition to secoisolariciresinol diglucoside.

Cardiovascular disease

Recent studies on the prevention of cardiovascular disease include studies on sesamin, a sesame lignan which is converted to enterolactone by intestinal bacteria. The results suggested that ingestion improved health in postmenopausal women by altering blood lipids favourably as well as improving antioxidant status and possibly sex hormone status (Wu et al. 2006), as has previously been described for other lignans and phytoestrogens.

Limited cardiovascular benefits of lignan intake were found, however, in Dutch postmenopausal women (Kreijkamp-Kaspers et al. 2005).

Breast cancer prevention

Recent studies, using a large (30 000) sample size of women aged 50–64 years in Denmark have confirmed that there is a tendency towards a lower risk of breast cancer with higher levels of enterolactone circulating in the bloodstream (Olsen et al., 2004), though this effect was found to be largely restricted to ERα-negative breast cancer. Results from studies on German women have also suggested that cytochrome P450c17alpha (CYP17) genotype modifies the protective effect of lignans on premenopausal breast cancer risk (Piller et al. 2006). It was found that women homozygous for the CYP17 A2 allele benefited most from high plasma enterolactone concentrations.

Prostate cancer prevention

As well as helping to prevent the development of oestrogen-dependent tumours, lignans are also thought to be useful in the prevention of male prostate cancer. In a recent Swedish study (Hedelin et al. 2006) no association between dietary intake of total or individual lignans or isoflavonoids and risk of prostate cancer was found, but more specifically intermediate serum levels of enterolactone were associated with a decreased risk of prostate cancer. Phytoestrogens are thought to protect against prostate cancer via modulation of circulating androgen concentrations. Recent studies (Low et al. 2005) have shown that enterolactone interactions with the CYP19 gene may be involved.

Prevention of other types of cancer

The health benefits of lignan consumption do not seem to be restricted to the prevention of breast or prostate cancers, but extend to other types. It has been found, for example, in a recent study on lung cancer (Schabath et al. 2005) that a high intake of lignans in women combined with the use of hormone therapy was associated with a 50% reduction in lung cancer.

Not all studies carried out have shown positive health promoting effects for lignans. Studies such as the Zupthen Elderly Study (Milder et al. 2006) were unable to associate total lignan intake and mortality. Similarly, another review (Boccardo et al. 2005) describes epidemicological evidence for enterolactone as a preventative agent for breast cancer as conflicting.

Other health benefits

Similar to isoflavones, a higher dietary intake of lignans has been found to be associated with better cognitive performance in postmenopausal women, the results being most pronounced in women who were 20- to 30-years postmenopausal (Franco et al. 2005).

Prenylflavonoids

Prenylated flavonoids are recognised as potent phytoestrogens, indeed, 8-prenylnaringenin has been described as the most potent phytoestrogen known (Milligan et al. 1999), although its oestrogenic activity is still less than 1% of that of 17 β-oestradiol (Milligan et al. 2000).

Beer is the most important source of prenylflavonoids. These compounds are found in the bitter flavouring agent, hops (*Humulus lupulus*), particularly the simple prenylated chalcone, xanthohumol; 8-prenylnaringenin is formed during the brewing process due to the isomerisation of desmethylxanthohumol in the brew kettle. The daily intake of 8-prenylnaringenin through beer per capita in the US ranges from 3.3 μg (lager/pilsner beers) to 54 μg (ales, porters and stouts). This level of intake is thought to represent no detriment to health (Stevens and Page 2004). Recent studies, however, suggest that isoxanthohumol is also converted into 8-prenylnaringenin in the human distal colon (Possemiers et al. 2006). Human intestinal microbiota may activate up to 4 mg/L isoxanthohumol in beer into 8-prenylnaringenin. Depending on interindividual differences this could increase the 8-prenylnaringenin tenfold upon beer consumption (Possemiers et al. 2005).

There has been much work carried out on the antioxidant properties of flavonoids, but less so on prenylated flavonoids. *In vitro* work using LDL oxidation assays concerning prenylated flavonoids has shown xanthohumol to be more effective than α-tocopherol and the isoflavone genistein, but less effective than the flavonol quercetin (Miranda et al. 2000a).

Phase I enzymes, for example Cyp1 A2 are thought to be inhibited by xanthohumol and 8-prenylnaringenin (Miranda et al. 2000b). Phase II enzymes by contrast have been shown to be induced *in vitro*. For example NAD(P)H: quinone reductase has been shown to be induced by xanthohumol and six other prenylated chalcones in cultured mouse hep- toma Hepa 1c1c7 cells (Miranda et al. 2000c). Xanthohumol could thus have beneficial effects on the detoxification of carcinogenic compounds by the inhibition of phase I and the induction of phase II enzymes.

Angiogenesis has shown to be inhibited by 8-prenylnaringenin in an *in vitro* model (Pepper et al. 2004) with IC_{50} values between 3 and $10\,\mu M$. Xanthohumol has been shown to inhibit the proliferation of MCF-7 breast cancer cells and A-2780 ovarian cancer cells in a dose-dependent manner with IC_{50} values of 17 and $42\,\mu M$, respectively (Miranda et al. 1999). Also prenylflavonoids have been shown to modulate aromatase (oestrogen synthase) activity in choriocarcinoma-derived JAR cells, indicating another potential mechanism for the prevention and treatment of oestrogen-dependent cancers such as breast cancer (Monteiro et al. 2006).

What is lacking for prenylated flavonoids in comparison with isoflavonoids and flavo- noids in general is epidemiological and feeding trial data. Until this is forthcoming it is unknown whether or not they will be regarded as such potential health maintaining agents as the isoflavonoids. Indeed, in view of the relatively high oestrogenicity of prenylated flavonoids, concern has been expressed over their potential adverse effect on health. Also the presence of 'feminising' agents in beer is not something most brewers would wish to promote.

The relative binding of 8-prenylnaringenin to the cytosolic ER of an MCF7 human breast cancer cell line has been found to be 45× (Matsumura et al. 2005); where relative binding was calculated as the molar excess needed for 50% inhibition of ^3H oestradiol. This compared with a figure of 1000× for genistein, showing the potency of 8-prenylnaringenin as a phytoestrogen. Cell-based assays measuring ligand ability to induce a stably transfected oestrogen-responsive ERE-CAT reporter gene, cell growth in terms of proliferation rate after 7 days, and cell growth in terms of saturation density after 14 days, have also been carried out (Matsumura et al. 2005) and calculated as IC_{50} values (the concentration needed to achieve a response equivalent to 50% of that found with 17βoestradiol). Using 8-prenylnaringenin the IC_{50} values for the respective assays were 1 $\times 10^{-9}$ M, 3×10^{-10} M and 3×10^{-10} M, which compared with 1×10^{-11} M, 1×10^{-11} M and 2×10^{-11} M, respectively for 17βoestradiol and 4×10^{-8} M, 2×10^{-8} M and 1×10^{-8} M, respectively for genistein. The results again showed the potency of 8-prenylnaringenin as a phytoestrogen, although it displayed a relatively potent ability to displace ^3H-oestradiol from cytosolic ER compared with its effect in cell-based assays.

Selectivity, as well as potency, differs for 8-prenylnaringenin binding to oestrogen receptors in comparison with isoflavonoids. 8-Prenylnaringenin was found to be a 100 times more potent ERα agonist than genistein, but a much weaker agonist of ERβ in fur- ther oestradiol-competition assays for receptor binding (Schaefer et al. 2003).

The prenyl group of 8-prenylnaringenin is crucial to its observed oestrogenicity as can be seen by the comparative lack of oestrogenicity of naringenin. Recent studies have investigated substituting the prenyl group (at C8) with alkyl chains of varying lengths and branching patterns (Roelens et al. 2006). The new alkylnaringenins were found to have an activity spectrum ranging from full agonist to partial agonism to agonism. Interestingly 8-(2,2-dimethylpropyl)naringenin showed full agonist characteristics using ERα activity assays, but pronounced antagonist characteristics using ERβ activity assays. This clearly showed the potential for the chemical optimisation of phytoestrogens, in particular the flavonoids, as potential selective oestrogen modulators (SERMs) of the future. The search for new natural prenylflavonoids also continues, in particular evaluating prenylflavonoids from tonics and herbal medicines for their oestrogenic properties (Wang et al. 2006).

Stilbenes

By far the most widely researched dietary stilbene is resveratrol or 3,5,4′-hydroxystilbene, which is found in plants mainly in the *trans* form. Like most polyphenols resveratrol is generally found conjugated, principally as 3-O-β-D-glucosides called piceids. Other minor conjugated forms contain 1–2 methyl groups (e.g. pterostilbene) a sulphate group or a fatty acid. *Trans* resveratrol is widely distributed in the plant kingdom, but the principle dietary sources are grapes (*Vitis* spp.), peanuts (*Arachis* spp.), berries (blueberries and cranberries, *Vaccinium* spp.) and rhubarb (*Rheum* spp.) (Signorelli and Ghidoni 2005). Recently resveratrol has been produced in transgenic apple fruit so in the future it may be present in even greater quantities in the diet (Ruhmann et al. 2006).

As with isoflavonoids, absorption of resveratrol in the human intestine is principally via the aglycone form and therefore there is a requirement for glycosidases, including bacterial types, in the intestine. As regards metabolism and excretion it is interesting that flavonoids such as quercetin inhibit the glucuronidation of resveratrol and may therefore increase its bioavailability (Signorelli and Ghidoni 2005).

The principle health benefits of resveratrol ingestion are seen as the prevention of cardiovascular disease and cancer. Proposed mechanisms for the promotion of cardiovascular health include, in common with other phytoestrogens, antioxidant action and the induction of nitrous oxide to maintain vasodilation (Orallo et al. 2002).

There has been particular interest, however, in resveratrol for its potential prevention of cancer. As for isoflavonoids and 8-prenylnaringenin, proposed mechanisms include the down-regulation of Phase I enzymes and up-regulation of Phase II enzymes (Szaefer et al. 2004). Interestingly resveratrol was found to inhibit nitric oxide production and iNOS (inducible nitric oxide synthase) expression in cancer cells, in contrast to its vasodilatory function, while it induced apoptosis in human B-cell lines derived from patients with chronic B-cell malignancies or lymphyocytic leukaemia (Roman et al. 2002).

Resveratrol has been noted for its ability to inhibit the activity of cyclooxygenases (COX) which catalyse the first committed steps of prostaglandin (PG) biosynthesis, known stimulators of cell proliferation and angiogenesis (Jang et al. 1997).

A number of studies have shown resveratrol able to arrest proliferative activity including at the G1/S boundary, in S phase or in the G2/M phase. Many authors also report that cell cycle arrest is followed by apoptosis (Signorelli and Ghidoni 2005). The p53 oncosuppressor is a DNA-binding protein that activates transcription of genes that induce cell cycle arrest due to acetylation and phosphorylation. In a variety of cell lines resveratrol has strongly up-regulated p53 (Orallo et al. 2002). The regulation of p53 by resveratrol occurs via MAP kinases, including p38 which is also activated by resveratrol (Woo et al. 2004).

Resveratrol inhibits DNA synthesis thereby impairing the normal course of the S phase of the cell cycle, in particular, resveratrol has been shown to inhibit ribonucleotide reductase activity in leukaemia cells (Fontecave et al. 1998).

Survivin, a member of the inhibitors of apoptosis proteins (IAPs) family is decreased by resveratrol by enhanced degradation as well as reduced transcription. This resulted in decreased cell proliferation and sensitisation to chemotherapy (Hayashibara et al. 2002). Similarly over-expression of members of the Bcl2 family impairs resveratrol induced apoptosis in T-acute lymphoblastic leukaemia (Tinhofer et al. 2001).

Sirtuins are a nicotinamide adenosine dinucleotide (NAD)-dependent class of deacetylases responsible for regulating the response to DNA damage and gene silencing process of ageing and survival. Resveratrol was found to activate human sirtuin 1 (SIRT 1) and sensitised cells to apoptosis (Yeung et al. 2004).

In addition to interfering with cell cycle control, resveratrol, like other phytoestrogens, is potentially able to overcome drug resistance of tumours, for example breast cancer, that express multidrug resistance associated proteins (ATP-dependent pumps that remove chemotherapeutics out of cells) (Cooray et al. 2004).

There therefore seems to be great potential for the use of resveratrol as a chemopreventative agent although, as for many other phytoestrogens, further specific feeding trials need to be carried out to determine more precisely potential health benefits.

Resveratrol is not a potent phytoestrogen as demonstrated by its relative binding to cytosolic ER of an MCF-7 human breast cancer cell line, which was undetermined on the scale used (Matsumura et al. 2005). Cell-based assays measuring ligand ability to induce a stably transfected oestrogen-responsive ERE-CAT reporter gene, cell growth in terms of proliferation rate after 7 days, and cell growth in terms of saturation density after 14 days, also showed resveratrol to be a very weak phytoestrogen (Matsumura et al. 2005). The IC_{50} values measured using resveratrol in the respective assays were 4×10^{-6} M, not achieved and not achieved, which compared with 1×10^{-11} M, 1×10^{-11} M and 2×10^{-11} M respectively for 17βoestradiol and 4×10^{-8} M, 2×10^{-8} M and 1×10^{-8} M respectively for genistein.

Further studies have been carried out in which MCF-7 cells were transiently transfected with ERα or ERβ and the oestrogenic response measured through an ERE-response element linked to a luciferase reporter gene (Harris et al. 2005). The EC_{50} values (effective concentration that elicits half the maximal response) values of resveratrol for ERα and ERβ were unachieved, compared with values, for example utilising ERβ, of 3.9×10^{-11} M for 17β-oestradiol and 3.4×10^{-9} M for genistein.

Another study that distinguished between resveratrol ERα and ERβ binding again showed resveratrol to be a weak phytoestrogen (Mueller et al. 2004). IC_{50} values calculated using flourescein-labelled 17β-oestradiol, gave values of 7.7×10^{-6} M for ERα compared with 29×10^{-6} M for ERβ indicating some differential binding to the different ER subtypes. This compared with EC_{50} values for genistein of 0.3×10^{-6} M for ERα and 15×10^{-6} M for ERβ, which clearly showed greater differential binding than resveratrol. EC_{50} values for 17β-oestradiol were 4.3×10^{-9} M for ERα and 5.7×10^{-9} M for ERβ. Studies on the induction/suppression of ERα and ERβ transactivation and coactivator recruitment in Ishikawa cells, showed that resveratrol was antagonistic on both ERα and ERβ at high concentrations. (Mueller et al. 2004).

It would seem therefore that oestrogenicity is not the most significant property of resveratrol in terms of human health and that properties such as the activation of human sirtuin 1 (SIRT 1) will prove more significant for this compound in the future.

Miroestrol

Miroestrol was isolated as the active oestrogenic agent from the Thai rejuvenating folk medicine 'Kwao Keur' (*Pueraria mirifica*) in 1960 (Cain 1960). More recently it has been suggested, however, that deoxymiroestrol is the actual oestrogenic principle found in *Pueraria mirifica* and that miroestrol is formed as an artefact following the oxidation of deoxymiroestrol (Chansakaow et al. 2000).

The relative binding of deoxymiroestrol and miroestrol to the cytosolic ER of an MCF7 human breast cancer cell line has been found to be 50× and 260× times, respectively (Matsumura et al. 2005); where relative binding was calculated as the molar excess needed for 50% inhibition of ^{3}H-oestradiol. This compared with a figure of 1000× for genistein, showing the potency of miroestrol and deoxymiroestrol, in particular deoxymiroestrol, as phytoestrogens. Cell-based assays measuring ligand ability to induce a stably transfected oestrogen-responsive ERE-CAT reporter gene, cell growth in terms of proliferation rate after 7 days, and cell growth in terms of saturation density after 14 days, have also been carried out (Matsumura et al. 2005) and calculated as IC_{50} values (the concentration needed to achieve a response equivalent to 50% of that found with 17βoestradiol). Using deoxymiroestrol the IC_{50} values for the respective assays were 1×10^{-10} M, 3×10^{-11} M and 2×10^{-11} M, and for miroestrol the respective IC_{50} values were, 3×10^{-10} M, 2×10^{-11} M and 8×10^{-11} M which compared with 1×10^{-11} M, 1×10^{-11} M and 2×10^{-11} M respectively for 17βoestradiol and 4×10^{-8} M, 2×10^{-8} M and 1×10^{-8} M, respectively for genistein. The results again showed the potency of miroestrol and deoxymiroestrol, in particular deoxymiroestrol, as phytoestrogens; indeed both of these compounds proved to show greater oestrogenicity than even 8-prenylnaringenin (see above).

Deoxybenzoins

Deoxybenzoins are intermediates in the synthesis of isoflavones whose oestrogenic activity has only recently been investigated (Fokialakis et al. 2004).

The affinity of deoxybenzoins for ERα and ERβ has been found to be similar to that of daidzein, although some types show selectivity and transcriptional bias towards ERβ (Fokialakis et al. 2004) as is typified by the isoflavone genistein. Molecular modelling has confirmed that deoxybenzoins fit well in the ligand binding pocket of ERβ and as such they represent a new class of ERβ selective phytoestrogen.

Coumestans

Coumestrol is a type of coumestan, a derivative of simple isoflavonoids. The main sources of coumestrol are alfalfa and clover, i.e. animal fodder, and as such any health benefits/risks relate more to veterinary science than human nutrition (Dixon 2004), although clover can be used as a medicinal plant (Nelson et al. 2002). Coumestrol shows strong oestrogenic activity, with binding for the oestrogen receptor higher than that of genistein. In the rat uterotrophic assay its oestrogen activity is similar to that of oestradiol (Tinwell et al. 2000). It has also been found that coumestrol can suppress oestrous cycles in rats and can negatively affect the sexual behaviour of male offspring (Whitten et al. 1995).

Phytoestrogens and human health: conclusions

The important question of whether phytoestrogens should be used to protect human health clearly requires much more information to be provided by appropriate studies. Factors such as age and biological responsiveness to the different potential protective or even harmful effects of phytoestrogens seem to play an important role.

In 1999, the US FDA allowed health claims (on food labels) on the association between soy protein and reduced risk of coronary heart disease, for foods containing ≥6.25 g of soya protein, assuming either four servings, or that a total of 25 g of soya protein are consumed daily. Furthermore, in 2002 the UK Joint Health Claims Initiative approved a health claim on the association between soya protein and cholesterol reduction, 'the inclusion of at least 25 g of soya protein per day, as part of a diet low in saturated fat, can help reduce blood cholesterol levels' and it is important to note that this claim relates to soya protein that has retained its naturally occurring isoflavones.

In conclusion, phytoestrogens have considerable potential in the field of health improvement. It is still unclear, however, whether phytoestrogens should be used as health-promoting foods or disease-preventing medicines (or both) but further large-scale human studies and the application of nutritional 'omics' technologies (Davis and Hord 2005) should provide a clearer picture in the near future. Furthermore, prospective studies of the effects of chronic consumption of high levels of phytoestrogens including soya isoflavones (Reinwald and Weaver 2006; Setchell 2006) at each stage of life to ascertain the risk to benefit ratio is an area of research that should be made a high priority, and that will also be of use to assessing their pharmaceutical potential (Usui 2006). However, it is likely that the greatest potential for phytoestrogens in the protection of human health, lies in including them in the diet early in life to help in the prevention of chronic diseases rather than attempting to use them to treat the pathogenic changes associated with disease that are usually irreversible.

References

Adams, N.R. (1995) Detection of the effects of phytoestrogens on sheep and cattle. *Journal of Animal Science* **73**, 1509–15.
Adlercreutz, H. (2002) Phyto-oestrogens and cancer. *Lancet Oncology* **3**, 32–40.

Adlercreutz, H., Markkanen, H. and Watanabe, S. (1993) Plasma concentrations of phytoestrogens in Japanese men. *Lancet* **342**, 1209–10.

Akiyama, T., Ishida, J., Nakagawa, S. et al. (1987) Genistein, a specific inhibitor of tyrosine-specific protein kinases. *Journal of Biological Chemistry* **262**, 5592–5.

Anderson, J.J. and Garner, S.C. (1998) Phytoestrogens and bone. *Ballieres Clinical Endocrinology and Metabolism* **12**, 543–57.

Anderson, J.W., Johnstone, B.M. and Cook-Newell, M.E. (1995) Meta-analysis of the effects of soy protein intake on serum lipids. *New England Journal of Medicine* **333**, 276–82.

Arora, A., Nair, N.G. and Strasburg, G.M. (1998) Antioxidant activities of isoflavones and their biological metabolites in a liposomal system. *Archives of Biochemistry and Biophysics* **356**, 133–41.

Arteaga, E., Villaseca, P., Rojas, A., Marshall, G. and Bianchi, M. (2004) Phytoestrogens possess a weak antioxidant activity on low density lipoprotein in contrast to the flavonoid quercetin *in vitro* in postmenopausal women. *Climacteric* **7**, 397–403.

Arts, J., Kuiper, G.G.J.M. and Janssen, J.M.M.F. (1997) Differential expression of estrogen receptors α and β mRNA during differentiation of human osteoblast SV-HFO cells. *Endocrinology* **138**, 5067–70.

Atkinson, C. and Bingham, S.A. (2002) Mammographic breast density as a biomarker of effects of isoflavones on the female breast. *Breast Cancer Research* **4**, 1–4.

Atkinson, C., Compston, J.E., Day, N.E., Dowsett, M. and Bingham, S.A. (2004a) The effects of phytoestrogen isoflavones on bone density in women: a double-blind, randomised, placebo-controlled trial. *American Journal of Clinical Nutrition* **79**, 326–33.

Atkinson, C., Oosthuizen, W., Scollen, S., Loktionov, A., Day, N.E. and Bingham, S.A. (2004b) Modest protective effects of isoflavones from a red clover-derived dietary supplement on cardiovascular diease risk factors in perimenopausal women, and evidence of an interaction with ApoE Genotype in 49–65 year-old women. *Journal of Nutrition* **134**, 1759–64.

Atkinson, C., Warren, R.M.L., Sala, E., Dowsett, M., Dunning, A.M., Healey, C.S., Runswick, S., Day, N.E. and Bingham, S.A. (2004c) Red clover-derived isoflavones and mammographic breast density: a double-blind, randomized, placebo-controlled trial. *Breast Cancer Research* **6**, R170–79.

Badger, T.M., Ronis, M.J., Hakkak, R., Rowlands, J.C. and Korourian, S. (2002) The health consequences of early soya consumption. *Journal of Nutrition* **132**, 559S–565S.

Bairey-Merz, C.N., Johnson, B.D., Braunstein, G.D., Pepine, C.J., Reis, S.E., Paul-Labrador, M., Hale, G., Sharaf, B.L., Bettner, V., Sopko, G. and Kelsey, S.F. (2006) Phytoestrogens and lipoproteins in women. *Journal of Clinical Endocrinology and Metabolism* **91**, 2209–13.

Barkhem, T., Carlsson, B. and Nilsson, Y. (1998) Differential response of estrogen receptor α and estrogen receptor β to partial estrogen agonists/antagonists. *Molecular Pharmacology* **54**,105–12.

Barnes, S. (1998) Phytoestrogens and breast cancer. *Ballieres Clinical Endocrinology and Metabolism* **12**, 559–79.

Bazzoli, D.L., Hill, S. and DiSilvestro, R.A. (2002) Soy protein antioxidant actions in active, young adult women. *Nutrition Research* **22**, 807–15.

Bhakta, D., Higgins, C.D., Sevak, L., Mangtani, P., Adlercreutz, H., McMichael, A.J. and dos Santos-Sliva, I. (2006) Phyto-oestrogen intake and plasma concentrations in South Asian and native British women resident in England. *British Journal of Nutrition* **95**, 1150–58.

Bingham, S.A., Atkinson, C., Liggins, J., Bluck, L. and Coward, A. (1998) Plant oestrogens: where are we now. *British Journal of Nutrition* **79**, 393–406.

Boccardo, F., Puntoni, M., Guglielmini, P. and Rubagotti, A. (2005) Enterolactone as a risk factor for breast cancer: a review of the published evidence. *Clinica Chimica Acta,* **365**, 58–67.

Boersma, B.J., D'Alessandro, T. and Benton, M.R. (2003) Neutrophil myeloperoxidase chlorinates and nitrates soy isoflavones and enhances their antioxidant properties. *Free Radical Biology and Medicine* **35**, 1417–30.

Boker, L.K., Van der Schouw, Y.T. and De Kleijn, M.J. (2002) Intake of dietary phytoestrogens by Dutch women. *Journal of Nutrition* **132**, 1319–28.

Bowey, E., Aldercreutz, A. and Rowland, I. (2003) Metabolism of isoflavones and lignans by the gut microflora: a study in germ-free and human flora associated rats. *Food and Chemical Toxicology* **41**, 631–6.

Boyd, N.F., Lockwood, G.A., Byng, J.W,, Tritchler, D.L. and Yaffe, M.J. (1998) Mammographic densities and breast cancer risk. *Cancer Epidemiology Biomarkers and Prevention* **7**, 1133–44.

Boyd, N.F., Lockwood, G.A.and Martin, L.J. (2001) Mammographic density as a marker of suscepti-bility to breast cancer: a hypothesis. *IARC Scientific Publications* **154**, 163–9.

Brosens, J.J. and Parker, M.G. (2003) Gene expression: oestrogen receptor hijacked. *Nature* **423**, 487–8.

Bruce, B., Messina, M. and Spiller, G.A. (2003) Isoflavone supplements do not affect thyroid function in iodine replete postmenopausal women. *Journal of Medicinal Food* **6**, 309–16.

Bruckdorfer, K.R. (1996) Antioxidants, lipoprotein oxidation, and arterial function. *Lipids* **31**, S83–5.

Bruner SD, Norman DPG, Verdine Gl. Structural basis for recognition and repair of the endogenous mutagen 8-oxoguanine in DNA. *Nature* **403**, 859–866, 2000.

Brzozowski, A.M., Pike, A.C.W. and Dauter, Z. (1997) Molecular basis of agonism and antagonism in the oestrogen receptor. *Nature* **389**, 753–8.

Buckley, C., Bund, S.J. and McTaggart, F. (1996) Oxidized low-density lipoproteins inhibit endothe-lium-dependent relaxations in isolated large and small rabbit coronary arteries. *Journal of Autonomic Pharmacology* **16**, 261–7.

Cain, J.C. (1960) Miroestrol: an oestrogen from the plant *Pueraria mirifica*. *Nature* **188**, 774–7.

Campbell, C.G., Brown, B.D., Dufner, D. and Thorland, W.G. (2006) Effects of soy or milk protein during a high-fat feeding challenge on oxidative stress, inflammation, and lipids in healthy men. *Lipids* **41**, 257–65.

Casini, M.L., Marelli, G., Papaleo, E., Ferrari, A., D'Ambroaio, F. and Unfer, V. (2006) Psycho-logical assessment of the effects of treatment with phytoestrogens on postmenopausal women: a randomized, double-blind, crossover, placebo-controlled study. *Fertility and Sterility* **85**, 972–8.

Cassidy, A., Brown, J.E., Hawdon, A., Faughnan, M.S., King, L.J., Millward, J., Zimmer-Nechemias, L., Wolfe, B. and Setchell, K.D. (2006) Factors affecting the bioavailability of soy isoflavones in humans after ingestion of physiologically relevant levels from different soy foods. *Journal of Nutrition* **136**, 45–51.

Chansakaow, S., Ishikawa, T., Seki, H., Sekine, K., Okada, M. and Chaichantipyuth, C. (2000) Identification of deoxymiroestrol as the actual rejuvenating principle of 'Kwao Keur', *Pueraria mirifica*. The known miroestrol may be an artefact. *Journal of Natural Products* **63**, 173–5.

Chen, Y.-M., Ho, S.C. and Lam, S.S.H. (2003) Soy isoflavones have a favourable effect on bone loss in Chinese postmenopausal women with lower bone mass: a double-blind, randomized, controlled trial. *Journal of Clinical Endocrinology and Metabolism* **88**, 4740–7.

Clarke, D.B. and Lloyd, A.S. (2004) Dietary exposure estimates of isoflavones from the 1998 UK Total Diet Study. *Food Additives and Contaminants* **21**, 305–16.

Clarke, D.B., Lloyd, A.S. and Botting, N.P. (2002) Measurement of intact sulfate and glucuron-ide phytoestrogen conjugates in human urine using isotope dilution liquid chromatography-tandem mass spectrometry with $[^{13}C_3]$ isoflavone internal standards. *Analytical Biochemistry* **309**, 158–72.

Clarkson, T.B. (2002) Soy, phytoestrogens and cardiovascular disease. *Journal of Nutrition* **132**, 566S–569S.

Clavel, T., Borrmann, D., Braune, A., Dore, J. and Blaut, M. (2006) Occurance and activity of human intestinal bacteria involved in the conversion of dietary lignans. *Anaerobe* **12**, 140–47.

Coldham, N.G., Darby, C. and Hows, M. (2002) Comparative metabolism of genistin by human and rat gut microflora: detection and identification of the end-products of metabolism. *Xenobiotica* **32**, 45–62.

Cooray, H.C., Janvilisri, T., van Ween, H.W., Hladky, S.B. and Barrand, M.A. (2004) Interaction of breast cancer resistance protein with plant polyphenols. *Biochemical and Biophysical Research Communications,* **317**, 269–75.

Cornwell, T., Cohick, W. and Raskin, I. (2004) Dietary phytoestrogens and health. *Phytochemistry* **65**, 995–1016.

Cotroneo, M.S., Wang, J., Fritz, W.A., Eltoum, I.E. and Lamartiniere, C.A. (2002) Genistein action in the prepubertal mammary gland in a chemoprevention model. *Carcinogenesis* **23**, 1467–74.

Coward, L., Barnes, N.C., Setchell, K.D.R. and Barnes, S. (1993) Genistein, daidzein and their β-glycoside conjugates: antitumor isoflavones in soybean foods from American and Asian diets. *Journal of Agricultural and Food Chemistry* **41**, 1961–7.

Crandall, D.L., Busler, D.E., Novak, T.J., Weber, R.V. and Kral, J.G. (1998) Identification of estrogen receptor beta RNA in human breast and abdominal subcutaneous adipose tissue. *Biochemical and Biophysical Research Communications* **248**, 523–6.

D'Alessandro, T., Prasain, J. and Benton, M.R. (2003) Polyphenols, inflammatory response, and cancer prevention: chlorination of isoflavones by human neutrophils. *Journal of Nutrition* **133**, 3773S–3777S.

Dahlman-Wright, K., Cavailles V., Fugua, S.A., Jordan, V.C., Katzenellenbogen J.A., Korach, K.S., Maggi, A., Muramatsu, M., Parker, M.G. and Gustafsson, J-A. (2006) International Union of Phamacology. LXIV. Estrogen receptors. *Pharmacological Reviews* **58**, 773–81.

Dalu, A., Haskell, J.F., Coward, L. and Lamartiniere, C.A. (1998) Genistein, a component of soy, inhibits the expression of the EGF and ErbB/Neu receptors in the rat dorsolatteral prostate. *Prostate* **37**, 36–43.

Davis, C.D. and Hord, N.G. (2005) Nutritional 'omics' technologies for elucidating the role(s) of bioactive food components in colon cancer prevention. *Journal of Nutrition* **135**, 2694–7.

Deavours, B.E. and Dixon, R. (2005) Metabolic engineering of isoflavonoid biosynthesis in alfalfa. *Plant Physiology* **138**, 2245–59.

Desroches, S., Mauger, J.F., Ausman, L.M., Lichtenstein, A.H. and Lamarche, B. (2004) Soy protein favourably affects LDL size independently of isoflavones in hypercholesterlemic men and women. *Journal of Nutrition* **134**, 574–9.

Divi, R.L., Chang, H.C. and Doerge, D.R. (1997) Anti-thyroid isoflavones from soybean: isolation, characterization and mechanisms of action. *Biochemical Pharmacology* **54**, 1087–96.

Dixon, R.A. (2004) Phytoestrogens. *Annual Review of Plant Biology* **55**, 225–61.

Djuric, Z., Chen, G., Doerge, D.R., Heilbrun, L.K. and Kucuk, O. (2001) Effect of soy isoflavone supplementation on markers of oxidative stress in men and women. *Cancer Letters* **172**, 1–6.

Dubey, R.K., Gillespie, D.G. and Imthurn, B. (1999) Phytoestrogens inhibit growth and MAP kinase activity in human aortic smooth muscle cells. *Hypertension* **33**, 177–82.

Duffy, R., Wiseman, H. and File, S. (2003) Improved cognitive function in postmenopausal women after 12 weeks of consumption of a soy extract containing isoflavones. *Pharmacology Biochemistry and Behavior* **75**, 721–9.

Eden, J. (1998) Phytoestrogens and the menopause. *Ballieres Clinical Endocrinology and Metabolism* **12**, 581–7.

Engelman, H.M., Alekel, D.L., Hanson, L.N., Kanthasamy, A.G. and Reddy, M.B. (2005) Blood lipid and oxidative stress responses to soy protein with isoflavones and phytic acid in postmenopausal women. *American Journal of Clinical Nutrition* **81**, 590–6.

Fam, S.S. and Morrow, J.D. (2003) The isoprostanes: unique products of arachidonic acid oxidation a review. *Current Medicinal Chemistry* **10**, 1723–40.

Fentiman, I.S., Wang, D.Y. and Allen, D.S. (1994) Bone density of normal women in relation to endogenous and exogenous oestrogens. *British Journal of Rheumatology* **33**, 808–15.

File, S.E., Duffy, R. and Wiseman, H. (2002) Soya improves human memory. In: *Soy and Health, Clinical Evidence and Dietetic Applications* (eds, C.K. Descheemaeter and I. Debruyre), pp. 167–73. Antwerp-Apeldoorn: Garant.

File, S.E., Hartley, D.E., Elsabagh, S., Duffy, R. and Wiseman, H. (2005) Cognitive improvement after 6 weeks of soy supplementation in postmenopausal women is limited to frontal lobe function. *Menopause* **12**, 193–201.

File, S.E., Jarrett, N., Fluck, E., Duffy, R., Casey, K. and Wiseman, H. (2001) Eating soya improves human memory. *Psychopharmacology* **157**, 430–6.

Fletcher, R.J. (2003) Food sources of phyto-oestrogens and their precursors in Europe. *British Journal of Nutrition* **89** (Suppl 1), S39–43.

Fokialakis, N., Lambrinidis, G., Mitsiou, D.J. Aligiannis, N., Mitakou, S., Skaltsounis, A.L., Pratsinis, H., Mikros, E. and Alexis, M.N. (2004) A new class of phytoestrogens; evaluation of the oestrogenic activity of deoxybenzoins. *Chemistry and Biology* **11**, 397–406.

Fontecave, M., Lepoivre, M., Elleingand, E., Gerez, C. and Guitter, O. (1998) Resveratrol, a remarkable inhibitor of ribonucleotide reductase. *FEBS Letters* **421**, 277–9.

Foti, P., Erba, D. and Riso, P. (2005) Comparison between daidzein and genistein antioxidant activity in primary and cancer lymphocytes. *Archives of Biochemistry and Biophysics* **433**, 431–27.

Fotsis, T., Pepper, M. and Adlercreutz, H. (1995) Genistein, a dietary ingested isoflavonoid, inhibits cell proliferation and *in vitro* angiogenesis. *Journal of Nutrition* **125**, 790S–797S.

Fotsis, T., Pepper, M., Adlercreutz, H., Fleischmann, G., Hase, T., Montesano, R. and Schweigerer, L. (1993) Genistein, a dietary-derived inhibitor of *in vitro* angiogenesis. *Proceedings of the National Academy of Sciences USA* **90**, 2690–4.

Franco, O.H., Burger, H., Lebrun, C.E., Peeters, P.H., Lamberts, S.W., Grobbee, D.E. and Van der Schouw, Y.T. (2005) Higher dietary intake of lignans is associated with better cognitive performance in postmenopausal women. *Journal of Nutrition* **135**, 1190–95.

Franke, A.A., Yu, M.C. and Maskarinec, G. (1999) Phytoestrogens in human biomatrices including breast milk. *Biochemical Society Transactions* **27**, 308–18.

Fritz, W., Wang, J., Coward, L. and Lamartiniere, C.A. (1998) Dietary genistein: perinatal mammary cancer prevention, bioavailability and toxicity testing in the rat. *Carcinogenesis* **19**, 2151–8.

Gambacciani, M., Ciaponi, M., Cappagli, B., Piaggesi, L. and Genazzani, A.R. (1997) Effects on combined low dose of the isoflavone derivative ipriflavone and estrogen replacement on bone mineral density and metabolism in postmenopausal women. *Maturitas* **28**, 75–81.

Gang, D.R., Kasahara, H., Xia, Z.Q., Mijnsbrugge, K.V. Bauw, G., Boerjan, W., Van Montagu, M., Davin, L.B. and Lewis, N.G. (1999) Evolution of plant defense mechansisms: relationships of phenylcoumaran benzylic ether reductases to pinoresinol-lariciresinol and isoflavone reductases. *Journal of Biological Chemistry* **274**, 7516–27.

Giampietro, P.G., Bruno, G. and Furcolo, G. (2004) Soy protein formulas in children: no hormonal effects in long term feeding. *Journal of Pediatric Endocrinology and Metabolism* **17**, 191–6.

Gotoh, T., Yamada, K. and Ito, A. (1998b) Chemoprevention of N-nitroso-N-methylurea-induced rat mammary cancer by miso and tamoxifen, alone and in combination. *Japanese Journal of Cancer Research* **89**, 487–95.

Gotoh, T., Yamada, K. and Yin, H. (1998a) Chemoprevention of N-nitroso-N-methylurea-induced rat mammary carcinogenesis by soy foods or biochanin A. *Japanese Journal of Cancer Research* **89**, 137–42.

Grainger, D.J. and Metcalfe, J.C. (1996) Tamoxifen: teaching an old drug new tricks. *Nature Medicine* **2**, 381–5.

Greene, G.L., Gilna, P., Waterfield, M., Baker, A., Hort, A. and Shine, J. (1986) Sequence and expression of human estrogen receptor complementary DNA. *Science* **231**, 1150–54.

Greenwald, P. (2004) Clinical trials in cancer prevention: current results and perspectives for the future. *Journal of Nutrition* **134** (12 Suppl), 3507S–3512S.

Guo, J.Y., Li, X. and Browning, J.D., Jr (2004) Dietary soy isoflavones and estrone protect ovariectomized ERalphaKO and wild-type mice from carcinogen-induced colon cancer. *Journal of Nutrition* **134**, 179–82.

Ha, T.C., Lyons-Wall, P.M., Moore, D.E., Tattam, B.N., Boyages, J., Ung, O.A. and Taylor, R.J. (2006) Phytoestrogens and indicators of breast cancer prognosis. *Nutrition and Cancer* **56**, 3–10.

Hall, W.L., Vafeiadou, K., Hallund, J., Bugel, S., Koebnick, C., Reimann, M., Ferrari, M., Branca, F., Talbot, D., Dadd, T., Nilsson, M., Dahlman-Wright, K., Gustafsson, J.A., Minihane, A.M. and Williams, C.M. (2005) Soy-isoflavone-enriched foods and inflammatory biomarkers of cardiovascular disease risk in postmenopausal women: interactions with genotype and equol production. *American Journal of Clinical Nutrition* **82**, 1260–68.

Hall, W.L., Vafeiadou, K., Hallund, J., Bugel, S., Reimann, M., Koebnick, C., Zunft, H.J., Ferrari, M., Branca, F., Dadd, T., Talbot, D., Powell, J., Minihane, A.M., Cassidy, A., Nilsson, M., Dahlman-Wright, K., Gustafsson, J.A. and Williams, C.M. (2006) Soy-iosflavone-enriched foods and markers of lipid and glucose metabolism in postmenopausal women: interactions with genotype and equol production. *American Journal of Clinical Nutrition* **83**, 592–600.

Halliwell, B., Rafter, J. and Jenner, A. (2005) Health promotion by flavonoids, tocopherols, tocotrienols, and other phenols: direct of indirect effects? Antioxidant or not? *American Journal of Clinical Nutrition* **81** (suppl) 268S–276S.

Halliwell, B. and Whiteman, M. (2004) Measuring reactive species and oxidative damage *in vivo* and in cell culture: how should you do it and what do the results mean? *British Journal of Pharmacology* **142**, 231–55.

Hanna, K., Wong, J., Patterson, C., O'Neill, S. and Lyons-Wall, P. (2004) Phytoestrogen intake, excretion and markers of bone health in Australian women. *Asia Pacific Journal of Clinical Nutrition* **13** (Suppl), S74.

Hargreaves, D.F., Potten, C.S. and Harding, C. (1999) Two-week soy supplementation has estrogenic effect on normal premenopausal breast. *Journal of Clinical Endocrinology and Metabolism* **84**, 4017–24.

Harris, D.M., Besselink, E., Henning, S.M., Go, V.L.W. and Heber, D. (2005) Phytoestrogens induce differential estrogen receptor alpha- or beta-mediated responses in transfected breast cancer cells. *Experimental Biology and Medicine* **230**, 558–68.

Hayashibara, T., Yamada, Y., Nakayama, S., Harasawa, H., Tsuruda, K., Sugahara, K., Miyanishi, T., Kamihira, S., Tomonaga, M. and Maita, T. (2002) Resveratrol induces downregulation in surviving in expression and apoptosis in HTLV-1 infected cell lines: a prospective agent for adult T cell leukaemia chemotherapy. *Nutrition and Cancer* **44**, 193–201.

Hedelin, M., Klint, A., Chang, E.T., Bellocco, R., Johansson, J.E., Andersson, S.O., Heinonen, S.M., Aldercreutz, H., Adami, H.O., Gronberg, H. and Balter K.A. (2006) Dietary phytoestrogen, serum enterolactone and risk of prostate cancer: the cancer prostate Sweden study (Sweden). *Cancer Causes and Control* **17**, 169–80.

Heinloth, A., Brune, B., Fischer, B. and Galle, J. (2002) Nitric oxide prevents oxidised LDL-induced p53 accumulation, cytochrome c translocation and apoptosis in macrophages via guanylate cyclase stimulation. *Atherosclerosis* **162**, 93–101.

Heneman, K.M., Chang, H.C., Prior, R.L. and Steinberg, F.M. (2007) Soy protein with and without isoflavones fails to substantially increase postprandial antioxidant capacity. *Journal of Nutritional Biochemistry* **18**, 46–53.

Hernandez-Montes, E., Pollard, S.E., Vauzour, D., Jofre-Montseny, L., Rota, C., Rimbach, G., Weinberg, P.D. and Spencer, J.P. (2006) Activation of glutathione peroxidase via Nrf1 mediates genistein's protection against oxidative endothelial cell injury. *Biochemical and Biophysical Research Communications* **346**, 851–9.

Hilakivi-Clarke, L., Cho, E. and Clarke, R. (1998) Maternal genistein exposure mimics the effects of oestrogen on mammary gland development in female mouse offspring. *Oncology Reports* **5**, 609–15.

Hilakivi-Clarke, L., Cho, E., Onojafe, I., Raygada, M. and Clarke, R. (1999a) Maternal exposure to genistein during pregnancy increases carcinogen-induced mammary tumorigenesis in female rat offspring. *Oncology Reports* **6**, 1089–95.

Hilakivi-Clarke, L., Onojafe, I., Raygada, M., Cho, E., Skaar, T., Russo, I and Clarke, R. (1999b) Prepubertal exposure to zearalenone or genistein reduces mammary tumorigenesis. *British Journal of Cancer* **80**, 1682–8.

Hodgson, J.M., Croft, K.D., Puddey, I.B., Mori, T.A. and Beilin, L.J. (1996) Soybean isoflavonoids and their metabolic products inhibit *in vitro* lipoprotein oxidation in serum. *Journal of Nutritional Biochemistry* **7**, 664–9.

Hodgson, J.M., Puddey, I.B. and Croft, K.D. (1999) Isoflavonoids do not inhibit *in vivo* lipid peroxidation in subjects with high-normal blood pressure. *Atherosclerosis* **145**, 167–2.

Hoey, L., Rowland, I.R., Lloyd, A.S., Clarke, D.B. and Wiseman, H. (2004) Influence of soya-based infant formula consumption on isoflavone and gut microflora metabolite concentrations in urine and on faecal microflora composition and metabolic activity in infants and children. *British Journal of Nutrition* **91**, 607–16.

Holzbeierlein, J.M., McIntosh, J. and Thrasher, J.B. (2005) The role of soy phytoestrogens in prostate cancer. *Current Opinion in Urology* **15**, 17–22.

Horn-Ross, P.L., Barnes, S., Lee, V.S., Collins, C.N., Reynolds, P., Lee, M.M., Stewart, S.L., Canchola, A.J., Wilson, L. and Jones, K. (2006) Reliability and validity of an assessment of usual phytoestrogen consumption (United States). *Cancer Causes and Control* **17**, 85–93.

Hsieh, C.Y., Santell, R.C., Haslam, S.Z. and Helferich, W.G. (1998) Estrogenic effects of genistein on the growth of estrogen receptor-positive human breast cancer (MCF-7) cells *in vitro* and *in vivo Cancer Research* **58**, 3833–8.

Huntley, A.L. and Ernst, E. (2004) Soy for the treatment of perimenopausal symptoms – a systematic review. *Maturitas* **47**, 1–9.

Hur, H.-G., Lay, J.L., Beger, R.D., Freeman, J.P. and Rafii, F. (2000) Isolation of human intestinal bacteria metabolising the natural isoflavone glycosides daidzin and genistin. *Archives of Microbiology* **174**, 422–8.

Ikeda, Y., Iki, M., Morita, A., Kajita, E., Kagamimori, S., Kagawa, Y. and Yoneshima, H. (2006) Intake of fermented soybeans, natto, is associated with reduced bone loss in postmenopausal women: Japanese population-based osteoporosis (JPOS) study. *Journal of Nutrition* **136**, 1323–8.

Ingram, D,, Sanders, K., Kolybaba, M. and Lopez, D. (1997) Case control study of phyto-oestrogens and breast cancer. *Lancet* **350**, 990–94.

Jang, M., Cai, L., Udeani, G.O., Slowing, K.V., Thomas, C.F., Beecher C.W., Fong, H.H., Farnsworth, N.R., Kinghorn, A.D., Mehta, R.G., Moon, R.C. and Pezzuto, J.M. (1997) Cancer chemopreventive activity of resveratrol, a natural product derived from grapes. *Science* **275**, 218–20.

Johnson, D.W., Berg, J.N. and Baldwin, M.A. (1996) Mutations in the activin receptor-like kinase I gene in hereditary haemorrhagic telangiectasia type 2. *Nature Genetics* **13**, 189–95.

Katzenellenbogen, J.A., O'Malley, B.W. and Katzenellenbogen, B.S. (1996) Tripartite steroid hormone receptor pharmacology: interaction with multiple effector sites as a basis for the cell- and promoter-specific action of these hormones. *Molecular Endocrinology* **10**, 119–31.

Kelly, G.E., Joannou, G.E., Reeder, A.Y., Nelson, C. and Waring, M.A. (1995) The variable metabolic response to dietary isoflavones in humans. *Proceedings of the Society for Experimental Biology and Medicine* **208**, 40–43.

Kim, H., Peterson, T.G. and Barnes, S. (1998) Mechanisms of action of the soy isoflavone genistein: emerging role of its effects through transforming growth facotr beta signaling pathways. *American Journal of Clinical Nutrition* **68**, 1418S–1425S.

Kim, H., Xu, J. and Su, Y. (2001) Actions of the soy phytoestrogen genistein in models of human chronic disease: potential involvement of transforming growth factor β. *Biochemical Society Transactions* **29**, 216–22.

Kim, J.W., Kim, Y.T. and Kim, D.K. (1996) Expression of epidermal growth factor receptor in carcinoma of the cervix. *Gynecologic Oncology* **60**, 283–287.

Kim, H., Deshane, J., Barnes, S. and Meleth, S. (2006) Protemics analysis of the actions of grape seed extract in rat brain: technological and biological implications for the study of the actions of psychoactive compounds. *Life Science* **78**, 2060–65.

King, R.A. and Bursill, D.B. (1998) Plasma and urinary kinetics of the isoflavones daidzein and genistein after a single soy meal in humans. *American Journal of Clinical Nutrition* **67**, 867–72.

Koehler, K.F., Helguero, L.A., Haldosen, L.-A., Warner, M. and Gustafsson, J.-A. (2005) Reflections on the discovery and significance of estrogen receptor β. *Endocrine Reviews* **26**, 465–78.

Kondo, K., Tsuneizumi, K., Watanabe, T. and Oishi, M. (1991) Induction of *in vivo* differentiation of mouse embryonal carcinoma (F9) cells by inhibitors of topoisomerases. *Cancer Research* **50**, 5398–404.

Krebs, E.E., Ensrud, K.E., MacDonald, R. and Wilt, T.J. (2004) Phytoestrogens for treatment of menopausal symptoms: a systematic review. *Obstetrics and Gynecology* **104**, 824–36.

Kreijkamp-Kaspers, S., Kok, L., Bots, M.L., Grobbee, D.E. and Van Der Schouwy, T. (2005) Dietary phytoestrognes and plasma lipids in Dutch postmenopausal women; a cross-sectional study. *Atherosclerosis* **178**, 95–100.

Kreijkamp-Kaspers, S., Kok, L. and Grobbee, D.E. (2004) Effect of soy protein containing isoflavones on cognitive function, bone mineral density and plasma lipids in postmenopausal women. *JAMA* **292**, 65–74.

Kritz-Silverstein, D., Von Muhlen, D., Barrett-Connor, E., Bressel, M.A. (2003) Isoflavones and cognitive function in older women: the SOy and Postmenopausal Health In Aging (SOPHIA) study. *Menopause* **10**, 196–202.

Kruse, F.E., Joussen, A.M. and Fotsis, T. (1997) Inhibition of neovacularizationof the eye by dietary factors exemplified by isoflavonoids. *Ophthalmologie* **94**, 152–6.

Kuiper, G.G.J.M., Carlsson, B., Grandien, K. (1997) Comparison of the ligand binding specificity and transcript tissue distribution of estrogen receptors α and β. *Endocrinology* **138**, 863–70.

Kuiper, G.G.J.M., Enmark, E., Pelto-Huikko, M., Nilsson, S. and Gustafsson, J.-A. (1996) Cloning of a novel estrogen receptor expressed in rat prostate and ovary. *Proceedings of the National Academy of Sciences USA* **93**, 5925–30.

Kuiper, G.G.J.M., Lemmen, J.G. and Carlsson, B.O. (1998) Interaction of estrogenic chemicals and phytoestrogens with estrogen receptor β. *Endocrinology* **139**, 4252–63.

Lamartiniere, C.A., Moore, J.B. and Brown, N.A. (1995) Genistein suppresses mammary cancer in rats. *Carcinogenesis* **16**, 2833–40.

Lampe, J.W., Karr, S.C., Hutchins, A.M. and Slavin, J.L. (1998) Urinary equol excretion with a soy challenge: influence of habitual diet. *Proceedings of the Society for Experimental Biology and Medicine* **217**, 335–9.

Lampe, J.W., Skor, H.E., Li, S. (2001) Wheat bran and soy protein do not alter urinary excretion of the isoflavan equol in premonopausal women. *Journal of Nutrition* **131**, 740–44.

Lapcik, O., Hill, M., Hampl, R., Wahala, K. and Adlercreutz, H. (1998) Identification of isoflavonoids in beer. *Steroids* **63**, 14–20.

Lephart, E.D., Porter, J.P., Hedges, D.W., Lund, T.D. and Setchell, K.D. (2004) Phytoestrogens: implications in neurovascular research. *Current Neurovascular Research* **1**, 455–64.

Leung, Y.-K, Mak, P., Hassan, S. and Ho, S.-M. (2006) Estrogen receptor (ER)-β isoforms: a key to understanding ER-β signalling. *PNAS* **103**, 13162–7.

Low, Y.L., Taylor, J.I., Grace, P.B., Dowsett, M., Folkerd, E., Doody, D., Dunning, A.M., Scollen, S., Mulligan, A.A., Welch, A.A., Luben, R.N., Khaw, K.T., Day, N.E., Wareham, N.J. and Bingham, S.A. (2005) Polymorphisms in the CYP19 gene may affect the positive correlations between serum and urine phytoestrogen metabolites and plasma androgen concentrations in men. *Journal of Nutrition* **135**, 2680–86.

Low, Y.L, Taylor, J.I., Grace, P.B., Mulligan, A.A., Welch, A.A., Scollen, S., Dunning, A.M., Lube, R.N., Khaw, K.T., Day, N.E., Wareham, N.J. and Bingham, S.A. (2006) Phytoestrogen exposure, polymorphisms in COMT, CYP19, ESR1, and SHBG genes, and their associations with prostrate cancer risk. *Nutrition Cancer* **56**, 31–9.

Lu, L.J. and Anderson, K.E. (1998) Sex and long-term diets affect the metabolism and excretion of soy isoflavones in humans. *American Journal of Clinical Nutrition* **68** (suppl), 1500S–1504S.

Lu, L.J., Grady, J.J., Marshall, M.V., Ramanujam, V.M. and Anderson, K.E. (1995) Altered time course of urinary daidzein and genistein excretion during chronic soya diet in healthy male subjects. *Nutrition and Cancer* **24**, 311–23.

Lu, L.J., Lin, S.N., Grady, J.J., Nagamani, M. and Anderson, K.E. (1996) Altered kinetics and extent of urinary daidzein and genestein excretion in women during chronic soy exposure. *Nutrition and Cancer* **26**, 289–302.

Lund, T.D., Munson, D.J. and Haldy, M.E. (2004) Equol is a novel anti-androgen that inhbits prostate growth and hormone feedback. *Biology of Reproduction* **70**, 1188–95.

Lydeking-Olsen, E., Beck-Jensen, J.E., Setchell, K.D. and Holm-Jensen, T. (2004) Soymilk or progesterone for prevention of bone loss: a 2 year randomised, placebo-controlled trial. *European Journal of Nutrition* **43**, 246–57.

McCarty, M.F. (2006) Isoflavones made simple – genistein's agonist activity for the beta-type estrogen receptor mediates their health benefits. *Medical Hypotheses* **66**, 1093–114.

Macready, A.L., Kennedy, O.B., Ellis, J.A., Williams, C.M., Spencer, J.P.E. and Butler, L.T. (2009) Flavonoids and cognitive function: a review of human randomized controlled trial studies and recommendations for future studies. *Genes and Nutrition* **4**, 227–42.

McVeigh, B.L., Dillingham, B.L., Lampe, J.W. and Duncan, A.M. (2006) Effect of soy protein varying isoflavone content on serum lipids in healthy young men. *American Journal of Clinical Nutrition* **83**, 244–51.

Magee, P.J. and Rowland, I.R. (2004) Phyto-oestrogens, their mechanism of action: current evidence for a role in breast and prostate cancer. *British Journal of Nutrition* **91**, 513–31.

Makela, S., Poutanen, M. and Kostlan, M.L. (1998) Inhibition of 17 beta-hydroxysteroid oxidoreductase by flavonoids in breast and prostate cancer cells. *Proceedings of the Society for Experimental Biology and Medicine* **217**, 310–16.

Makela, S., Savolainen, H. and Aavik, E. (1999) Differentiation between vasculoprotective and uterotrophic effects of ligands with different binding affinities to estrogen receptors α and β. *Proceedings of the National Academy of Sciences USA* **96**, 7077–72.

Markiewicz, L., Garey, J., Aldercreutz, H. and Gurpide, E. (1993) *In-vitro* bioassays of non-steroidal phytoestrogens. *Journal of Steroid Biochemistry* **45**, 399–405.

Matsumura, A., Ghosh, A., Pope, G.S. and Darbre, P.D. (2005) Comparative study of oestrogenic properties of eight phytoestrogens in MCF7 human breast cancer cells. *Journal of Steroid Biochemistry and Molecular Biology* **94**, 431–43.

Mendez, M.A., Anthony, M.S. and Arab, L. (2002) Soy-based formulae and infant growth and development. *Journal of Nutrition* **132**, 2127–30.

Meng, Q.H., Hockerstedt, A. and Heinonen, S. (1999) Antioxidant protection of lipoproteins containing estrogens: *in vitro* evidence for low- and high-density lipoproteins as estrogen carriers. *Biochimica et Biophysica Acta* **1439**, 331–40.

Merritt, R.J. and Jenks, B.H. (2004) Safety of soy-based infant formulas containing isoflavones: the clinical evidence. *Journal of Nutrition* **134**, 1220S–1224S.

Messina, M. (2010) Insights gained from 20 years of soy research. *Journal of Nutrition* **140**, 2289S–2295S.

Messina, M., Ho, S. and Alekel, D.L. (2004) Skeletal benefits of soy isoflavones: a review of the clinical trial epidemiologic data. *Current Opinion in Clinical Nutrition and Metabolic Care* **7**, 649–58.

Messina, M., Persky, V., Setchell, K.D.R. and Barnes, S. (1994) Soy intake and cancer risk: a review of the *in vitro* and *in vivo* data. *Nutrition and Cancer* **21**, 113–31.

Messina, M. and Redmond, G. (2006) Effects of soy protein and soybean isoflavones on thyroid function in healthy adults and hypothyroid patients: a review of the relevant literature. *Thyroid* **16**, 249–58.

Miksicek, R.J. (1995) Estrogenic flavonoids. structural requirements for biological activity. *Proceedings of the Society for Experimental Biology and Medicine* **208**, 44–50.

Milder, I.E.J., Feskens, E.J.M., Arts, I.C.W., Bueno-de-Mesquita, H.B., Hollman, P.C.H. and Kromhout, D. (2006) Intakes of 4 dietary lignans and cause-specific and all-cause mortality in the Zutphen Elderly Study. *American Journal of Clinical Nutrition* **84**, 400–5.

Milligan, S.R., Kalita, J.C., Heyerick, A., Rong, H., De Cooman, L. and De Keukeleire, D. (1999) Identification of a potent phytoestrogen in hops (*Humulus lupulus* L.) and beer. *Journal of Clinical Endocrinology and Metabolism* **84**, 2249–52.

Milligan, S.R., Kalita, J.C., Pocock, V., Van De Kauter, V., Stevens, J.F., Deinzer, M.L., Rong, H. and De Keukeleire, D. (2000) The endocrine activities of 8-prenylnaringenin and related hop (*Humulus lupulus* L.) flavonoids. *Journal of Clinical Endocrinology and Metabolism* **85**, 4912–15.

Miquel, J., Ramirez-Bosca, A., Ramirez-Bosca, J.V. and Alperi, J.D. (2006) Menopause: a review on the role of oxygen stress and favourable effects of dietary antioxidants. *Archives of Gerontology and Geriatrics* **42**, 289–306.

Miranda, C.L., Aponso, G.L., Stevens, J.F., Deinzer, M.L. and Buhler, D.R. (2000c) Prenylated chalcones and flavonones as inducers of quinone reductase in mouse Hepa 1c1c7 cells. *Cancer Letters* **149**, 21–9.

Miranda, C.L, Stevens, J.F., Helmrich, A., Henderson, M.C., Rodriguez, R.J., Yang, Y.H., Deinzer, M.L., Barnes, D.W. and Buhler, D.R. (1999) Antiproliferative and cytotoxic effects of prenylated flavonoids from hops (*Humulus lupulus*) in human cancer cell lines. *Food and Chemical Toxicology* **37**, 271–85.

Miranda, C.L., Stevens, J.F., Ivanov, V., McCall, M., Frei, B., Deinzer, M.L. and Buhler, D.R. (2000a) Antioxidant and prooxidant actions of prenylated and nonprenylated chalcones and flavanones *in vitro*. *Journal of Agricultural and Food Chemistry* **48**, 3876–84.

Miranda, C.L., Yang, Y.H., Henderson, M.C., Stevens, J.F., Santana-Rios, G., Deinzer, M.L. and Buhler, D.R. (2000b) Prenylated flavonoids from hops inhibit the metabolic acitivation of the carcinogenic heterocyclic amine 2-amino-3-methylimidazo[4,5-*f*]quinoline, mediated by cDNA-expressed human CYP1A2. *Drug Metabolism and Disposition* **28**, 1297–302.

Mitchell, J.H., Gardner, P.T. and Mcphail, D.B. (1998) Antioxidant efficacy of phytoestrogens in chemical and biological model systems. *Archives of Biochemistry and Biophysics* **360**, 142–8.

Monteiro, R., Becker, H., Azevedo, I. and Calhau, C. (2006) Effect of hop (*Humulus lupulus* L.) flavonoids on aromatase (oestrogen synthase) activity. *Journal of Agricultural and Food Chemistry* **54**, 2938–43.

Morton, M.S., Matos-Ferreira, A. and Abranches-Monteiro, L. (1997) Measurement and metabolism of isoflavonoids and lignans in the human male. *Cancer Letters* **114**, 145–51.

Morton, M.S., Wilcox, G., Wahlqvist, M.L. and Griffiths, K. (1994) Determination of lignans and isoflavonoids in human female plasma following dietary supplementation. *Journal of Endocrinology* **142**, 251–9.

Mueller, S.O., Simon, S., Chae, K., Metzier, M. and Korach, K.S. (2004) Phytoestrogens and their human metabolites show distinct agonistic and antagonistic properties on estrogen receptor alpha (ERalpha) and ERbeta in human cells. *Toxicological Sciences* **80**, 14–25.

Mulligan, A.A., Welch, A.A., McTaggart, A.A., Bhaniani, A. and Bingham, S.A. (2007) Intakes and sources of soya foods and isoflavones in a UK population cohort study (EPIC-Norfolk). *European Journal of Clinical Nutrition* **61**, 248–54.

Munro, I.C., Harwood, M. and Hlywka, J.J. (2003) Soy Isoflavones: a safety review. *Nutrition Reviews* **61**, 1–33.

Murkies, A.L., Lombard, C. and Strauss, B.I.G. (1995) Dietary flour supplementation decreases post-menopausal hot flushes: effect of soy and wheat. *Maturitas* **21**, 189–95.

Nelson, H.D., Vesco, K.K., Haney, E., Fu, R., Nedrow, A., Miller, J., Nicolaidis, C., Walker, M. and Humphrey, L. (2006) Nonhormonal therapies for menopausal hot flushes: systematic review and meta-analysis. *Journal of the American Medical Association* **295**, 2057–71.

Nelson, J., Barrette, E.P., Tsouronis, C., Basch, S. and Bent, S. (2002) Red clover (*Trifolium pratense*) monograph: a clinical decision support tool. *Journal of Herbal Pharmacotherapy* **2**, 49–72.

Nestel, P.J., Yamashita, T., Sasahara, T., Pomeroy, S., Dart, A., Komesaroff, P., Owen, A. and Abbey, M. (1997) Soy isoflavones improve systemic arterial compliance but not plasma lipid in menopausal and perimenopausal women. *Arteriosclerosis Thrombosis and Vascular Biology* **17**, 3392–8.

Newton, K.M., Lacroix, A.Z., Levy, L., Li, S.S., Qu, P., Potter, J.D. and Lampe, J.W. (2006) Soy protein and bone mineral density in older men and women: a randomized trial. *Maturitas* **55**, 270–77.

Nguyen, D.T., Hernandez-Montes, E., Vauzour, D., Schonthal, A.H., Rice-Evans, C., Cadenas, E. and Spencer, J.P. (2006) The intracellular genistein metabolite 5,7,3′,4′-tetrahydroxyisoflavone mediates G2-M cell cycle arrest in cancer cells via modulation of the p38 signaling pathway. *Free Radical Biology and Medicine* **41**, 1225–39.

Nhan, S., Anderson, K.E., Nagamani, M., Grady, J.J. and Lu, L.J. (2005) Effect of soymilk supplement containing isoflavones on urinary F2 isoprostane levels in premenopausal women. *Nutrition and Cancer* **53**, 73–81.

O'Reilly, J.D., Mallet, A.I. and McAnlis, G.T. (2001) Consumption of flavonoids in onions and black tea: lack of effect on F_2-isoprostanes and autoantibodies to oxidized LDL in healthy humans. *American Journal of Clinical Nutrition* **73**, 1040–44.

O'Reilly, J.D., Sanders, T.A.B. and Wiseman, H. (2000) Flavonoids protect against oxidative damage to LDL *in vitro*: use in selection of a flavonoid rich diet and relevance to LDL oxidation resistance *ex vivo? Free Radical Research* **33**, 419–26.

Olsen, A., Knudsen, K.E., Thomsen, B.L., Loft, S., Stripp, C., Overvad, K., Moller, S. and Tjonneland, A. (2004) Plasma enterolactone and breast cancer incidence by oestrogen receptor status. *Cancer Epidemiology Biomarkers and Prevention,* **13**, 2084–9.

Onoe, Y., Miyaura, C., Ohta, H., Nozawa, S. and Suda, T. (1997) Expression of estrogen receptor β in rat bone. *Endocrinology* **138**, 4509–12.

Orallo, F., Alvarez, E., Camina, M., Leiro, J.M., Gomez, E. and Fernandez, P. (2002) The possible implication of trans-resveratrol in the cardioprotective effects of long-term moderate wine consumption. *Molecular Pharmacology* **61**, 294–302.

de Pascual-Teresa, S., Hallund, J., Talbot, D., Schroot, J., Williams, C.M., Bugel, S. and Cassidy, A. (2006) Absorption of isoflavones in humans: effects of food matrix and processing. *Journal of Nutritional Biochemistry* **17**, 257–64.

Peeters, P.H., Slimani, N, van der Schouw, Y.T., Grace, P.B., Navarro, C., Tjonneland, A., Olsen, A., Clavel-Chapelon, F., Touillaud, M., Boutron-Ruault, M.C., Jenab, M., Kaaks, R., Linseisen, J., Trichopoulou, A., Trichopoulos, D., Dilis, V., Boeing, H., Weikert, C., Overad, K., Pala, V., Gils, C.H., Skeie, G., Jakszyn, P., Hallmans, G., Berglund, G., Key, T.J., Travis, R., Riboli, E. and Bingham, S.A. (2007) Variations in plasma phytoestrogen concentrations in European adults. *Journal of Nutrition* **137**, 1294–300.

Pepper, M.S., Hazel, S.J., Humpel, M. and Schleuning, W.D. (2004) 8-Prenylnaringenin, a novel phytoestrogen, inhibits angiogenesis *in vitro* and *in vivo*. *Journal of Cell Physiology* **199**, 98–107.

Peterson, T.G. and Barnes, S. (1991) Genistein inhibition of the growth of human breast breast cancer cells: independence from estrogen receptors and the multi-drug resistance gene. *Biochemical and Biophysical Research Communications* **179**, 661–7.

Peterson, T.G. and Barnes, S. (1996) Genistein inhibits both estrogen and growth factor stimulated proliferation of human breast cancer cells. *Cell Growth and Differentiation* **7**, 1345–51.

Petrakis, N., Barnes, S. and King, E.B. (1996) Stimulatory influence of soy protein isolate on breast secretion in pre- and postmenopausal women. *Cancer Epidemiology Biomarkers and Prevention* **5**, 785–94.

Pike, A.C.W., Brzozowski, A.M. and Hubbard, R.E. (1999) Structure of the ligand-binding domain of oestrogen receptor beta in the presence of a partial agonist and a full antagonist. *EMBO Journal* **18**, 4608–18.

Piller, R., Veria-Tebit, E., Wang-Gohrke, S., Linseisen, J. and Chang-Claude, J. (2006) CYP17 genotype modifies the association between lignan supply and premenopausal breast cancer risk in humans. *Journal of Nutrition* **136**, 1596–603.

Possemiers, S., Bolca, S., Grootaert, C., Heyerick, A., Decross, K., Dhooge, W., De Keukeleire, D., Rabot, S., Verstraete, W. and Van der Wiele, T. (2006) The prenylatedflavonoid Isoxanthohumol from hops (*Humulus lupulus* L.) is activated into the potent phytoestrogen 8-prenylnaringenin *in vitro* and in the human intestine. *Journal of Nutrition* **136**, 1862–7.

Possemiers, S., Heyerick, A., Robbens, V., De Keukeleire, D. and Verstraete, W. (2005) Activation of proestrogens from hops (*Humulus lupulus* L.) by intestinal microbiota; conversion of isoxanthohumol into 8-prenylnaringenin. *Journal of Agricultural and Food Chemistry* **53**, 6281–8.

Potter, S.M., Baum, J.A. and Teng, H. (1998) Soy protein and isoflavones: their effects on blood lipids and bone density in postmenopausal women. *American Journal of Clinical Nutrition* **68** (suppl), 1375S–1379S.

Pratico, D., Lawson,, J.A., Rokach, J. and Fitzgerald, G.A. (2001) The isoprostanes in biology and medicine. *Trends in Endocrinology and Metabolism* **12**, 243–7.

Raines, E.W. and Ross, R. (1995) Biology of atherosclerotic plaque formation: possible role of growth factors in lesion development and the potential impact of soy. *Journal of Nutrition* **125**, 624S–630S.

Ramanathan, L. and Gray, W.G. (2003) Identification and characterization of a phytoestrogen-specific gene from the MCF-7 human breast cancer cell. *Toxicology and Applied Pharmacology* **191**, 107–17.

Raschke, M., Rowland, I.R., Magee, P.J. and Pool-Zobel, B.L. (2006) Genistein protects prostate cells against hydrogen peroxide-induced DNA damage and induces expression of genes involved in the defence against oxidative stress. *Carcinogenesis* **27**, 2322–30.

Reinli, K. and Block, G. (1996) Phytoestrogen content of foods – a compendium of literature values. *Nutrition and Cancer* **26**, 123–48.

Reinwald, S. and Weaver, C.M. (2006) Soy isoflavones and bone health: a double-edged sword? *Journal of Natural Products* **69**, 450–9.

Rimbach, G., de Pascual-Teresa, S. and Ewins, B.A. (2003) Antioxidant and free radical scavenging activity of isoflavone metabolites. *Xenobiotica* **33**, 913–25.

Rimbach, G., Weinberg, P.D. and de Pascual-Teresa, S. (2004) Sulfation of genistein alters its anti-oxidant properties and its effect on platelet aggregation and monocyte and endothelial function. *Biochimica et Biophysica Acta* **1670**, 229–37.

Ritchie, M.R., Cummings, J.H., Morton, M.S., Michael-Steel, C., Bolton-Smith, C. and Ritches, A.C. (2006) A newly constructed and validated isoflavone database for the assessment of total genistien and daidzein intake. *British Journal of Nutrition* **95**, 204–13.

Ritchie, M.R., Morton, M.S., Deighton, N., Blake, A. and Cummings, J.H. (2004) Plasma and urinary phyto-oestrogens as biomarkers of intake: validatity by dublicate diet analysis. *British Journal of Nutrition* **91**, 447–57.

Roelens, F., Heldring, N., Dhooge, W., Bengtsson, M., Comhaire, F., Gustafsson, J.A., Treuter,E. and De Keukeleire, D. (2006) Subtle side-chain modifications of the hop phytoestrogen 8-prenylnarin-genin result in distinct agonist/antagonist activity profiles for oestrogen receptors alpha and beta. *Journal of Medicinal Chemistry* **49**, 7357–65.

Roman, V., Billard, C., Kern, C., Ferry-Dumazet, H., Izard, J.C., Mohammad, R., Mossalayi, D.M. and Kolb, J.P. (2002) Analysis of resveratrol-induced apoptosis in human B-cell chronic leukaemia. *British Journal of Haematology* **117**, 842–51.

Rowland, I., Faughnan, M. and Hoey, L. (2003) Bioavailability of phyto-oestrogens. *British Journal of Nutrition* **89** (Suppl 1), S45–58.

Rowland, I.R., Wiseman, H., Sanders, T.A.B., Aldercreutz, H. and Bowey, E.A. (2000) Interindividual variation in metabolism of soy isoflavones and lignans: influence of habitual diet on equol produc-tion by the gut microflora. *Nutrition and Cancer* **36**, 27–32.

Rufer, C.E. and Kulling, S.E. (2006) Antioxidant activity of isoflavones and their major metabolites using different *in vitro* assays. *Journal of Agricultural and Food Chemistry* **54**, 2926–31.

Ruhmann, S., Treutter, D., Fritsche, S., Briviba, K. and Szankowski, I. (2006) Piceid (resveratrol glucoside) synthesis in stilbene synthase transgenic apple fruit. *Journal of Agricultural and Food Chemistry* **54**, 4633–40.

Ryan-Borchers, T.A., Park, J.S., Chew, B.P., McGuire, M.K., Fournier, L.R. and Beerman, K.A. (2006) Soy isoflavones modulate immune function in healthy postmenopausal women. *American Journal of Clinical Nutrition* **83**, 1118–25.

Sacks, F.M., Lichtenstein, A., Van Horn, L., Harris, W., Kris-Etherton, P., Winston, M.; American Heart Association Nutrition Committee (2006). Soy protein, isoflavones, and cardiovascular health: an American Heart Association Science Advisory for professionals from the Nutrition Committee. *Circulation* **113**, 1034–44.

Sagara, M., Kanda, T. and Njelekera, M. (2004) Effects of dietary intake of soy protein and isofla-vones on cardiovascular disease risk factors in high risk, middle-aged men in Scotland. *Journal of the American College of Nutrition* **23**, 85–91.

Saji, S., Jensen, E.V., Nilsson, S., Rylander, T., Warner, M. and Gustafsson, J.-A. (2000) Estrogen receptors α and β in the rodent mammary gland. *PNAS* **97**, 337–42.

Sanders, T.A.B., Dean, T.S., Grainger, D., Miller, G.J. and Wiseman, H. (2002) Moderate intakes of soy isoflavones increase HDL but do not influence transforming growth factor β concentrations and haemostatic risk factors for coronary heart disease in healthy subjects. *American Journal of Clinical Nutrition* **76**, 373–7.

Sarker, F.H., Adsule, S., Padhye, S., Kulkarni, S. and Li, Y. (2006) The role of genistein and synthetic derivatives of isoflavone in cancer prevention and therapy. *Mini Reviews in Medicinal Chemistry* **6**, 401–7.

Sathyamoorthy, N., Gilsdorf, J.F. and Wang, T.T.Y. (1998) Differential effects of genistein on trans-forming growth factor beta-1 expression in normal and malignant mammary epithelial cells. *Anticancer Research* **18**, 2449–53.

Sathyamoorthy, N. and Wang, T.T. (1997) Differential effects of dietary phyto-oestrogens daidzein and equol on human breast cancer MCF-7 cells. *European Journal of Cancer* **33**, 2384–9.

Schabath, M.B., Hernandez, L.M., Wu, X., Pillow, P.C. and Spitz, M.R. (2005) Dietary phytoestrogens and lung cancer risk. *Journal of the American Medical Association* **294**, 1493–504.

Schaefer, O., Humpel, M., Fritzemeier, K.H., Bohlmann, R. and Schleuning, W.D. (2003) 8-Prenyl naringenin is a potent ERalpha selective phytoestrogen present in hops and beer. *Journal of Steroid Biochemistry and Molecular Biology* **84**, 359–60.

Scheiber, M.D., Liu, J.H., Subbiah, M.T.R., Rebar, R.W. and Setchell, K.D.R. (2001) Dietary inclusion of whole soy foods results in significant reductions in clinical risk factors for osteoporosis and cardiovascular disease in normal postmenopausal women. *Menopause* **8**, 384–92.

Setchell, D.R., Brown, N.M. and Lydeking-Olsen, E. (2002) The clinical importance of the metabolite equol – a clue to the effectiveness of soy and its isoflavones. *Journal of Nutrition* **132**, 3577–84.

Setchell, K.D. (2006) Assessing risks and benefits of genistein and soy. *Environmental Health Perspectives* **114**, A332–3.

Setchell, K.D. and Cassidy, A. (1999) Dietary isoflavones: biological effects and relevance to human health. *Journal of Nutrition* **129**, 758S–767S.

Setchell, K.D. and Cole, S.J. (2003) Variations in isoflavone levels in soy foods and soy protein isolates and issues related to isoflavone databases and food labelling. *Journal of Agricultural and Food Chemistry* **51**, 4146–55.

Setchell, K.D., Faughnan, M.S. and Avades, T. (2003b) Comparing the pharmacokinetics of daidzein and genistein with the use of ^{13}C-labelled tracers in premenopausal women. *American Journal of Clinical Nutrition* **77**, 411–19.

Setchell, K.D., Gosselin, S.J. and Welsh, M.B. (1987) Dietary oestrogens – a probable cause of infertility and liver disease in captive cheetahs. *Gastroenterology* **93**, 225–33.

Setchell, K.D., Zimmer-Nechemias, L., Cai, J. and Heubi, J.E. (1997) Exposure of infants to phyto-oestrogens from soy-based infant formula. *Lancet* **350**, 23–7.

Setchell, K.D.R., Brown, N.M., Desai, P.B., Zimmer-Nechemias, L., Wolfe, B., Jakate, A.S., Creutzinger, V. and Heubi, J.E. (2003a) Bioavailability, disposition and dose–response effects of soy isoflavones when consumed by healthy women at physiologically typical dietary intakes. *Journal of Nutrition* **133**, 1027–35.

Sfakianos, J., Coward, L., Kirk, M. and Barnes, S. (1997) Intestinal uptake and biliary excretion of the isoflavone genistein in the rat. *Journal of Nutrition* **127**, 1260–8.

Shimizu, H., Ross, R.K., Bernstein, L., Yatani, R., Henderson, B.E. and Mack, T.M. (1991) Cancers of the prostate and breast among Japanese and white immigrants in Los Angeles County. *British Journal of Cancer* **63**, 963–6.

Signorelli, P. and Ghidoni, R. (2005) Resveratrol as an anticancer nutrient: molecular basis, open questions and promises. *Journal of Nutritional Biochemistry* **16**, 449–66.

Simons, L.A., von Konigsmark, M., Simons, J. and Celermajer, D.S. (2000) Phytoestrogens do not influence lipoprotein levels or endothelial function in healthy, postmenopausal women. *American Journal of Cardiology* **85**, 1297–301.

Sirtori, C.R. and Lovati, M.R. (2001) Soy proteins and cardiovascular disease. *Current Atherosclerosis Reports* **3**, 47–53.

So, F.V., Guthrie, N., Chambers, A.F. and Carroll, K.K. (1997) Inhibition of proliferation of estrogen receptor-positive MCF-7 human breast cancer cells by flavonoids in the presence and absence of excess estrogen. *Cancer Letters* **112**, 127–33.

Song, K.B., Atkinson, C., Frankenfeld, C.L., Jokela, T., Wahala, K., Thomas, W.K. and Lampe, J.W. (2006) Prevalence of diadzein-metabolising phenotypes differs between Caucasian and Korean American women and girls. *Journal of Nutrition* **136**, 1347–51.

Soung do, Y., Patade, A., Khalil, D.A., Lucas, E.A., Devereddy, L., Greaves, K.A. and Arjmandi, B.H. (2006) Soy protein supplementation does not cause lymphocytopenia in postmenopausal women. *Nutrition Journal* **11**, 5–12.

Steinberg, F.M., Guthrie, N.L., Villablanca, A.C., Kumar, K. and Murray, M.J. (2003) Soy protein with isoflavones has favourable effects on endothelia function that are independent of lipid and antioxidant effect in health postmenopausal women. *American Journal of Clinical Nutrition* **78**, 123–30.

Stevens, J.F. and Page, J.E. (2004) Xanthohumol and related prenylflavonoids from hops to beer: to your good health! *Phytochemistry* **65**, 1317–30.

Stossi, F., Barnett, D.H. and Frasor, J. (2004) Transcriptional profiling of oestrogen-regulated gene expression via estrogen receptor (ER) α or ERβ in human osteosarcoma cells: distinct and common target genes for these receptors. *Endocrinology* **145**, 3473–86.

Strom, B.L., Schinnar, R. and Ziegler, E.E. (2001) Exposure to soy-based formula in infancy and endocrinological and reproductive outcomes in young adulthood. *Journal of the American Medical Association* **286**, 807–14.

Su, S.J., Yeh, T.M. and Chuang, W.J. (2005) The novel targets for anti-angiogenesis of genistein on human cells. *Biochemical Pharmacology* **69**, 307–18.

Szaefer, H., Cichocki, M., Brauze, D. and Baer-Dubowska, W. (2004) Alteration in phase I and phase II enzyme activities and polycyclic aromatic hydrocarbons – DNA adduct formation by plant phenolics in mouse epidermis. *Nutrition and Cancer,* **48**, 70–77.

Tanaka, H., Arakawa, H. and Yamaguchi, T. (2000) A ribonucleotide reductase gene involved in a p53-dependent cell-cycle checkpoint for DNA damage. *Nature* **404**, 42–9.

Teede, H.J., Dalais, F.S. and Kotsopulos, D. (2001) Dietary soy has both beneficial and potentially adverse cardiovascular effects: a placebo-controlled study in men and postmenopausal women. *Journal of Clinical Endocrinology and Metabolism* **86**, 3053–60.

Thomsen, A.R., Almstrup, K., Nielsen, J.E., Sorensen, I.K., Petersen, O.W., Leffers, H. and Breinholt, V.M. (2006) Estrogenic effect of soy isoflavones on mammary gland morphogenesis and gene expression profile. *Toxicological Sciences* **93**, 357–68.

Thorneycroft, I,H. (1989) The role of oestrogen replacement therapy in the prevention of osteoporosis. *American Journal of Obstetrics and Gynecology* **160**, 1306–10.

Tian, L. and Dixon, R.A. (2006) Engineering isoflavone metabolism with an artificial bifunctional enzyme. *Planta* **224**, 496–507.

Tikkanen, M.J., Wahala, K., Ojala, S., Vihma, V. and Adlercreutz, H. (1998) Effect of soybean phytoestrogen intake on low density lipoprotein oxidation resistance. *Proceedings of the National Academy of Sciences USA* **95**, 3106–10.

Tinhofer, I., Bernhard, D., Denfter, M., Anether, G., Loeffler, M. and Kroemer, G. (2001) Resveratrol, a tumor-suppressive compound from grapes, induces apoptosis via a novel mitochondrial pathway controlled by Bcl-2. *FASEB Journal* **15**, 1613–15.

Tinwell, H., Soames, A.R., Foster, J.R. and Ashby, J. (2000) Estradiol-type activity of coumestrol in mature and immature ovariectomized rat uterotrophic assays. *Environmental Health Perspectives* **108**, 631–4.

Totta, P., Acconcia, F. and Virgili, F. (2005) Daidzein-sulphate metabolites affect transcriptional and antiproliferative activities of estrogen receptor-beta in cultured human cancer cells. *Journal of Nutrition* **135**, 2687–93.

Tsuchiya, H., Nagayama, M. and Tanaka, T. (2002) Membrane-rigidifying effects of anti-cancer dietary factors. *Biofactors* **16**, 45–56.

Turner, R., Baron, T. and Wolffram S. (2004) Effect of circulating forms of soy isoflavones on the oxidation of low density lipoprotein. *Free Radical Reearch* **38**, 209–16.

Ueno, T. and Uchiyama, S. (2001) Identification of the specific intestinal bacteria capable of metabolizing soy isoflavone to equol. *Annals of Nutrition and Metabolism* **45**, 114 (abstract).

Uesugi, T., Fukui, Y. and Yamori, Y. (2002) Beneficial effects of soybean isoflavone supplementation on bone metabolism and serum lipids in postmenopausal Japanese women: a four-week study. *Journal of the American College of Nutrition* **21**, 97–102.

Usui, T. (2006) Pharmaceutical prospects of phytoestrogens. *Endocrine Journal* **53**, 7–20.

Van Der Weijer, P. and, Barentsen, R. (2002) Isoflavones from red clover (Promensil(R)) significantly reduce menopausal hot flush symptoms compared with placebo. *Maturitas* **42**, 187.

Van Popele, N.M., Grobbee, D.E. and, Bots, M.L. (2001) Association between arterial stiffness and atherosclerosis: the Rotterdam Study. *Stroke* **32**, 454–60.

Vega-Lopez, S., Yeum, K.J. and Lecker, J.L. (2005) Plasma antioxidant capacity in response to diets high in soy or animal protein with or without isoflavones. *American Journal of Clinical Nutrition* **81**, 43–9.

Verheus, M., van Gils, C.H., Keinan-Boker, L., Grace, P.B., Bingham, S.A. and Peeters, P.H. (2007) Plasma phytoestrogens and subsequent breast cancer risk. *Journal of Clinical Oncology* **25**, 648–55.

Wang, C. and Kurzer, M,S. (1997) Phytoestrogen concentration determines effects on DNA synthesis in human breast cancer cells. *Nutrition and Cancer* **28**, 236–47.

Wang, T.T.Y., Sathymoorthy, N. and Phang, J.M. (1996) Molecular effects of genistein on estrogen receptor-mediated pathways. *Carcinogenesis* **17**, 271–5.

Wang, Y., Jones, P.J., Ausman, L.M. and Lichtenstein, A.H. (2004) Soy protein reduces triglyceride levels and triglyceride fatty acid fractional synthesis rate in hypercholesterolemic subjects. *Atherosclerosis* **173**, 269–75.

Wang, Z.Q., Weber, N., Lou, Y.J. and Proksch, P. (2006) Prenylflavonoids as nonsteroidal phytoestrogens and related structure–activity relationships. *ChemMedChem* **1**, 482–8.

Wantanabe, S., Yamaguchi, M. and Sobue, T. (1998) Pharmacokinetics of soybean isoflavones in plasma, urine and feces of men after ingestion of 60 g baked soybean powder (Kinako). *Journal of Nutrition* **128**, 1710–15.

Wei, H., Bowen, R. and Cai, Q. (1995) Antioxidant and antipromotional effects of the soybean isoflavone genistein. *Proceedings of the Society for Experimental Biology and Medicine* **208**, 124–30.

Whitten, P.L., Lewis, C., Russel, E. and Naftolin, F. (1995) Potential adverse effects of phytoestrogens. *Journal of Nutrition* **125**, 771S–716S.

Wiseman, H. (1994) *Tamoxifen: Molecular Basis of Use in Cancer Treatment and Prevention.* Chichester: John Wiley & Sons Ltd.

Wiseman, H. (1999) The bioavailability of non-nutrient plant factors: dietary flavonoids and phyto-oestrogens. *Proceedings of the Nutrition Society* **58**, 139–46.

Wiseman, H. (2000a) Dietary phytoestrogens, oestrogens and tamoxifen: mechanisms of action in modulation of breast cancer risk and in heart disease prevention. In: *Biomolecular Free Radical Toxicity: Causes and Prevention* (eds H. Wiseman, P. Goldfarb, T.J. Ridgway and A. Wiseman), pp. 170–208. Chichester: John Wiley & Sons Ltd.

Wiseman, H. (2000b) The therapeutic potential of phytoestrogens. *Expert Opinion on Investigational Drugs* **9**, 1829–40.

Wiseman, H. (2005) Phytochemicals (b) Epidemiological factors. In: *Encyclopedia of Human Nutrition* (eds B. Caballero, L. Allen and A. Prentice). London: Academic Press.

Wiseman, H. (2006) Isoflavonoids and human health. In: *Flavonoids: Chemistry, Biochemistry and Applications* (eds O.M. Andersen and K.R. Markham), pp. 371–96. Boca Raton, FL: CRC Press.

Wiseman, H. (in press) Phytochemicals: health effects. In: *Encylopedia of Human Nutrition*, 3rd edn (ed. B. Caballero). Oxford: Elsevier UK.

Wiseman, H., Cannon, M., Arnstein, H.R.V. and Halliwell, B. (1990) Mechanism of inhibition of lipid peroxidation by tamoxifen and 4-hydroxytamoxifen introduced into liposomes. Similarity to cholesterol and ergosterol. *FEBS Letters* **274**, 107–10.

Wiseman, H., Casey, K., Bowey, E.A., Duffy, R., Davies, M., Rowland, I.R., Lloyd A.S., Murray A., Thompson R. and Clarke D.B. (2004) Influence of 10 wk of soy consumption on plasma concentrations and excretion of isoflavonoids and on gut microflora metabolism in healthy adults. *American Journal of Clinical Nutrition* **80**, 692–9.

Wiseman, H., Casey, K., Clarke, D.B., Barnes, K.A. and Bowey, E. (2002) Isoflavone aglycone and glucoconjugate content of high- and low-soy U.K. foods used in nutritional studies. *Journal of Agricultural and Food Chemistry* **50**, 1404–10.

Wiseman, H. and Halliwell, B. (1996) Damage to DNA by reactive oxygen and nitrogen species: role in inflammatory disease and progression to cancer. *Biochemical Journal* **313**, 17–29.

Wiseman, H., O'Reilly, J.D., Adlercreutz, H., Mallet, I., Bowey, E.A., Rowland, I.R. and Sanders, T.A. (2000) Isoflavone phytoestrogens consumed in soy decrease F_2–isoprostane concentrations and increase resistance of low-density lipoprotein to oxidation in humans. *American Journal of Clinical Nutrition* **72**, 395–400.

Wiseman, H., O'Reilly, J. and Lim, P. (1998) Antioxidant properties of the isoflavone phytoestrogen functional ingredient in soy products. In: *Functional Foods, the Consumer, the Products and the Evidence* (eds M. Sadler and M. Saltmarsh), pp. 80–6. Cambridge: Royal Society of Chemistry.

Wiseman, H., Quinn, P. and Halliwell, B. (1993) Tamoxifen and related compounds decrease membrane fluidity in liposomes. Mechanism for the antioxidant action of tamoxifen and relevance to its anticancer and cardioprotective actions? *FEBS Letters* **330**, 53–6.

Witzum, J.L. (1994) The oxidation hypothesis of atherosclerosis. *Lancet* **344**, 793–5.

Wong, M.C.Y., Wheeler, J., Lilley, K.S., Emery P.W., Preedy, V.R. and Wiseman H. (2008) Identification of putative protein biomarkers of dietary supplementation with soya foods. *Proceedings of the Nutrition Society* **16**, 235–9.

Woo, J.H., Lim, J.H., Kim, Y.K., Suh,S.I., Min do, S. and Chang, J.S. (2004) Resveratrol inhibits phorbol myristate acetate-induced matrix metalloproteinase-9 expression by inhibiting JNK and PKC delta signal transduction. *Oncogene* **23**, 1845–53.

Wu, W.H., Kang, Y.P., Wang, N.H., Jou, H.J. and Wang, T.A. (2006) Sesame ingestion affects sex hormones, antioxidant status, and blood lipids in postmenopausal women. *Journal of Nutrition* **135**, 1270–75.

Xu, X., Harris, K.S., Wang, H.-J., Murphy, P.A. and Hendrich, S. (1995) Bioavailability of soybean isoflavones depends upon gut microflora in women. *Journal of Nutrition* **125**, 2307–15.

Yamamoto, H., Senda, M. and Inoue, K. (2000) Flavanone 8-dimethylallytransferase in *Sophora flavescens* cell suspension cultures. *Phytochemistry* **54**, 649–55.

Yan, C.H. and Han, R. (1998) Genistein supresses adhesion-induced protein tyrosine phosphorylation and invasion of B16-BL6 melanoma cells. *Cancer Letters* **129**, 117–24.

Yasuda, T., Mizunuma, S. and Kano, Y. (1996) Urinary and biliary metabolites of genistein in rats. *Biological and Pharmaceutical Bulletin* **19**, 413–17.

Yeung, F., Hoberg, J.E., Ramsey, C.S., Keller, M.D., Jones, D.R., Frye, R.A. and Mayo, M.W. (2004) Modulation of NF-kappaB-dependent transcription and cell survival by the SIRT 1 deacetylase. *EMBO Journal* **23**, 2369–80.

Yeung, J. and Yu, T.F. (2003) Effects of isoflavones (soy phyto-estrogens) on serum lipids: analysis of randomized controlled trials. *Nutrition Journal* **2**, 15–22.

Yu, O., Shi, J., Hession, A.O., Maxwell, C.A., McGonigle, B. and Odell, J.T. (2003) Metabolic engineering to increase isoflavone biosynthesis in soybean seed. *Phytochemistry* **63**, 753–63.

Zava, D.T. and Duwe, G. (1997) Estrogenic and antiproliferative properties of genistein and other isoflavonoids in human breast cancer cells *in vitro*. *Nutrition and Cancer* **27**, 31–40.

Zhuo, X.-G., Melby, M.K. and Wantanabe, S. (2004) Soy isoflavone intake lowers serum LDL cholesterol: a meta-analysis of 8 randomized controlled trials in humans. *Journal of Nutrition* **134**, 2395–400.

Chapter 8

Plant minerals

Martin R. Broadley and Philip J. White

Introduction

Humans require more than 20 essential mineral elements. Several of these minerals are not thought to be essential for plants. Nevertheless, all occur naturally in plant tissues (Figure 8.1; Table 8.1). Therefore, adequate human mineral nutrition can be achieved by an appropriate diet. However, over half of the world's 6 billion people are likely to be deficient in one or more of the following elements: iron (Fe), zinc (Zn), iodine (I), selenium (Se), calcium (Ca), magnesium (Mg) and copper (Cu). Dietary mineral deficiencies are caused by the consumption of plants – either directly or indirectly via the livestock food chain containing insufficient minerals. Crop mineral concentrations are driven by soil factors, including the phyto-availability of minerals in the soil, and by genetic factors, whereby species and cultivars differentially accumulate and metabolise minerals. In plants, some essential mineral elements (e.g. K and Na) occur solely in ionic form. However, most mineral elements occur in inorganic and organic forms of varying solubility and bioavailability. Uptake and assimilation of dietary minerals across the human gut depends not only on the concentration and chemical form of minerals in plants, but also on the concentration of 'promoter' compounds, such as certain organic and amino acids, that stimulate gut absorption, and 'anti-nutrients', such as polyphenolics (e.g. tannins) or phytate (IP_6), that inhibit gut absorption. In humans, mineral malnutrition can be addressed through dietary diversification, food fortification, human/livestock supplementation, and/or by increasing the bioavailable mineral content of crops through fertiliser (agronomic biofortification) and crop-improvement-based (genetic biofortification) strategies. Whilst dietary refinement requires the total amount of each element delivered to be considered within a context of its chemical form, and its interactions with other compounds in food, this chapter will focus on the mineral concentration of plants per se.

The first section of this chapter ('Genetic variation in plant mineral concentration') provides a review of the variation in plant mineral concentrations at the species and cultivar levels. Between-species genetic variation in mineral concentrations is illustrated first at the leaf-organ scale, whereby genetic variation in leaf mineral concentrations

Phytonutrients, First Edition. Edited by Andrew Salter, Helen Wiseman and Gregory Tucker.
© 2012 Blackwell Publishing Ltd. Published 2012 by Blackwell Publishing Ltd.

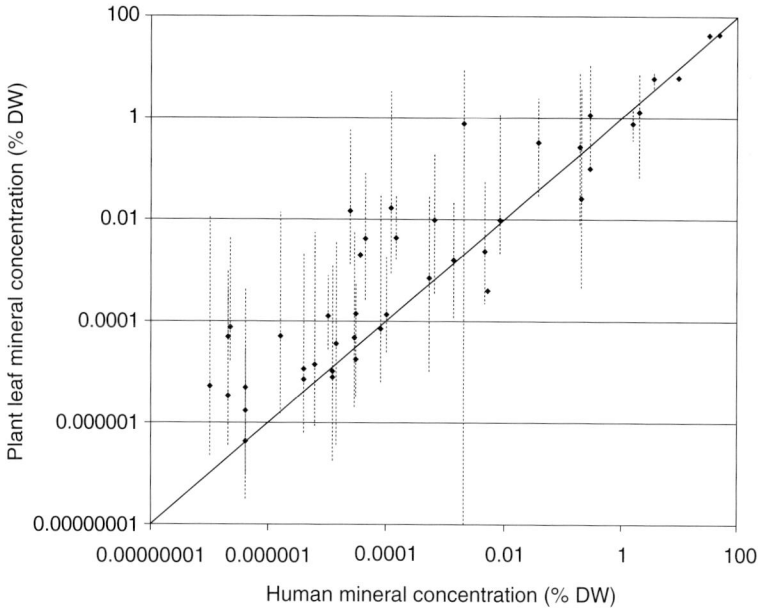

Figure 8.1 Concentrations of mineral elements in humans and plants. Data are given in Table 8.1. Human data are from Emsley (1997). Plant data are from Broadley et al. (2004), Epstein (1972), Hodson et al. (2005), Kay et al. (1975), Marschner (1995), and Watanabe et al. (2007); arithmetic means ± range. Solid line represents unity.

(leaf-MC) occurs *between* plant species for all elements and this variation is associated with both recent (species-level) and ancient (family-level) selection pressures. In contrast, most of the published data on the within-species genetic variation in mineral concentrations has focused on the carbohydrate-rich edible fractions of staple crops (e.g. grain, roots and tubers). Crop varieties with higher mineral concentrations in their edible portions are already available, and improved varieties are being developed for genetic biofortification strategies.

The second section of the chapter ('Has the mineral concentration of crops declined due to breeding for increased yield?') provides a critical assessment of the claim, expressed in the recent literature, that modern cultivars and/or agronomic practices has caused reductions in the concentrations of essential mineral elements in the edible portions of many crops. Literature-based evidence for a decline in mineral concentration in fruit and vegetable crops is inconclusive. However, recent experimental studies have shown that, when grown under identical conditions, concentrations of several mineral elements are lower in genotypes yielding more grain or shoot biomass than in older, lower-yielding genotypes. A detailed case study is presented, summarising a recently published study on potato (*Solanum tuberosum* L.; White et al. 2009). Whilst there is considerable genotypic variation in tuber mineral concentration between potato genotypes, and variation in tuber mineral concentration induced by agronomic interventions, the mineral concentration of potato tubers is not consistently correlated negatively with yield.

Table 8.1 Concentrations of mineral elements in humans and plants

Element	Chemical symbol	Mass of element (g) in 49 kg dry body tissue (Emsley 1997)	Mean concentration of element in humans (% DW)	Mean concentration of element in plant leaves (% DW)	Minimum concentration among 670 species of plant (mg/kg DW; Watanabe et al. 2007)	Maximum concentration among 670 species of plant (mg/kg DW; Watanabe et al. 2007)	Source of plant data (Watanabe et al. 2007, unless stated)
Oxygen	O	24333	50	44	–	–	Epstein et al. (1972)
Carbon	C	16000	33	43	–	–	Broadley et al. (2004)
Hydrogen	H	4667	9.5	6.2	–	–	Epstein et al. (1972)
Nitrogen	N	1800	3.7	6.1	–	–	Broadley et al. (2004)
Calcium	Ca	1000	2.0	1.3	668	76420	
Phosphorus	P	780	1.6	0.78	–	–	Broadley et al. (2004)
Potassium	K	140	0.29	1.15	1080	114234	
Sulfur	S	140	0.29	0.10	–	–	Marschner (1995)
Sodium	Na	100	0.20	0.03	4.11	39498	
Chlorine	Cl	95	0.19	0.27	78.6	81879	
Magnesium	Mg	19	0.039	0.33	268	24005	
Iron	Fe	4.2	0.0086	0.010	19.6	12296	
Fluorine	F	2.6	0.0053	0.000	–	–	Kay et al. (1975)
Zinc	Zn	2.3	0.0047	0.002	2.21	611	
Silicon	Si	1	0.0020	0.770	–	–	Hodson et al. (2005)
Rubidium	Rb	0.68	0.0014	0.0016	1.17	239	
Strontium	Sr	0.32	0.00065	0.0097	3.40	2010	
Bromine	Br	0.26	0.00053	0.0007	0.0958	290	
Lead	Pb	0.12	0.00024	–	–	–	
Copper	Cu	0.07	0.00015	0.0043	16.4	288	
Aluminum	Al	0.06	0.00012	0.0167	8.49	33390	
Cadmium	Cd	0.05	0.00010	0.00013	0.2380	19.8	
Cerium	Ce	0.04	0.000082	0.00007	0.0631	291	
Barium	Ba	0.02	0.000045	0.00417	2.3	792	
Iodine	I	0.02	0.000041	–	–	–	
Tin	Sn	0.02	0.000041	–	–	–	
Titanium	Ti	0.02	0.000041	–	–	–	
Boron	B	0.018	0.000037	0.00200	–	–	Marschner (1995)

Nickel	Ni	0.015	0.000031	0.00014	0.0818	5.76
Selenium	Se	0.015	0.000031	0.00002	0.0297	1.49
Chromium	Cr	0.014	0.000029	0.00005	0.0194	54.6
Manganese	Mn	0.012	0.000024	0.01466	12.6	5687
Arsenic	As	0.007	0.000014	0.00004	0.0032	38.5
Lithium	Li	0.007	0.000014	–	–	–
Cesium	Cs	0.006	0.000012	0.000010	0.0018	13.5
Mercury	Hg	0.006	0.000012	0.000008	0.0030	1.28
Germanium	Ge	0.005	0.000010	–	–	–
Molybdenum	Mo	0.005	0.000010	0.000126	0.2595	7.71
Cobalt	Co	0.003	0.0000061	0.000014	0.0084	54.7
Antimony	Sb	0.002	0.0000041	0.000007	0.0063	20.7
Silver	Ag	0.002	0.0000041	0.000011	0.0154	1.92
Niobium	Nb	0.002	0.0000031	–	–	–
Zirconium	Zr	0.001	0.0000020	–	–	–
Lanthanium	La	0.0008	0.0000016	0.000050	0.0145	139
Gallium	Ga	0.0007	0.0000014	–	–	–
Tellurium	Te	0.0007	0.0000014	–	–	–
Yttrium	Y	0.0006	0.0000012	–	–	–
Bismuth	Bi	0.0005	0.0000010	–	–	–
Thallium	Tl	0.0005	0.0000010	–	–	–
Indium	In	0.0004	0.00000082	–	–	–
Gold	Au	0.0002	0.00000041	0.0000004	0.0003	0.2859
Scandium	Sc	0.0002	0.00000041	0.0000017	0.0009	4.39
Tantalum	Ta	0.0002	0.00000041	0.0000049	0.0063	1.41
Vanadium	V	0.0001	0.00000022	0.0000758	0.1530	48.3
Thorium	Th	0.0001	0.00000020	0.0000034	0.0034	4.32
Uranium	U	0.0001	0.00000020	0.0000491	0.0432	9.48
Samarium	Sm	0.00005	0.00000010	0.0000051	0.0020	116
Beryllium	Be	0.00004	0.00000007	–	–	–
Tungsten	W	0.00002	0.00000004	–	–	–
Dysprosium	Dy	–	–	0.0000801	0.0115	76.4778
Europium	Eu	–	–	0.0000026	0.0015	4.8988
Gadolinium	Gd	–	–	0.0000980	0.0765	24.3785
Hafnium	Hf	–	–	0.0000026	0.0024	3.4418
Lutetium	Lu	–	–	0.0000023	0.0030	0.3094
Neodymium	Nd	–	–	0.0005802	0.0028	709.1024
Terbium	Tb	–	–	0.0000041	0.0029	2.1576
Ytterbium	Yb	–	–	0.0000078	0.0060	3.1456

Genetic variation in plant mineral concentration

Introduction

Plants require at least 17 mineral elements to complete their life cycles (Marschner 1995). Except for carbon (C), these elements are acquired primarily from the soil solution. Plants are sessile, thus, plant mineral concentrations are influenced strongly by the surrounding environment. The effects of the soil, and the phyto-availability of mineral elements, on plant mineral concentrations have been studied intensively in crops of agricultural importance so that crop yields can be optimised with fertilisers (Mengel and Kirkby 2001). In contrast, genetic factors that influence plant mineral concentrations have received far less attention, even for important crop species. Genetic sources of variation in plant mineral concentration can be used to optimise crop yields under low-fertility, i.e. to improve nutrient-use efficiency, and to breed crops with higher mineral concentrations in their edible portions and thereby improve human dietary mineral intakes, i.e. genetic biofortification (Grusak and DellaPenna 1999; Welch and Graham 2004; White and Broadley 2005a).

Between-species genetic variation in plant mineral concentration

Genetic variation in plant mineral concentration between species is associated with: (1) plant size and growth rate, (2) biomass partitioning between leaves, stems, roots, and reproductive organs, and (3) concentration, morphology and function of different organs (Grime 2001; Kerkhoff et al. 2006; Watanabe et al. 2007). At an organ level, genetic variation in leaf-MC varies between plant species for all elements (Thompson et al. 1997; Broadley et al. 2004; Kerkhoff et al. 2006; Watanabe et al. 2007). For example, species-differences in leaf-N and P – the two elements most likely to limit plant growth – correlate with leaf morphology (Ågren 2004; Wright et al. 2005; Kerkhoff et al. 2006). Other differences between plant species in leaf-MC are more extreme. For example, some 'hyperaccumulator' species can have leaf metal (e.g. Al, Cd, Ni, Zn) or metalloid (e.g. As, Se) concentrations up to three orders of magnitude greater than closely-related species when these plants are grown in the same substrate (Reeves and Baker 2000; Broadley et al. 2001, 2007; Jansen et al. 2002; Macnair 2003; White et al. 2007).

Selenium is an element with no proven role in plant nutrition, yet there is a substantial literature on the differing accumulation and assimilation capacities of different flowering plant (angiosperm) species (White et al. 2004, 2007). This is because Se is an essential nutrient for animals, and because Se is a potential toxin if consumed in excess. For Se, species are typically divided into three categories: 'non-accumulator', 'Se-indicator' and 'Se-accumulator' plants. Non-accumulator plants rarely contain over 100 µg Se/g dry matter, Se-indicator plants can contain up to 1000 µg Se/g dry matter, and Se-accumulator plants can contain up to 40 000 mg Se/g dry matter when sampled from Se-rich environments in which they occur, for example, in areas of Western USA where soils have been derived from seleniferous shale and sedimentary materials. In Se accumulators, Se predominantly occurs as non-protein amino acid forms Se-methylselenocysteine, and in a conjugated form as γ-glutamyl-methylselenocysteine, but also as selenocystathione, selenohomocysteine, γ-glutamyl-selenocystathione, methyl selenol and selenate (Pickering et al. 2000, 2003). Extreme Se accumulation (as high as 2.2% on a dry matter basis) has also been reported in the fruit of some species within the Lecythidaceae family, including the Brazil nut (*Bertholletia excelsa* Humb. & Bonpl.), Paradise nut (*Lecythis zabucaja* Aubl.), Coco de Mono (*L. ollaria* Loefl.) and Sapucaia nut (*L. elliptica* Kunth). The consumption of *Lecythis* has been reported to induce acute selenosis in humans, characterised by symptoms of hair and nail loss, alongside other dermatological, neurological and gastric disorders (Kerdel-Vegas 1966; Dickson 1969). In *B. excelsa,* the dominant form of Se is selenomethionine, which is the predominant form of organic Se to be found in most non-accumulator species (Vonderheide et al. 2002; Kannamkumarath et al. 2005). Overall, leaf-Se is significantly greater in Se-accumulator plants than in other angiosperms. However, concentrations of S, a plant macronutrient of similar chemistry to Se, are unremarkable, leading to a discontinuous distribution of leaf Se/S quotient among angiosperm species, i.e. the leaf Se/S quotient of Se-accumulator species is significantly greater than those in other angiosperms (White et al. 2007). This observation suggests either that the transporters responsible for the uptake or translocation of Se and S, are selective for either sulphate (in non-accumulator plants) or selenate (in Se-accumulator plants).

Whilst there is considerable variation between plant species in terms of their Se concentration, there is little variation in shoot-Se concentrations between angiosperm families and orders (White et al. 2004). However, for many other elements, species-differences in leaf-MC can also be associated with higher-level evolutionary processes, i.e., present-day species-differences in the leaf concentration of some elements are, in part, due to ancestral selection pressures which can be seen at the family or higher-level scales (Broadley et al. 2003, 2004; Kerkhoff et al. 2006; Watanabe et al. 2007). For example, leaf-Ca and Mg are typically lower (Thompson et al. 1997; Broadley et al. 2003, 2004), and leaf-Si is higher (Hodson et al. 2005), in commelinid monocotyledon species – which include grasses and cereals – than in species from other angiosperm families. Differences in tissue Ca and Mg between species of different families, when grown under comparable conditions, has been attributed to family-level differences in cell wall chemistry and cation-exchange capacity (Broadley et al. 2003, 2004; White and Broadley 2003). These observations are consistent with an increased risk of Ca- and Mg-related deficiency disorders in populations changing from bean-rich to cereal-rich diets (Graham et al. 2001; Welch and Graham 2004). Similarly, there has been an increase in Fe-deficiency anaemia and Zn-deficiency as cereals have replaced traditional, more mineral-rich dicotyledonous crops such as pulses, vegetables and fruits (Welch and Graham 2004). This highlights the importance of the choice of plant species in strategies to increase the delivery of mineral elements to vulnerable populations.

Within-species genetic variation in plant mineral concentration

Most within-species surveys of plant mineral concentration have focused on carbohydrate-rich fractions of staple crops. These fractions include rice (*Oryza sativa* L.), wheat (*Triticum* spp.) and maize (*Zea mays* L.) grains, common bean (*Phaseolus vulgaris* L.) and pea (*Pisum sativum* L.) seeds, and cassava (*Manihot esculenta* Crantz) and yam

(*Dioscorea alata* L.) roots (reviewed by Grusak and Cakmak 2005; White and Broadley 2005a). This is because a large proportion of the world's population subsists on cereal-based diets, including diets based primarily on rice or wheat in Asia and maize in sub-Saharan Africa and Latin America. In addition, the common bean supplies significant amounts of minerals to Africa and Latin America and cassava is a widely consumed root crop in tropical America, sub-Saharan Africa and parts of Asia. Considerable within-species genetic variation has been observed in the elements most frequently lacking in human diets – notably Ca, Fe, Mg, Se, and Zn – in all of these crops, and this is described in detail in the subsequent sections of this chapter. Within-species genetic variation in plant mineral concentration informs genetic biofortification strategies.

In contrast, surveys of natural genetic variation in leaf-MC within species are relatively scarce in the published literature. However, among 322 accessions of spinach (*Spinacia oleracea* L.), leaf-MC has been reported to be: Ca (0.3–1.2%), Cu (2.2–11.0 µg/g dry weight), Fe (50.4–138.6 µg/g dry weight), K (5.6–11.3%), Ni (0.07–5.44 µg/g dry weight), Mg (0.5–1.5%), Mn (29.8–427.0 µg/g dry weight), Mo (0.20–8.62 µg/g dry weight), P (0.4–1.0%), and Zn (31.4–386.8 µg/g dry weight; Grusak and Cakmak 2005; USDA, ARS, National Genetic Resources Program 2007; M.A. Grusak, personal communication). In other studies, leaf-B, Ca, Cu, Fe, K, Mg, Mn, Ni, P, and Zn varied between 1.3-fold and 2.4-fold among 19 chickpea (*Cicer arietinum* L.) accessions (Ibrikci et al. 2003). Among 111 accessions of *Brassica rapa* L., leaf-MC varied: Zn (23–156 µg/g dry weight), Fe (60–350 µg/g dry weight), and Mn (21–53 µg/g dry weight) (Vreugdenhil et al. 2005). Among 22 accessions of *B. oleracea* L. var. *acephala* (kale/collards) leaf-MC varied: Ca (1.2–3.1%), Fe (53.1–114.2 µg/g dry weight), K (2.1–3.5%), Mg (0.3–0.6%), and Zn (29.1–79.9 µg/g dry weight) and leaf-MC rankings of cultivars were consistent between years despite substantial year-to-year variability in leaf-Ca, Mg, Fe, and Zn (Kopsell et al. 2004). In *B. oleracea* var. *italica* (broccoli/calabrese), non-genetic sources of variation were found to dominate inflorescence head Ca and Mg concentrations, although significant genetic variation was observed (Farnham et al. 2000; Rosa et al. 2002). Among 70 accessions of *Arabidopsis thaliana* (L.) Heynh., leaf-K varied from 2.78–4.85% (Harada and Leigh 2006) and leaf Pi ranged from 2.0–12.8 mg/g fresh weight (Bentsink et al. 2003; D. Vreugdenhil, personal communication). Genomic regions (quantitative trait loci, QTL) associated with several leaf- and seed-MC have been mapped in *A. thaliana* (Loudet et al. 2003; Payne et al. 2004; Vreugdenhil et al. 2005; Harada and Leigh 2006). Recently, large-scale ionomic profiling programs have released data on natural variation in leaf-MC of diversity collections of *A. thaliana* and rapid progress in associating genomic regions with leaf-MC is envisaged in these populations (Baxter et al. 2007; Zhao et al. 2007).

Iron and zinc

Iron and Zn are the two most abundant transition metals in the human body, with the typical adult comprising 4.2 and 2.3 g of Fe and Zn, respectively (Emsley 1997). Humans require Fe and Zn to maintain the activities of numerous enzymes. Iron is a critical component of haem proteins, such as haemoglobin, myoglobin and cytochromes which are involved in oxygen transport and energy metabolism (NRC 1989). Zinc is potentially a constituent of up to 10% of all human proteins and it is likely to be involved in most metabolic pathways (Beyersmann and Haase 2001; Andreini et al. 2006). Both Fe and Zn are under tight homeostatic control (NRC 1989), yet Fe and Zn deficiency are extremely common, affecting over half of the world's population (Kennedy et al. 2003; Welch and Graham 2004). Populations especially affected include those reliant on staple crops for the bulk of their calorie intake, although the prevalence of Fe and Zn deficiency is probably far more widespread. For example, the 2003 UK National Diet and Nutrition Survey estimated that 25% of women had inadequate Fe nutrition, and this value rose to >40% amongst 18- to 34-year-olds (Henderson et al. 2003; Marriott and Buttriss 2003). Notably, total Fe intake was not related to the Fe status of an individual, rather, Fe status was positively associated with haem-Fe and vitamin C intake, and negatively associated with susceptibility to blood loss.

To address low Fe and Zn intakes amongst populations reliant on staple crops, the Consultative Group on International Agricultural Research (CGIAR; www.cgiar.org), launched the HarvestPlus Challenge Program (www.harvestplus.org) with the aim of increasing the concentration of bioavailable Fe and Zn in rice, wheat, maize, common bean and cassava through genetic improvement. The initial priorities of HarvestPlus are to determine: (1) the genetic variability and heritability of Fe and Zn traits, (2) the stability of these traits across diverse soil conditions and climactic zones, (3) the number of genes impacting on these traits, and (4) the feasibility of breeding for increased concentrations of Fe and Zn (and potentially other minerals) in edible tissues without affecting yields or other quality characteristics (Bouis 2003). Clearly, fertilisers containing Fe and Zn can also be used to boost the concentrations of these minerals in staple crops (e.g. for review of Zn see Broadley et al. 2007), but, a review of agronomic biofortification is outside the scope of the chapter.

Fourfold variation in grain Fe and Zn concentrations occurs between rice (Gregorio et al. 2000; Table 8.2) and wheat (Monasterio and Graham 2000; Bálint et al. 2001; Cakmak et al. 2004; Grusak and Cakmak 2005; Table 8.2) cultivars. In wheat, grain Fe and Zn concentrations are generally lower, and show less genetic variability, among cultivated tetraploid (ssp. *durum*) and hexaploid (ssp. *aestivum*) varieties than among wild diploid (ssp. *urartu,* ssp. *boeoticum,* ssp. *monococcum*) and tetraploid (ssp. *dicoccoides*) wheats and close relatives (*Aegilops tauschii* Coss.). In maize, kernel Fe and Zn concentrations also vary substantially (Bänziger and Long 2000; Maziya-Dixon et al. 2000; Oikeh et al. 2003a, b; Table 8.2). For all three cereals, accessions with grain Fe and Zn concentrations at least twofold higher than the most widely grown varieties are available (White and Broadley 2005a). In general, seeds of legumes such as common bean and pea have higher Zn and Fe concentrations than cereal grain, which can vary more widely than in cereals (Islam et al. 2002, 2004; Hacisalihoglu et al. 2004; Table 8.2). In legumes, seed Fe and Zn concentration behave as quantitative traits which can be mapped to genetic loci using quantitiative trait loci (QTL) analyses (Guzmán-Maldonado et al. 2003; Ghandilyan et al. 2006). QTL for seed Fe and Zn have also been mapped in *A. thaliana* (Vreugdenhil et al. 2004). Following the identification of QTL, candidate genes or loci can be resolved through fine mapping and map-based cloning, and this information could be used for gene-based selection or marker-assisted breeding strategies. An advantage of this strategy is that knowledge of the genes and/or chromosomal loci controlling Fe or Zn concentration

Table 8.2   Iron and zinc concentrations in edible portions of crops

	Trial	*n*	Iron (mg/kg)	Zinc (mg/kg)
Rice *(Oryza sativa)* grain				
Core collection	Field	1138	6–24	14–58
Wheat (*Triticum* spp) grain				
Selected genotypes	Field	324	25–73	25–92
T. dicoccoides	Field	518	15–94	30–98
T. dicoccoides	Glasshouse	111	21–91	14–190
Selected genotypes	Hydroponic	28	80–368	33–149
Maize (*Zea mays*) grain				
Core collection	Field	1814	10–63	13–58
Mid-altitude inbred lines	Field	60	15–159	12–96
Low-altitude inbred lines	Field	49	14–134	24–95
Selected genotypes	Field	90	14–26	17–32
Advanced lines	Field	20	16–19	17–21
Elite varieties	Field	49	17–24	17–25
Bean (*Phaseolus vulgaris*) seed				
Core collection	Field	1072	34–92	21–59
Cultivated genotypes	Field	1031	34–89	21–54
Wild genotypes	Field	119	<96	<43
Selected genotypes	Glasshouse	35	ND	24–57
Mapping population	Glasshouse	120	41–142	27–67
Cultivated genotypes	Hydroponic	24	52–157	30–62
Pea (*Pisum sativum*) seed				
Core collection	Glasshouse	500	23–105	16–107
Cassava (*Manihot esculenta*) root				
Core collection	Field	162	4–49	4–18
Yam (Dioscorea alata) root				
Core collection	Field	23	9–176	8–25
***Brassica oleracea* shoot**				
Core collection	Glasshouse	424	59–1089	8–229
***Brassica rapa* leaves**				
Core collection	Glasshouse	111	60–350	23–156
Spinach (*Spinacea oleracea*) leaves				
Core collection	Glasshouse	327	50–139	31–387

Reproduced and edited from White and Broadley (2005a).

in one plant species could be used in a different target crop species by exploiting gene homology and/or genome collinearity.

The Zn and Fe concentrations in roots of cassava and yam, and in leaves of spinach and brassicas, are also higher than in cereal grains, which again illustrates the genetic potential to breed for increased Fe and Zn concentrations in crops (Table 8.2). For example, there is 14-fold variation in root Fe and 4-fold variation in root Zn amongst cassava genotypes (Chavez et al. 2000; Maziya-Dixon et al. 2000) and 3-fold variation in root Fe and 19-fold variation in root Zn in yam (Frossard et al. 2000). In spinach, leaf-Fe varied 2.7-fold, and leaf-Zn varied 12-fold (Guzmán-Maldonado et al. 2003; Grusak and

Cakmak 2005). In *Brassica oleracea,* leaf-Fe and Zn varied both varied >10-fold (White and Broadley 2005a).

Genetic modification is also being used in an attempt to increase the accumulation of iron in rice (Lucca et al. 2002). A twofold enhancement of iron concentration was achieved by the expression of a gene for ferritin in rice. In addition to enhancing mineral levels, factors that influence bioavailability, either positively or negatively, may also be manipulated. The manipulation of phytase activity is one such approach to enhance mineral bioavailability. Phytic acid, a storage form of phosphorus in plant tissue, binds several minerals, including iron and zinc very strongly. Phytate is poorly digested and thus prevents absorption of these minerals. The expression of phytase in crops enhances the breakdown of phytic acid and releases minerals. In rice the bioavailability of iron has been targeted by introducing a gene for phytase which resulted in a 130-fold increase in the expression of this enzyme in rice. Cysteine-rich peptides, in comparison, are thought to enhance bioavailability of iron; the expression of a cysteine-rich metallothionein-like protein gene in rice may also assist absorption of this mineral (Lucca et al. 2002).

Iodine and selenium

Iodine and Se are essential micronutrients for all animal species although neither element has been proven to be essential for higher plants. A typical adult human contains *ca.* 20 and 15 mg of I and Se, respectively (Emsley 1997). Iodine is a component of the hormones thyroxine (T_4) and triiodothyronine (T_3), which are integral to metabolic functions. Selenium is incorporated into selenoproteins as the 21st amino acid selenocysteine (Sec), or during non-specific replacement of cysteine with Sec (Castellano et al. 2004). To date, *ca.* 25 mammalian selenoproteins have been identified and several have been characterised (Rayman 2002). Some selenoproteins are antioxidants (e.g. glutathione peroxidase; GSH-Px), whilst others contribute to protein stability, transcription of mRNA and other biochemical functions. Sub-optimal Se intake and status is associated with impaired immune function, increased risk of cancers, increased oxidative stress-related disorders and reduced fertility (Rayman 2000, 2002, 2004). At least a quarter of the world's population is thought to be I and Se deficient, including populations in developed and developing countries (Lyons et al. 2004). For example, in the UK, Se intake in humans has declined from 60 µg/day in the 1970s to 1980s to <39 µg/day in the 1990s to 2000s with a concomitant decline in Se status (reviewed by Broadley et al. 2006b). This decline has been primarily attributed to the changes in wheat consumption patterns, with UK-grown milling wheat largely replacing milling wheat sourced from North America. UK soils are extremely low in Se in comparison with North America.

Although it may be possible to increase the consumption of foodstuffs which naturally contain more I and Se, dietary diversification is not always feasible (Rayman 2002). Similarly, the use of I supplementation through the use of iodised salt is not always an appropriate long-term solution to dietary I deficiency (Lyons et al. 2004). However, some notable agronomic biofortification case studies have succeeded in increasing the dietary delivery of I and Se to humans. These include the use of irrigation water supplemented with I (fertigation; Lyons et al. 2004), and the Finnish nationwide Se fertilisation programme which has now been running continuously for >20 years (reviewed by Broadley et al. 2006b). However, there is also the – as yet unexploited – prospect of harnessing within-species genetic variation to increase the delivery of Se to human diets through genetic biofortification (Lyons et al. 2004; Broadley et al. 2006b). In the first instance, it may be possible to simply select existing varieties of crops which accumulate more I and/or Se. In the longer term, it may be possible to breed crops for increased I and/or Se concentration.

Published data on between- or within-species genetic variation in the I concentration of plants are scarce. In perennial rye grass (*Lolium perenne* L.), the leaf-I of individual plants sampled randomly from a homogeneous soil varied from 0.185 to 2.47 µg I/g dry weight and leaf-I was shown to be inherited (Butler and Johnson 1957; Johnson and Butler 1957; Butler and Glenday 1962; Gerloff 1963). Further, variation in leaf-I was greater between species than it was between soils of different I contents or between seasons. Since these studies provide strong evidence that leaf-I is under genetic control, there is a need to establish within-species genetic variation in the I concentration of edible portions of staple crops and other dietary plant components and such data are not currently available (Lyons et al. 2004).

In the most detailed study of within-species genetic variation in Se of a crop, Lyons et al. (2005) reported Se concentrations in a range of cereal grains, including those from modern wheats (*Triticum aestivum* L.), durum wheats (*Triticum dicoccum* (Schrank) Schubl.), wheat landrace accessions, ancestral diploid relatives (*Aegilops tauschii* (Coss.) Schmal.), wheat recombinant inbred and doubled haploid mapping populations, and also grains from barley (*Hordeum valgare*), triticale (× *Triticosecale* Wittmack ex A. Camus.) and rye (*Secale cereale* L.). Whilst grain Se varied from 0.005–0.720 mg Se/kg, most of the variation was due to soil factors. However, *A. tauschlii* accumulated most grain Se, thus providing the genetic potential to breed for increased grain Se in wheat. In non-cereals, shoot-Se varied significantly between *Lycopersicon* taxa (tomatoes and relatives; Shennan et al. 1990; Pezzarossa et al. 1999). Soybean (Yang et al. 2003; Zhang et al. 2003) and onion (Kopsell and Randle 1997) genotypes also vary significantly in their Se concentration, and leaf-Se is moderately heritable in *Brassica oleracea* L. (Kopsell and Randle 2001). Therefore, there is a case that genetic biofortification strategies could increase the delivery of dietary I and Se, possibly in combination with agronomic interventions (Lyons et al. 2004; Broadley et al. 2006b).

Calcium and magnesium

The typical adult contains >1.0 kg Ca, 99% of which is associated with bones and teeth (NRC 1989). The remainder occurs in soft tissues where it is involved in signalling, maintenance of cell structure and other metabolic functions. Under Ca deficiency, soft tissue Ca is maintained at the expense of hard tissues, thereby reducing bone strength and increasing the risk of Ca-related clinical symptoms including osteoporosis (NRC 1989). Dietary Ca deficiency is the major cause of nutritional rickets affecting rural populations (Thacher et al. 2006). The increased prevalence of nutritional rickets has been attributed to a change from bean-rich to cereal-rich diets in many areas (Graham et al. 2001; Welch and Graham 2004). For Mg, the average adult typically contains 25 g Mg, 60% of which is in hard tissues, 40% of Mg in muscles and soft tissues, and 1% in extracellular fluids, where it is also under tight homeostatic control (NRC, 1989). Magnesium is a component of numerous enzymatic reactions, including energy, protein and fatty acid metabolism, and in maintenance of cell ionic balance (Gums 2004). Human Mg deficiency is linked to numerous conditions including hypertension, heart dysfunction, diabetes and preeclampsia. It is difficult to determine the proportion of the world's population affected by Ca and Mg deficiency, but it is likely to be a significant problem in populations reliant on staple cereal crops, and more generally among older people (NRC 1989).

As discussed previously, plant Ca and Mg concentration are under strong genetic control with leaf-Ca and Mg typically lower in commelinid monocotyledon species – which include grasses and cereals – than in species from other angiosperm families (Broadley et al. 2003, 2004). This is likely to be due to family-level differences in cell wall chemistry and cation-exchange capacity (Broadley et al. 2003, 2004; White and Broadley 2003). Furthermore, Ca is also almost immobile in the phloem of plants, and therefore source-to-sink transfer rates are invariable low (Marschner 1995). Cereal grain thus has low Ca concentrations, as typically do fruits and root storage organs (White and Broadley 2005a, b). In contrast, leafy vegetables are a rich source of Ca. However, the bioavailability of leaf-Ca depends on whether the leaves also contain oxalate, since Ca oxalate is not readily absorbed. For example, there are edible species from the Oxalidaceae family (e.g. oca, *Oxalis tuberosa*), and from the orders Caryophyllales (e.g. beet, *Beta vulgaris* L., rhubarb, *Rheum rhabarbarum* L.; spinach, *Spinacia oleracea*) and Malpighiales (e.g. castor bean, *Ricinus communis* L.; linseed, *Linum usitatissimum* L.) that often contain high Ca concentrations, yet their Ca-bioavailability is potentially very low (White and Broadley 2003; White 2005).

Substantial genetic variation and high heritability values have been reported for the Ca and Mg concentrations for several species of edible crops, making these two elements attractive targets for genetic biofortification strategies (White and Broadley 2005a). For example, grain-Ca varied almost threefold among wild and cultivated wheats (Graham et al. 1999; Bálint et al. 2001). In legumes, seed-Ca varied more than ninefold among wild and cultivated beans and peas (Guzmán-Maldonado et al. 2000, 2003; Islam et al. 2002, 2004; Grusak and Cakmak 2005) and more than fourfold among chickpea (Guzmán-Maldonado et al. 2003). In edible leaves, Ca and Mg concentrations varied up to threefold among diverse *B. oleracea* (Kopsell et al. 2004; Broadley et al. 2008), spinach (Grusak and Cakmak 2005) and chickpea (Ibrikci et al. 2003) accessions. Whilst non-genetic sources dominated variation in Ca and Mg concentrations in inflorescences of *B. oleracea* var. *italica* (broccoli/calabrese) accessions, significant genetic variation was also observed (Farnham et al. 2000; Rosa et al. 2002). Tissue Ca and Mg concentrations are often correlated, with tissue Mg concentrations often showing less, but still significant, variation among genotypes than for Ca (reviewed by White and Broadley 2005a). Intriguingly, correlations between Ca and Mg within a species may be constrained by higher level evolutionary effects. For example, species from families within the angiosperm order Caryophyllales (e.g. including the families Amaranthaceae, Caryophyllaceae) seem to have a tendency towards higher leaf-Mg, and thereby lower leaf-Ca:leaf-Mg ratios, than most other terrestrial plants (Broadley et al. 2004; Watanabe et al. 2007). Notably, Ca:Mg ratios across 322 spinach accessions of spinach (family Amaranthaceae) are typically fivefold lower than Ca:Mg ratios observed in >400 accessions of *B. oleracea* (Broadley et al. 2008).

Copper

Copper is an essential micronutrient for animals and plants. A typical adult human contains *ca.* 70 mg of Cu (Emsley 1997). As with the other major transition elements Fe and Zn, Cu is a major component of numerous enzymes (FSA 2003). These include cytochrome *c* oxidase, amino acid oxidase, and superoxide dismutase. Enzymes containing Cu include those involved in synthesis of neuroactive amines and peptides (e.g. catecholamines and enkephalins). Copper is also involved in host defence, red and white blood-cell maturation, Fe-transport, cholesterol and glucose metabolism, myocardial contractility, bone strength and brain development. Copper deficiency symptoms include cardiovascular dysfunction in adults, and leucopenia, skeletal fragility, and respiratory tract infections in infants (COMA 1994). It is not clear how widespread Cu-deficiency is globally. However, it is likely that subclinical Cu deficiency will be prevalent throughout the developed and developing world as a consequence of poor diet. In the UK, the Food Standards Agency Expert Group on Vitamins and Minerals concluded that Cu deficiency would be rare in the UK (FSA 2003), although it may occur in individuals with rare genetic defects, such as Menkes' steely hair disease (NRC 1989).

As with other minerals, there is considerable variation in tissue Cu concentrations both between and within angiosperm species. For example, grain-Cu varied *ca.* threefold between wheat species (Bálint et al. 2001). Within-species, leaf-Cu varied tenfold among pea accessions, and up to fivefold among *B. oleracea* and spinach (Grusak and Cakmak 2005; Broadley et al. 2008) genotypes. Leaf-Cu varied 1.3-fold and root-Cu varied 2.1-fold in cassava (Chavez et al. 2000) and 5.5-fold in roots of yam (Frossard et al. 2000). Therefore, there is potential for breeding increased Cu in edible fractions of numerous crop species.

Has the mineral concentration of crops declined due to breeding for increased yield?

Evidence for a decline in mineral concentration of horticultural crops

Using published UK food concentration tables (McCance and Widdowson 1960; Holland et al. 1991), Mayer (1997) reported a potential decline in the mean dry matter (DM) content and mean concentrations of Ca, Cu, Mg and Na in raw vegetables and Cu, Fe, K and Mg concentrations in fresh fruits between the 1930s and 1980s. Subsequently, White and Broadley (2005b) observed that the mean concentrations of Cu, Mg and Na in the DM of vegetables and the mean concentrations of Cu, Fe and K in the DM of fruits available in the UK had decreased between the 1930s and the 1980s. Based on comparable data from the USA, White and Broadley (2005b) also suggested that the mean Ca, Cu and Fe concentrations in the DM of vegetables and the mean concentrations of Cu, Fe and K in the DM of fruits had decreased between the 1930s and 1980s in the USA. Both Mayer (1997) and White and Broadley (2005b) used geometric means and *t*-tests to support their conclusions. Davis et al. (2004) used medians and sign (quantile) tests to conclude that the moisture-adjusted concentrations of Ca, Fe and P in horticultural produce available in the USA had declined between 1950 and 1999. Davis (2006) noted that the conclusions of White and Broadley (2005b) depended critically on the statistical method employed. He concluded that only Cu and Na concentrations in the DM of UK vegetables had decreased significantly, and that there had been no change in the mineral concentrations in the DM of fruits, between the 1930s and the 1980s using non-parametric tests. Unfortunately, it is not possible to determine whether mineral concentrations of any single vegetable or fruit has altered significantly over time either in the UK or in the USA using data from food composition tables. Ultimately, different varieties and/or cultivation practices must be compared directly under the same environmental conditions to determine whether mineral concentrations in a particular crop have been affected by changing cultivars or agricultural practices (Davis et al. 2004; Broadley et al. 2006a; Davis 2006).

Is there evidence for a decline in mineral concentration of staple crops?

Since horticultural products in general are likely to be relatively small contributors of minerals to the average diet in the UK and USA (Henderson et al. 2003), changes in mineral concentration of these crop groups are unlikely to be significant in overall dietary terms (White and Broadley 2005b). However, the preliminary evidence of a decline in the mineral concentration of vegetables in both the UK and USA, which have shared similar horticultural and consumer practices since the 1930s, suggests that this phenomenon might be a consequence of changing horticultural practices and/or the adoption of modern higher-yielding varieties (Davis et al. 2004; Davis 2006; White and Broadley 2005b). The phenomenon warrants further exploration and comparison with more widely-consumed staple crop species.

It has been hypothesised that increasing crop yields has led to a decline in crop mineral concentration as a consequence of the 'dilution effect'. In other words, the growth rate of the plant exceeds the ability of plants to acquire these elements (Davis et al. 2004; Davis 2006). Dilution effects could be due to environmental (e.g. improved agronomy, climate change) or genetic factors (i.e. higher-yielding cultivars). Environmental factors such as higher temperatures, light intensity, irrigation – and even mineral fertilisation – can increase plant growth rates and reduce the mineral concentrations of plant tissues (Jarrell and Beverly 1981).

Several recent studies have reported that higher-yielding crop genotypes have lower concentrations of various minerals in their tissues (Monasterio and Graham 2000; Davis et al. 2004; Garvin et al. 2006; White et al. 2009). For example, when a historical set of 26 bread wheat cultivars were grown together at two locations over 3 years (Monasterio and Graham 2000), a positive linear relationship was observed between year of release and grain yield, with a negative trend occurring between date of release and grain Fe, Zn and P concentrations. In a study of 14 US hard red winter wheat varieties, which were also grown together at two locations, Garvin et al. (2006) observed negative relationships between seed Fe, Zn and Se concentrations and both grain yields and date of release. The strength of the relationship was influenced strongly by environmental effects. In leafy vegetables, Farnham et al. (2000) found a strong negative relationship between head weight and Ca and Mg concentrations among 27 broccoli genotypes.

Table 8.3 The mineral content of 200 g fresh weight of potatoes and its potential contribution to the US diet calculated as a percentage of the US Dietary Reference Intake (DRI) for a 31- to 50-year-old male

		DRI	US potatoes	UK potatoes	% DRI
N	(mg)	ns		660	–
S	(mg)	ns		60	–
K	(mg)	4700	850	720	18.1
Cl	(mg)	2300		132	–
Ca	(mg)	1000	22	10	2.2
P	(mg)	700	118	74	16.8
Na	(mg)	1500	12	14	0.8
Mg	(mg)	420	45	34	10.6
Fe	(mg)	8	1.4	0.8	18.1
Zn	(mg)	11	0.6	0.6	5.5
Mn	(mg)	2.3	0.3	0.2	13.0
Cu	(μg)	900	231	160	25.6
I	(μg)	150	37	6	24.9
Se	(μg)	55	0.8	2	1.4

ns = not specified.
Reproduced entirely from White et al. (2009).

A case study on potatoes; a précis of White et al. (2009)

White et al. (2009) recently published a detailed survey of the mineral concentration of potato tubers, to test the hypothesis that increased yields, produced either by the application of mineral fertilisers and/or by growing higher-yielding varieties, leads to decreased mineral concentrations in potato tubers. Potato (*Solanum tuberosum*) tubers provide a substantial fraction of dietary proteins, carbohydrates, vitamins and minerals in many populations (White et al. 2009). Potato tubers are rich in Cu, K, P, Fe, moderately rich in Zn, Mg and Mn, and low in Ca and Na (Table 8.3). Potato tubers also have relatively high concentrations of promoter compounds, including ascorbate (vitamin C), protein cysteine and various organic and amino acids, and low concentrations of anti-nutrients such as phytate and oxalate. The study of White et al. (2009) is précised here.

Potato tuber yields can be increased significantly using fungicides, fertilisers and irrigation, with varying effects on tuber mineral concentration reported as a consequence. For example, irrigation can increase tuber P concentration and reduce tuber Ca and Mg concentrations, whilst having little effect on tuber N or K concentrations (Simpson 1962; Asfary et al. 1983). Unsurprisingly, the use of N fertilisers increases tuber N concentrations (e.g. Augustin 1975; Eppendorfer et al. 1979; Sen Tran and Giroux 1991; Harris 1992), P fertilisers increase tuber P concentrations (Simpson 1962; Rocha et al. 1997; Alvarez-Sánchez et al. 1999; Allison et al. 2001a; Trehan and Sharma 2003), K fertilisers increase tuber K concentrations (Addiscott 1976; Maier 1986; Harris 1992; Allison et al. 2001b) and Ca or Mg fertilisers increase tuber Ca (McGuire and Kelman 1984, 1986; Simmons and Kelling 1987; Bamberg et al. 1993, 1998; Clough 1994; Karlsson et al. 2006) and Mg concentrations (Allison et al. 2001c), respectively. However, fertiliser use alters tuber concentration of other minerals as a consequence of complex interactions between minerals in the soil and affects on internal redistribution of minerals within the plant. Thus, N fertilisers can decrease tuber Fe and P concentrations yet often have little effect on tuber K, Ca and Mg concentrations (Simpson 1962; Augustin 1975; Harris 1992; Allison et al. 2001c), P fertilisers can increase tuber N and Mg concentrations but reduce tuber Mn concentrations (J.P. Hammond and P.J. White, unpublished observations), K fertilisers can increase tuber Mg but reduce tuber Ca and P concentrations (Addiscott 1974, 1976; Maier 1986; Allison et al. 2001c), and Ca fertilisers can increase tuber P, S and K concentrations but decrease tuber Mg concentrations (Simmons and Kelling 1987; Clough 1994). Increasing yield through elevated CO_2 has been found to reduce the concentrations of N, K and Mg in tubers at crop maturity (Fangmeier et al. 2002). Taken together, these studies suggest that increased tuber yield can be associated with a reduction in the concentrations of some, but not all, mineral elements in the tubers.

White et al. (2009) also considered the literature evidence for an association between genetic variation in tuber mineral concentrations and tuber yield within *S. tuberosum*. When grown under identical conditions, *S. tuberosum* genotypes can differ in tuber N, P, S, K, Mg, Ca, Fe, Zn, Mg, Cu (White et al. 2009 and references therein). Further, systematic differences in tuber K, Mg, Fe, Zn, Mn and Cu concentrations have also been observed between potato varieties obtained commercially (Casañas Rivero et al. 2003; Di Giacomo et al. 2007). Tuber Ca, Fe and Zn concentrations also vary significantly between *Solanum* species with *S. gourlayi* Hawkes and *S. microdontum* Bitter having the highest tuber Ca concentrations, whilst *S. kurtzianum* Bitter & Wittm. and *S. tuberosum* had the lowest tuber Ca concentrations (Bamberg et al. 1993). Although tuber skins generally contain higher Ca concentrations than the flesh (McGuire and Kelman 1984, 1986; Ereifej et al. 1998; Wszelaki et al. 2005), differences in tuber Ca concentration between *Solanum* species were not associated simply with differences in skin-to-flesh ratios. In 74 Andean landraces of *Solanum*, correlations were observed between tuber Ca, Fe and Zn concentrations (Andre et al. 2007). It is likely, therefore, that tuber mineral concentrations can be manipulated genetically through commercial breeding programmes.

There is some evidence in the literature to suggest that higher-yielding potato genotypes have lower concentrations of mineral elements in their tubers than lower-yielding genotypes when grown in the same environment. For example, tuber P, S, K, Mg and Zn concentrations are lower in higher-yielding varieties than in lower-yielding varieties grown in the same trial (Tekalign and Hammes 2005). However, in other studies, no such relationship between yield and mineral concentration has been observed. For example, among eight potato varieties there was no relationship between tuber fresh weight and tuber K, Ca, Mg, Fe, Zn or Cu concentrations (Randhawa et al. 1984). In the study of Andre et al. (2007), tuber size explained about 13% of the variability in tuber Fe concentrations (Andre et al. 2007). Finally, in field trials of 26 commercial potato varieties, higher-yielding varieties did not have lower tuber concentrations of any mineral than lower-yielding varieties (Figure 8.2; White et al. 2009). In contrast, tuber P and Cu concentrations increased with increasing tuber FW yield.

In summary, White et al. (2009) concluded from the literature evidence that the mineral concentration of potato tubers is influenced by both genetic and environmental factors. There is some evidence in the literature to support the hypothesis that increasing tuber

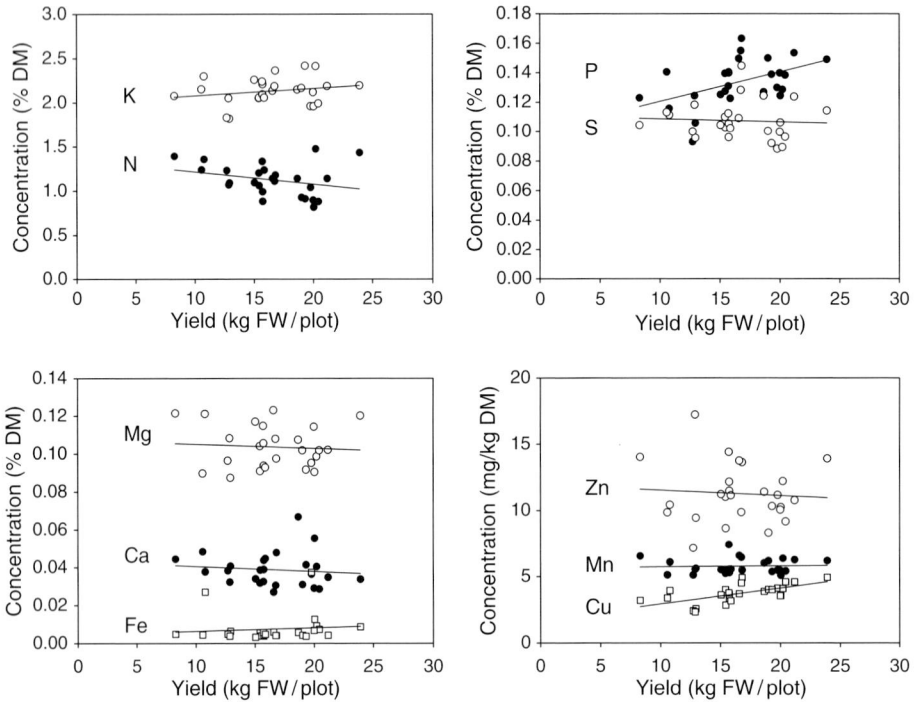

Figure 8.2 Relationships between tuber mineral concentrations and tuber yield in a core collection of 26 commercial *Solanum tuberosum* varieties trialed in the field at SCRI in 2006. Data are means of two replicate plots each containing eight plants at 40 cm spacing (reproduced from White et al. 2009).

yields, either by elevating CO_2 concentrations or by growing higher-yielding varieties, results in a decrease in the tuber concentration of some minerals. However, complex interactions between mineral elements in the soil–plant system will affect the concentrations of mineral elements in tubers independently of any 'yield dilution' phenomenon. Consequently, the optimal strategy for improving the delivery of minerals to the human diet via potato tubers is likely to benefit from combining genotypes that have naturally higher tuber mineral concentrations with appropriate fertilisation strategies to deliver more essential minerals to the diet without compromising yield. This case study provides a clear illustration of the likely benefits of an integrated approach to biofortification, which combines both agronomic and genetic solutions.

References

Addiscott, T.M. (1974) Potassium and the distribution of calcium and magnesium in potato plants. *Journal of the Science of Food and Agriculture* **25**, 1173–83.

Addiscott, T.M. (1976) Nutrient concentrations and interactions in young leaves of potato plants growing with and without tubers. *Annals of Botany* **40**, 65–72.

Ågren, G.I. (2004) The C: N: P stoichiometry of autotrophs – theory and observations. *Ecology Letters* **7**, 185–91.

Allison, M.F., Fowler, J.H. and Allen, E.J. (2001a) Effects of soil- and foliar-applied phosphorus fertilizers on the potato (*Solanum tuberosum*) crop. *Journal of Agricultural Science* **137**, 379–95.

Allison, M.F., Fowler, J.H. and Allen, E.J. (2001b) Responses of potato (*Solanum tuberosum*) to potassium fertilizers. *Journal of Agricultural Science* **136**, 407–26.

Allison, M.F., Fowler, J.H. and Allen, E.J. (2001c) Factors affecting the magnesium nutrition of potatoes (*Solanum tuberosum*). *Journal of Agricultural Science* **137**, 397–409.

Alvarez-Sánchez, E., Etchevers, J.D., Ortiz, J, Núñez, R., Volke, V., Tijerina, L. and Martínez, A. (1999) Biomass production and phosphorus accumulation of potato as affected by phosphorus nutrition. *Journal of Plant Nutrition* **22**, 205–17.

Andre, C.M., Ghislain, M., Bertin, P., Oufir, M., del Rosario Herrera, M., Hoffmann, L., Hausman, J.-F., Larondelle, Y. and Evers, D. (2007) Andean potato cultivars (*Solanum tuberosum* L.) as a source of antioxidant and mineral micronutrients. *Journal of Agricultural and Food Chemistryistry* **55**, 366–78.

Andreini, C., Banci, L., Bertini, I. and Rosato, A. (2006) Counting the zinc-proteins encoded in the human genome. *Journal of Proteome Research* **5**, 196–201.

Asfary, A.F., Wild, A. and Harris, P.M. (1983) Growth, mineral nutrition and water use by potato crops. *Journal of Agricultural Science* **100**, 87–101.

Augustin, J. (1975) Variations in the nutritional concentration of fresh potatoes. *Journal of Food Science* **40**, 1295–99.

Bálint, A.F., Kovács, G., Erdei, L. and Sutka, J. (2001) Comparisons of the Cu, Zn, Fe, Ca and Mg contents of the grains of wild, ancient and cultivated wheat species. *Cereal Research Communications* **29**, 375–82.

Bamberg, J.B., Palta, J.P., Peterson, L.A., Martin, M. and Krueger, A.R. (1993) Screening tuber-bearing *Solanum* (potato) germplasm for efficient accumulation of tuber calcium. *American Potato Journal* **70**, 219–26.

Bamberg, J.B., Palta, J.P., Peterson, L.A., Martin, M. and Krueger, A.R. (1998) Fine screening potato (*Solanum*) species germplasm for tuber calcium. *American Journal of Potato Research* **75**, 181–6.

Bänziger, M. and Long, J. (2000) The potential for increasing the iron and zinc density of maize through plant-breeding. *Food and Nutrition Bulletin* **21**, 397–400.

Baxter, I., Ouzzani, M., Orcun, S., Kennedy, B., Jandhyala, S.S. and Salt, D.E. (2007) Purdue Ionomics Information Management System. An integrated functional genomics platform. *Plant Physiology* **143**, 600–11.

Bentsink, L., Yuan, K., Koornneef, M. and Vreugdenhil, D. (2003) The genetics of phytate and phosphate accumulation in seeds and leaves of *Arabidopsis thaliana*, using natural variation. *Theoretical and Applied Genetics* **106**, 1234–43.

Beyersmann, D. and Haase, H. (2001) Functions of zinc in signaling, proliferation and differentiation of mammalian cells. *BioMetals* **14**, 331–41.

Bouis, H.E. (2003) Micronutrient fortification of plants through plant breeding: can it improve nutrition in man at low cost? *Proceedings of the Nutrition Society* **62**, 403–11.

Broadley, M.R., Bowen, H.C., Cotterill, H.L., Hammond, J.P., Meacham, M.C., Mead, A. and White, P.J. (2003) Variation in the shoot calcium content of angiosperms. *Journal of Experimental Botany* **54**, 1431–46.

Broadley, M.R., Bowen, H.C., Cotterill, H.L., Hammond, J.P., Meacham, M.C., Mead, A. and White, P.J. (2004) Phylogenetic variation in the shoot mineral concentration of angiosperms. *Journal of Experimental Botany* **55**, 321–36.

Broadley, M.R., Hammond, J.P., King, G.J., Astley, D., Bowen, H.C., Meacham, M.C., Mead, A., Pink, D.A.C., Teakle, G.R., Hayden, R.M., Spracklen, W.P. and White, P.J. (2008) Shoot calcium

(Ca) and magnesium (Mg) concentrations differ between subtaxa, are highly heritable, and associate with potentially pleiotropic loci in *Brassica oleracea*. *Plant Physiology* **146**, 1707–20.

Broadley, M.R., Mead, A. and White, P.J. (2006a) Reply to Davis (2006) commentary. *Journal of Horticultural Science and Biotechnology* **81**, 554–5.

Broadley, M.R., White, P.J., Bryson, R.J., Meacham, M.C., Bowen, H.C., Johnson, S.E., Hawkesford, M.J., McGrath, S.P., Zhao, F.-J., Breward, N., Harriman, M. and Tucker, M. (2006b) Biofortification of UK food crops with selenium. *Proceedings of the Nutrition Society* **65**, 169–81.

Broadley, M.R., White, P.J., Hammond, J.P., Zelko, I. and Lux, A. (2007) Zinc in plants. *New Phytologist* **173**, 677–702.

Broadley, M.R., Willey, N.J., Wilkins, J.C., Baker, A.J.M., Mead, A. and White, P.J. (2001) Phylogenetic variation in heavy metal accumulation in angiosperms. *New Phytologist* **152**, 9–27.

Butler, G.W. and Glenday, A.C. (1962) Iodine content of pasture plants. 2. Inheritance of leaf iodine content of perennial ryegrass (*Lolium perenne* L.). *Australian Journal of Biological Sciences* **15**, 183–7.

Butler, G.W. and Johnson J.M. (1957) Factors influencing the iodine content of pasture herbage. *Nature* **179**, 216–7.

Cakmak, I., Torun, A., Millet, E., Feldman, M., Fahima, T., Korol, A., Nevo, E., Braun, H.J. and Özkan, H. (2004) *Triticum dicoccoides*: an important genetic resource for increasing zinc and iron concentration in modern cultivated wheat. *Soil Science and Plant Nutrition* **50**, 1047–54.

Casañas Rivero, R., Suárez Hernández, P., Rodríguez Rodríguez, E.M., Darias Martín J. and Díaz Romero C.D. (2003) Mineral concentrations in cultivars of potatoes. *Food Chemistry* **83**, 247–53.

Castellano, S., Novoselov, S.V., Kryukov, G.V., Lescure, A., Blanco, E., Krol, A., Gladyshev, V.N. and Guigó, R. (2004) Reconsidering the evolution of eukaryotic selenoproteins: a novel non-mammalian family with scattered phylogenetic distribution. *EMBO Reports* **5**, 71–7.

Chavez, A.L., Bedoya, J.M., Sánchez, T., Iglesias, C., Ceballos, H. and Roca, W. (2000) Iron, carotene, and ascorbic acid in cassava roots and leaves. *Food and Nutrition Bulletin* **21**, 410–3.

Clough, H.G. (1994) Potato tuber yield, mineral concentration and quality after calcium fertilization. *Journal of the American Society for Horticultural Science* **119**, 175–9.

COMA (Committee on Medical Aspects of Food Policy) (1994) *Dietary reference values for food energy and nutrients for the United Kingdom*. Report of the Panel on Dietary Reference Values of the Committee on Medical Aspects of Food Policy, Report on Health and Social Subjects 41. London: HMSO.

Davis, D.R. (2006) Commentary on: 'Historical variation in the mineral concentration of edible horticultural products' [White, P.J. and Broadley, M.R. (2005) *Journal of Horticultural Science and Biotechnology,* 80, 660–667.]. *Journal of Horticultural Science and Biotechnology* **81**, 553–4.

Davis, D.R., Epp, M.D. and Riordan, H.D. (2004) Changes in USDA food concentration data for 43 garden crops, 1950 to 1999. *Journal of the American College of Nutrition* **23**, 669–82.

Di Giacomo, F., Del Signore, A. and Giaccio, M. (2007) Determining the geographic origin of potatoes using mineral and trace element content. *Journal of Agricultural and Food Chemistry* **55**, 860–66.

Dickson, J.D. (1969) Notes on hair and nail loss after ingesting Sapucaia Nuts (*Lecythis elliptica*). *Economic Botany* **23**, 133–4.

Emsley, J. (1997) *The Elements*, 3rd edn. Oxford: Clarendon Press.

Eppendorfer, W.H., Eggum, B.O. and Bille, S.W. (1979) Nutritive value of potato crude protein as influenced by manuring and amino acid concentration. *Journal of the Science of Food and Agriculture* **30**, 361–8.

Epstein, E. (1972) Mineral nutrition of plants: principles and perspectives. New York: John Wiley & Sons.

Ereifej, K.I., Shibli, R.A., Ajlouni, M.M. and Hussein, A. (1998) Mineral contents of whole tubers and selected tissues of ten potato cultivars grown in Jordan. *Journal of Food Science Technology* **35**, 55–8.

Fangmeier, A., De Temmerman, L., Black, C., Persson, K. and Vorne, V. (2002) Effects of elevated CO_2 and/or ozone on nutrient concentrations and nutrient uptake of potatoes. *European Journal of Agronomy* **17**, 353–68.

Farnham, M.W., Grusak, M.A. and Wang, M. (2000) Calcium and magnesium concentration of inbred and hybrid broccoli heads. *Journal of the American Society for Horticultural Science* **125**, 344–9.

FSA (2003) *Safe upper levels for vitamins and minerals*. Report of the Expert Group on Vitamins and Minerals. London; Food Standards Agency.

Frossard, E., Bucher, M., Mächler, F., Mozafar, A. and Hurrell, R. (2000) Potential for increasing the content and bioavailability of Fe, Zn and Ca in plants for human nutrition. *Journal of the Science of Food and Agriculture* **80**, 861–79.

Garvin, D.F., Welch, R.M. and Finley, J.W. (2006) Historical shifts in the seed mineral micronutrient concentration of US hard red winter wheat germplasm. *Journal of the Science of Food and Agriculture* **86**, 2213–20.

Gerloff, G.C. (1963) Comparative mineral nutrition of plants. *Annual Review of Plant Physiology* **14**, 107–24.

Ghandilyan, A., Vreugdenhil, D. and Aarts, M.G.M. (2006) Progress in the genetic understanding of plant iron and zinc nutrition. *Physiologia Plantarum* **126**, 407–17.

Graham, R., Sendadhira, D., Beebe, S., Iglesias, C. and Monasterio, I. (1999) Breeding for micronutrient density in edible portions of staple food crops: conventional approaches. *Field Crops Research* **60**, 57–80.

Graham, R.D., Welch, R.M. and Bouis, H.E. (2001) Addressing micronutrient malnutrition through enhancing the nutritional quality of staple foods: principles, perspectives and knowledge gaps. *Advances in Agronomy* **70**, 77–142.

Gregorio, G.B., Senadhira, D., Htut, H. and Graham, R.D. (2000) Breeding for trace mineral density in rice. *Food and Nutrition Bulletin* **21**, 382–6.

Grime, J.P. (2001) *Plant Strategies, Vegetation Processes, and Ecosystem Properties*, 2nd edn. Chichester: John Wiley & Sons.

Grusak, M.A. and Cakmak, I. (2005) Methods to improve the crop-delivery of minerals to humans and livestock. In: *Plant Nutritional Genomics* (eds Broadley, M.R. and White, P.J.), pp. 265–86. Oxford: Blackwell.

Grusak, M.A. and DellaPenna, D. (1999) Improving the nutrient concentration of plants to enhance human nutrition and health. *Annual Review of Plant Physiology and Plant Molecular Biology* **50**, 133–61.

Gums, J.G. (2004) Magnesium in cardiovascular and other disorders. *American Journal of Health-System Pharmacy* **61**, 1569–76.

Guzmán-Maldonado, S.H., Acosta-Gallegos, J. and Paredes-López, O. (2000) Protein and mineral content of a novel collection of wild and weedy common bean (*Phaseolus vulgaris* L). *Journal of the Science of Food and Agriculture* **80**, 1874–81.

Guzmán-Maldonado, S.H., Martínez, O., Acosta-Gallegos, J.A., Guevara-Lara, F. and Paredes-López, O. (2003) Putative quantitative trait loci for physical and chemical components of common bean. *Crop Science* **43**, 1029–35.

Hacisalihoglu, G., Ozturk, L., Cakmak, I., Welch, R. M. and Kochian, L. (2004) Genotypic variation in common bean in response to zinc deficiency in calcareous soil. *Plant and Soil* **259**, 71–83.

Harada, H. and Leigh, R.A. (2006) Genetic mapping of natural variation in potassium concentrations in shoots of *Arabidopsis thaliana*. *Journal of Experimental Botany* **57**, 953–60.

Harris, P.M. (1992) Mineral nutrition. In: *The Potato Crop: the Scientific Basis for Improvement* (ed. P.M. Harris), pp. 162–213. London: Chapman and Hall.

Henderson, L., Irving, K., Gregory, J., Bates, C.J., Prentice, A., Perks, J., Swan, G. and Farron, M. (2003) *The National Diet and Nutrition Survey: Adults aged 19–64 years, Volume 3: Vitamin and Mineral Intake and Urinary Analysis*. London: HMSO.

Hodson, M.J., White, P.J., Mead, A. and Broadley, M.R. (2005) Phylogenetic variation in the silicon concentration of plants. *Annals of Botany* **96**, 1027–46.

Holland, B., Welch, A.A., Unwin, I.D., Buss, D.H., Paul, A.A. and Southgate, D.A.T. (1991) *McCance and Widdowson's The Concentration of Foods*, 5th edn. Cambridge: The Royal Society of Chemistry.

Ibrikci, H., Knewtson, S.J.B. and Grusak, M.A. (2003) Chickpea leaves as a vegetable green for humans: evaluation of mineral concentration. *Journal of the Science of Food and Agriculture* **83**, 945–50.

Islam, F.M.A., Basford, K.E., Jara, C., Redden, R.J. and Beebe, S. (2002) Seed concentrational and disease resistance differences among gene pools in cultivated common bean. *Genetic Resources and Crop Evolution* **49**, 285–93.

Islam, F.M.A., Beebe, S., Muñoz, M., Tohme, J., Redden, R.J. and Basford, K.E. (2004) Using molecular markers to assess the effect of introgression on quantitative attributes of common bean in the Andean gene pool. *Theoretical and Applied Genetics* **108**, 243–52.

Jansen, S., Broadley, M.R., Robbrecht, E. and Smets, E. (2002) Aluminum hyperaccumulation in angiosperms: A review of its phylogenetic significance. *Botanical Review* **68**, 235–269.

Jarrell, W.M. and Beverly, R.B. (1981) The dilution effect in plant nutrition studies. *Advances in Agronomy* **34**, 197–225.

Johnson, J.M. and Butler, G.W. (1957) Iodine content of pasture plants. I. Method of determination and preliminary investigation of species and strain differences. *Physiologia Plantarum* **10**, 100–11.

Kannamkumarath, S.S., Wrobel, K. and Wuilloud, R.G. (2005) Studying the distribution pattern of selenium in nut proteins with information obtained from SEC-UV-ICP-MS and CE-ICP-MS. *Talanta* **66**, 153–9.

Karlsson, B.H., Palta, J.P. and Crump, P.M. (2006) Enhancing tuber calcium concentration may reduce incidence of blackspot bruise injury in potatoes. *Hortscience* **41**, 1213–21.

Kay, C.E., Tourangeau, P.C. and Gordon, C.C. (1975) Fluoride levels in indigenous animals and plants collected from uncontaminated ecosystems. *Fluoride* **8**, 125–33.

Kennedy, G., Nantel, G. and Shetty, P. (2003) The scourge of 'hidden hunger': global dimensions of micronutrient deficiencies. *Food Nutrition and Agriculture* **32**, 8–16.

Kerdel-Vegas, F. (1966) The depilatory and cytotoxic actions of 'Coco de Mono' (*Lecythis ollaria*) and its relationship to chronic selenosis. *Economic Botany* **23**, 133–4.

Kerkhoff, A.J., Fagan, W.F., Elser, J.J., Enquist, B.J. (2006) Phylogenetic and growth form variation in the scaling of nitrogen and phosphorus in the seed plants. *American Naturalist* **168**, E103–22.

Kopsell, D.A. and Randle, W.M. (1997) Short-day onion cultivars differ in bulb selenium and sulfur accumulation which can affect bulb pungency. *Euphytica* **96**, 385–90.

Kopsell, D.A. and Randle, W.M. (2001) Genetic variances and selection potential for selenium accumulation in a rapid-cycling *Brassica oleracea* population. *Journal of the American Society for Horticultural Science* **126**, 329–35.

Kopsell, D.E., Kopsell, D.A., Lefsrud, M.G. and Curran-Celentano, J. (2004) Variability in elemental accumulations among leafy *Brassica oleracea* cultivars and selections. *Journal of Plant Nutrition* **27**, 1813–26.

Loudet, O., Chaillou, S., Merigout, P., Talbotec, J. and Daniel-Vedele, F. (2003) Quantitative trait loci analysis of nitrogen use efficiency in *Arabidopsis*. *Plant Physiology* **131**, 345–50.

Lucca, P, Hurrell, R. and Potrykus, I. (2002) Fighting iron deficiency anemia with iron-rich rice. *Journal of the American College of Nutrition* **21**, 184S–190S.

Lyons, G., Ortiz-Monasterio, I., Stangoulis, J. and Graham, R. (2005) Selenium concentration in wheat grain: Is there sufficient genotypic variation to use in breeding? *Plant and Soil* **269**, 269–380.

Lyons, G.H., Stangoulis, J.C.R. and Graham, R.D. (2004) Exploiting micronutrient interaction to optimize biofortification programs: the case for inclusion of selenium and iodine in the *HarvestPlus* program. *Nutrition Reviews* **62**, 247–52.

McCance, R.A. and Widdowson, E.M. (1960) *The Concentration of Foods*, 3rd edn. Special Report Series No. 297. London: Medical Research Council.

McGuire, R.G. and Kelman, A. (1984) Reduced severity of *Erwinia* soft rot in potato tubers with increased calcium content. *Phytopathology* **74**, 1250–6.

McGuire, R.G. and Kelman, A. (1986) Calcium in potato tuber cell walls in relation to tissue maceration by *Erwinia carotovora* pv. *atroseptica*. *Phytopathology* **76**, 401–6.

Macnair, M.R. (2003) The hyperaccumulation of metals by plants. *Advances in Botanical Research* **40**, 63–105.

Maier, N.A. (1986) Potassium nutrition of irrigated potatoes in South Australia. 2. Effect on chemical concentration and the prediction of tuber yield response by plant analysis. *Australian Journal of Experimental Agriculture* **26**, 727–36.

Marriott, H. and Buttriss, J. (2003) Key points from the National Diet and Nutrition Survey of adults aged 19–64 years. *Nutrition Bulletin* **28**, 355–63.

Marschner, H. (1995) *Mineral Nutrition of Higher Plants*, 2nd edn. London: Academic Press.

Mayer, A.-M. (1997) Historical changes in the mineral content of fruits and vegetables. *British Food Journal* **99**, 207–11.

Maziya-Dixon, B., Kling, J.G., Menkir, A. and Dixon, A. (2000) Genetic variation in total carotene, iron, and zinc contents of maize and cassava genotypes. *Food and Nutrition Bulletin* **21**, 419–22.

Mengel, K. and Kirkby, E.A. (2001) *Principles of Plant Nutrition*, 5th edn. Dordrecht, The Netherlands: Kluwer Academic Press.

Monasterio, I. and Graham, R.D. (2000) Breeding for trace minerals in wheat. *Food and Nutrition Bulletin* **21**, 392–6.

NRC (1989) *Recommended Dietary Allowances*, 10th edn. Subcommittee on the Tenth Edition of the RDAs, Food and Nutrition Board, Commission on Life Sciences, National Research Council. Washington, DC: National Academy Press.

Oikeh, S.O., Menkir, A., Maziya-Dixon, B., Welch, R. and Glahn, R.P. (2003a) Assessment of concentrations of iron and zinc and bioavailable iron in grains of early-maturing tropical maize varieties. *Journal of Agricultural and Food Chemistry* **51**, 3688–94.

Oikeh, S.O., Menkir, A., Maziya-Dixon, B., Welch, R. and Glahn, R.P. (2003b) Genotypic differences in concentration and bioavailability of kernel-iron in tropical maize varieties grown under field conditions. *Journal of Plant Nutrition* **26**, 2307–19.

Payne, K.A., Bowen, H.C., Hammond, J.P., Hampton, C.R., Lynn, J.R., Mead, A., Swarup, K., Bennett, M.J., White, P.J. and Broadley, M.R. (2004) Natural genetic variation in caesium (Cs) accumulation by *Arabidopsis thaliana*. *New Phytologist* **162**, 535–48.

Pezzarossa, B., Piccotino, D., Shennan, C. and Malorgio, F. (1999) Uptake and distribution of selenium in tomato plants as affected by genotype and sulphate supply. *Journal of Plant Nutrition* **22**, 1613–35.

Pickering, I.J., Prince, R.C., Salt, D.E. and George, G.N. (2000) Quantitative, chemically specific imaging of selenium transformation in plants. *Proceedings of the National Academy of Sciences USA* **97**, 10717–22.

Pickering, I.J., Wright, C., Bubner, B., Ellis, D., Persans, M.W., Yu, E.Y., George, G.N., Prince, R.C. and Salt, D.E. (2003) Chemical form and distribution of selenium and sulfur in the selenium hyperaccumulator *Astragalus bisulcatus*. *Plant Physiology* **131**, 1460–7.

Randhawa, K.S., Sandhu, K.S., Kaur, G. and Singh, D. (1984) Studies of the evaluation of different genotypes of potato (*Solanum tuberosum* L.) for yield and mineral contents. *Qualitas Plantarum* **34**, 239–42.

Rayman, M.P. (2000) The importance of selenium to human health. *Lancet* **356**, 233–41.

Rayman, M.P. (2002) The argument for increasing selenium intake. *Proceedings of the Nutrition Society* **61**, 203–15.

Rayman, M.P. (2004) The use of high-selenium yeast to raise selenium status: how does it measure up? *British Journal of Nutrition* **92**, 557–73.

Reeves, R.D. and Baker, A.J.M. (2000) Metal-accumulating plants. In: *Phytoremediation of Toxic Metals: Using Plants to Clean Up the Environment* (eds I. Raskin and B.D. Ensley), pp. 193–229. New York: John Wiley & Sons.

Rocha, F.A.T., Fontes, P.C.R., Fontes, R.L.F. and Reis, F.P. (1997) Critical phosphorus concentrations in potato plant parts at two growth stages. *Journal of Plant Nutrition* **20**, 573–9.

Rosa, E.A.S., Haneklaus, S.H. and Schug, E. (2002) Mineral content of primary and secondary inflorescences of eleven broccoli cultivars grown in early and late seasons. *Journal of Plant Nutrition* **25**, 1741–51.

Sen Tran, T. and Giroux, M. (1991) Effects of N rates and harvest dates on the efficiency of 15N-labelled fertilizer on early harvested potatoes (*Solanum tuberosum* L.). *Canadian Journal of Soil Science* **71**, 519–32.

Shennan, C., Schachtman, D.P. and Cramer, G.R. (1990) Variation in [^{75}Se]selenate uptake and partitioning among tomato cultivars and wild species. *New Phytologist* **115**, 523–30.

Simmons, K.E. and Kelling K.A. (1987) Potato responses to calcium application on several soil types. *American Potato Journal* **64**, 119–36.

Simpson, K. (1962) Effects of soil-moisture tension and fertilizers on the yield, growth and phosphorus uptake of potatoes. *Journal of the Science of Food and Agriculture* **13**, 236–48.

Tekalign, T. and Hammes P.S. (2005) Growth and productivity of potato as influenced by cultivar and reproductive growth. II. Growth analysis, tuber yield and quality. *Scientia Horticulturae* **105**, 29–44.

Thacher, T.D., Fischer, P.R., Strand, M.A. and Pettifor, J.M. (2006) Nutritional rickets around the world: causes and future directions. *Annals of Tropical Paediatrics* **26**, 1–16.

Thompson, K., Parkinson, J.A., Band, S.R. and Spencer, R.E. (1997) A comparative study of leaf nutrient concentrations in a regional herbaceous flora. *New Phytologist* **136**, 679–89.

Trehan, S.P. and Sharma, R.C. (2003) External phosphorus requirement of different potato (*Solanum tuberosum*) cultivars resulting from different internal requirements and uptake efficiencies. Indian *Journal of Agricultural Science* **73**, 54–6.

USDA, ARS, National Genetic Resources Program (2007) Germplasm Resources Information Network—(GRIN). [Online Database] National Germplasm Resources Laboratory, Beltsville, Maryland. http://www.ars-grin.gov/cgi-bin/npgs/html/listdsc.pl?SPINACH, 19 February 2007.

Vonderheide, A.P., Wrobel, K., Kannamkumarath, S.S., B'Hymer, C., Montes-Bayón, M., de León, C.P. and Caruso, J.A. (2002) Characterization of selenium species in Brazil nuts by HPLC-ICP-MS and ES-MS. *Journal of Agricultural and Food Chemistry* **50**, 5722–8.

Vreugdenhil, D., Aarts, M.G.M. and Koornneef, M. (2005) Exploring natural genetic variation to improve plant nutrient content. In: *Plant Nutritional Genomics* (eds Broadley, M.R. and White, P.J.), pp. 201–19. Oxford: Blackwell.

Vreugdenhil, D., Aarts, M.G.M., Koornneef, M., Nelissen, H. and Ernst, W.H.O. (2004) Natural variation and QTL analysis for cationic mineral content in seeds of *Arabidopsis thaliana*. *Plant Cell and Environment* **27**, 828–39.

Watanabe, T., Broadley, M.R., Jansen, S., White, P.J., Takada, J., Satake, K., Takamatsu, T., Tuah, S.J. and Osaki, M. (2007) Evolutionary control of leaf element concentration in plants. *New Phytologist* **174**, 516–23.

Welch, R.M. and Graham, R.D. (2004) Breeding for micronutrients in staple food crops from a human nutrition perspective. *Journal of Experimental Botany* **55**, 353–64.

White, P.J. (2005) Calcium. In: *Plant Nutritional Genomics* (eds Broadley, M.R. and White, P.J.), pp. 66–86. Oxford: Blackwell.

White, P.J., Bradshaw, J.E., Dale, M.F.B., Ramsay, G., Hammond, J.P. and Broadley, M.R. (2009) Relationships between yield and mineral concentrations in potato tubers. *Hortscience* **44**, 6–11.

White, P.J. and Broadley, M.R. (2003) Calcium in plants. *Annals of Botany* **92**, 487–511.

White, P.J. and Broadley, M.R. (2005a) Biofortifying crops with essential mineral elements. *Trends in Plant Science* **10**, 586–93.

White, P.J. and Broadley, M.R. (2005b) Historical variation in the mineral concentration of edible horticultural products. *Journal of Horticultural Science and Biotechnology* **80**, 660–7.

White, P.J., Bowen, H.C., Marshall, B. and Broadley, M.R. (2007) Extraordinarily high leaf selenium to sulphur ratios define 'Se-accumulator' plants. *Annals of Botany* **100**, 111–8.

White, P.J., Bowen, H.C., Parmaguru, P., Fritz, M., Spracklen, W.P., Spiby, R.E., Meacham, M.C., Harriman, M., Trueman, L.J., Smith, B.M., Thomas, B. and Broadley, M.R. (2004) Interactions between selenium and sulphur nutrition in *Arabidopsis thaliana*. *Journal of Experimental Botany* **55**, 1927–37.

Wright, I.J., Reich, P.B., Cornelissen, J.H.C., Falster, D.S., Garnier, E., Hikosaka, K., Lamont, B.B., Lee, W., Oleksyn, J., Osada, N., Poorter, H., Villar, R., Warton, D.I. and Westoby, M. (2005) Assessing the generality of global leaf trait relationships. *New Phytologist* **166**, 485–96.

Wszelaki, A.L., Delwiche, J.F., Walker, S.D., Liggett, R.E., Scheerens, J.C. and Kleinhenz, M.D. (2005) Sensory quality and mineral and glycoalkaloid concentrations in organically and conventionally grown redskin potatoes (*Solanum tuberosum*). *Journal of the Science of Food and Agriculture* **85**, 720–26.

Yang, F.M., Chen, L.C., Hu, Q.H. and Pan, G.X. (2003) Effect of the application of selenium on selenium content of soybean and its products. *Biological Trace Element Research* **93**, 249–56.

Zhang, Y., Pan, G., Chen, J. and Hu, Q. (2003) Uptake and transport of selenite and selenate by soybean seedlings of two genotypes. *Plant and Soil* 253, 437–43.

Zhao, K.Y., Aranzana, M.J., Kim, S., Lister, C., Shindo, C., Tang, C.L., Toomajian, C., Zheng, H.G., Dean, C., Marjoram, P. and Nordborg, M. (2007) An *Arabidopsis* example of association mapping in structured samples. *PLOS Genetics* **3**, e4.

Index

Note: page numbers in italics refer to figures; page numbers in bold refer to tables.

Phytonutrients, First Edition. Edited by Andrew Salter, Helen Wiseman and Gregory Tucker.
© 2012 Blackwell Publishing Ltd. Published 2012 by Blackwell Publishing Ltd.